Quality of Care for
Women

A Review of Selected Clinical Conditions
and Quality Indicators

Elizabeth A. McGlynn • Eve A. Kerr
Cheryl L. Damberg • Steven M. Asch

Editors

RAND Health

Supported by the Health Care Financing Administration,
U.S. Department of Health and Human Services

Principal funding for this report was provided by a cooperative agreement from the Health Care Financing Administration, U.S. Department of Health and Human Services.

ISBN: 0-8330-2923-1

Published 2000 by RAND
1700 Main Street, P.O. Box 2138, Santa Monica, CA 90407-2138
1200 South Hayes Street, Arlington, VA 22202-5050
RAND URL: http://www.rand.org/
To order RAND documents or to obtain additional information, contact Distribution Services: Telephone: (310) 451-7002;
Fax: (310) 451-6915; Internet: order@rand.org

PREFACE

This report is one of a series of volumes describing the QA Tools, a comprehensive, clinically based system for assessing care for children and adults. The quality indicators that comprise these Tools cover 46 clinical areas and all 4 functions of medicine—screening, diagnosis, treatment, and follow-up. The indicators also cover a variety of modes of providing care, including history, physical examination, laboratory study, medication, and other interventions and contacts.

Development of each indicator was based on a review of the literature. Each volume documents the literature on which the indicators were based, explains how the clinical areas and indicators were selected, and describes what is included in the overall system.

The QA Tools were developed with funding from public and private sponsors—the Health Care Financing Administration, the Agency for Healthcare Research and Quality, the California HealthCare Foundation, and the Robert Wood Johnson Foundation.

The other four volumes in this series are:

Quality of Care for General Medical Conditions: A Review of the Literature and Quality Indicators. Eve A. Kerr, Steven M. Asch, Eric G. Hamilton, and Elizabeth A. McGlynn, eds. MR-1280-AHRQ, 2000.

Quality of Care for Oncologic Conditions and HIV: A Review of the Literature and Quality Indicators. Steven M. Asch, Eve A. Kerr, Eric G. Hamilton, Jennifer L. Reifel, and Elizabeth A. McGlynn, eds. MR-1281-AHRQ, 2000.

Quality of Care for Cardiopulmonary Conditions: A Review of the Literature and Quality Indicators. Eve A. Kerr, Steven M. Asch, Eric G. Hamilton, and Elizabeth A. McGlynn, eds. MR-1282-AHRQ, 2000.

Quality of Care for Children and Adolescents: A Review of Selected Clinical Conditions and Quality Indicators. Elizabeth A. McGlynn, Cheryl L. Damberg, Eve A. Kerr, and Mark A. Schuster, eds. MR-1283-HCFA, 2000.

These volumes should be of interest to clinicians, health plans, insurers, and health services researchers. At the time of publication, the QA Tools system was undergoing testing in managed care plans,

medical groups, and selected communities. For more information about the
QA Tools system, contact RAND_Health@rand.org.

CONTENTS

TABLES

FIGURES

ACKNOWLEDGMENTS

Funding for this work was provided by a Cooperative Agreement (No. 18-C-90315/9-02, "Development of a Global Quality Assessment Tool") from the Health Care Financing Administration, U.S. Department of Health and Human Services. We appreciate the continued and enthusiastic support of our project offer, Beth Benedict, Ph.D.

We are indebted to our expert panelists:

Elizabeth A. Alexander, M.D., M.S.
Professor
Medical Director, Managed Care Programs
Michigan State University
East Lansing, Michigan

Virginia L. Ambrosini, M.D. (Chair)
Kaiser Permanente
Panorama City, California

Bruce Bagley, M.D.
Latham Medical Group
Latham, New York

Carolyn M. Clancy, M.D.
Agency for Health Care Policy and Research
Rockville, Maryland
Assistant Clinical Professor
George Washington University
Washington, D.C.

Michelle, G. Cyr, M.D.
Rhode Island Hospital
Providence, Rhode Island
Associate Professor
Brown University
Providence, Rhode Island

Kathleen Fitzgerald, M.D.
Women's Care, Inc.
Providence, Rhode Island
Senior Clinical Instructor
Clinical Assistant Professor
Brown University
Providence, Rhode Island

Melvin D. Gerald, M.D., M.P.H.
Gerald Family Care Associates, P.C.
Washington, D.C.
Clinical Assistant Professor
Howard University
Washington, D.C.

Richard A. Johnson, M.D.
University of California Los Angeles Primary Care Group
Los Angeles, California
Associate Professor
Associate Chief
University of California Los Angeles
Los Angeles, California

A. Clinton MacKinney, M.D.
Mercy Family Care - Cresco
Cresco, Iowa

Edward C. Maeder, Jr., M.D.
Park Nicollet Clinic
Minneapolis, Minnesota
Clinical Professor
University of Minnesota
Minneapolis, Minnesota

We are also indebted to the project staff:

Landon Donsbach
Tamara Majeski
Paul Murata, M.D.
Eve Schenker, M.P.H.

INTRODUCTION

Developing and implementing a valid system of quality assessment is essential for effective functioning of the health care system. Although a number of groups have produced quality assessment tools, these tools typically suffer from a variety of limitations. Information is obtained on only a few dimensions of quality, the tools rely exclusively on administrative data, they examine quality only for users of services rather than the population, or they fail to provide a scientific basis for the quality indicators.

Under funding from public and private sponsors, including the Health Care Financing Administration (HCFA), the Agency for Healthcare Research and Quality (AHRQ), the California HealthCare Foundation, and the Robert Wood Johnson Foundation (RWJ), RAND has developed and tested a comprehensive, clinically based system for assessing quality of care for children and adults. We call this system QA Tools.

In this introduction, we discuss how the clinical areas were selected, how the indicators were chosen, and what is included in the overall system. We then describe in detail how we developed the indicators for children and adolescents.

ADVANTAGES OF THE QA TOOLS SYSTEM

QA Tools is a comprehensive, clinically based system for assessing the quality of care for children and adults. The indicators cover 46 clinical areas and all four functions of medicine including screening, diagnosis, treatment, and follow-up. The indicators also cover a variety of modes of providing care, such as history, physical examination, laboratory study, medication, and other interventions and contacts. Initial development of indicators for each clinical area was based on a review of the literature.

The QA Tools system addresses many limitations of current quality assessment tools by offering the following:

- They are clinically detailed and require data typically found in the medical record rather than just relying exclusively on data from administrative records.

- They examine quality for a population-based sample rather than for a more restricted sample of those who use care or have insurance.

- They document the scientific basis for developing and choosing the indicators.

- The QA Tools system is designed to target populations vulnerable to underutilization.

- Because of the comprehensiveness of the system, it is difficult for health care organizations to focus on a few indicators to increase their quality scores.

- QA Tools is a system that can be effective for both internal and external quality reviews. Health care organizations can use the system in order to improve the overall quality of the care provided.

- Because of the simple summary scores that will be produced, it will be an important tool for purchasers and consumers who are making choices about health care coverage and which provider to see.

Given its comprehensiveness, the QA Tools system contrasts with *leading indicators*, the most common approach to quality measurement in use today. Under the leading indicators approach, three to five specific quality measures are selected across a few domains (for example, rates of mammography screening, prevalence of the use of beta blockers among persons who have recently had a heart attack, and appropriateness of hysterectomy).

Leading indicators may work well for drawing general conclusions about quality when they correlate highly with other similar but unmeasured interventions and when repeated measurement and public reporting does not change the relationship of those indicators to the related interventions. However, to date no real evaluation of the utility of leading indicators in assessing health system performance has

been done. We also do not know whether the selected indicators
currently in use consistently represent other unmeasured practices.

By contrast, a comprehensive system can represent different
dimensions of quality of care delivery by using a large number of
measures applied to a population of interest and aggregated to produce
index scores to draw conclusions about quality. A comprehensive system
works well when evidence exists of variability within and between the
diagnosis and management of different conditions and when the question
being asked is framed at a high level (for instance, how well is the
health system helping the population stay healthy, or how much of a
problem does underuse present?).

In the 46 clinical areas they encompass, the QA Tools adequately
represent scientific and expert judgment on what constitutes quality
care. However, both the science and the practice of medicine continue to
evolve. For the QA Tools to remain a valid tool for quality assessment
over time, the scientific evidence in each area needs to be reviewed
annually to determine if new evidence warrants modifying the indicators
and/or clinical areas included in the system.

SELECTING CLINICAL AREAS FOR THE QA TOOLS

We reviewed Vital Statistics, the National Health Interview Survey,
the National Hospital Discharge Survey, and the National Ambulatory
Medical Care Survey to identify the leading causes of morbidity and
mortality and the most common reasons for physician visits in the United
States. We examined statistics for different age and gender groups in
the population (0-1, 1-5, 6-11, 12-17, 18-50 [men and women], 50-64,
65-75, over 75).

We selected topics that reflected these different areas of
importance (death, disability, utilization of services) and that covered
preventive care as well as care for acute and chronic conditions. In
addition, we consulted with a variety of experts to identify areas that
are important to these various populations but that may be
underrepresented in national data sets (for example, mental health
problems). Finally, we sought to select enough clinical areas to
represent a majority of the health care delivery system.

Table I.1 lists the 46 clinical areas included in the QA Tools system by population group; 20 include indicators for children and 36 for adults. The clinical areas, broadly defined, represent about 55 percent of the reasons for ambulatory care visits among children, 50 percent of the reasons for ambulatory care visits for the entire population, and 46 percent of the reasons for hospitalization among adults.

Note: Table I.1 reflects the clinical areas that were included in the system currently being tested. Several clinical areas (e.g., lung cancer, sickle cell disease) for which indicators were developed were not incorporated into the current tool due to budgetary constraints.

Table I.1

Clinical Areas in QA Tools System By Covered Population Group

Clinical Areas	Children	Adults
Acne	X	
Adolescent preventive services	X	
Adult screening and prevention		X
Alcohol dependence		X
Allergic rhinitis	X	
Asthma	X	X
Atrial fibrillation		X
Attention deficit/hyperactivity disorder	X	
Benign prostatic hyperplasia		X
Breast cancer		X
Cataracts		X
Cerebrovascular disease		X
Cervical cancer		X
Cesarean delivery	X	X
Chronic obstructive pulmonary disease		X
Colorectal cancer		X
Congestive heart failure		X
Coronary artery disease		X
Depression	X	X
Developmental screening	X	
Diabetes Mellitus	X	X
Diarrheal disease	X	
Family planning and contraception	X	X
Fever of unknown origin	X	
Headache		X
Hip fracture		X
Hormone replacement therapy		X
Human immunodeficiency virus		X
Hyperlipidemia		X
Hypertension		X
Immunizations	X	X
Low back pain		X
Orthopedic conditions		X
Osteoarthritis		X
Otitis media	X	
Pain management for cancer		X
Peptic ulcer disease & dyspepsia		X
Pneumonia		X
Prenatal care and delivery	X	X
Prostate cancer		X
Tuberculosis	X	X
Upper respiratory tract infections	X	
Urinary tract infections	X	X
Uterine bleeding and hysterectomy		X
Vaginitis and sexually transmitted diseases	X	X
Well child care	X	
Total number of clinical areas	**20**	**36**

SELECTING QUALITY INDICATORS

In this section, we describe the process by which indicators were chosen for inclusion in the QA Tools system. This process involved RAND staff drafting proposed indicators based on a review of the pertinent clinical literature and expert panel review of those indicators.

Literature Review

For each clinical area chosen, we reviewed the scientific literature for evidence that effective methods of prevention, screening, diagnosis, treatment, and follow-up existed (Asch et al., 2000; Kerr et al., 2000a; Kerr et al., 2000b; McGlynn et al., 2000). We explicitly examined the continuum of care in each clinical area. RAND staff drafted indicators that

- addressed an intervention with potential health benefits for the patient
- were supported by scientific evidence or formal professional consensus (guidelines, for example)
- can be significantly influenced by the health care delivery system
- can be assessed from available sources of information, primarily the medical record.

The literature review process varied slightly for each clinical area, but the basic strategy involved the following:

- Identify general areas in which quality indicators are likely to be developed.
- Review relevant textbooks and review articles.
- Conduct a targeted MEDLINE search on specific topics related to the probable indicator areas.

The levels of evidence for each indicator were assigned to three categories: randomized clinical trial; nonrandomized controlled trials, cohort or case analysis, or multiple time series; and textbooks, opinions, or descriptive studies. For each proposed indicator, staff noted the highest level of evidence supporting the indicator.

Because of the breadth of topics for which we were developing indicators, some of the literature reviews relied exclusively on textbooks and review articles. Nonetheless, we believe that the reviews adequately summarize clinical opinion and key research at the time that they were conducted. The literature reviews used to develop quality indicators for children and adolescents, and for women, were conducted between January and July 1995. The reviews for general medical conditions, oncologic conditions, and cardiopulmonary conditions were conducted between November 1996 and July 1997.

For each clinical area, we wrote a summary of the scientific evidence and developed tables of the proposed indicators that included the level of evidence, specific studies in support of the indicator, and the clinical rationale for the indicator. Because the organization of care delivery is changing so rapidly, we drafted indicators that were not in most cases inextricably linked to the place where the care was provided.

Types of Indicators

Quality of care is usually determined with three types of measures:

- *Structural measures* include characteristics of clinicians (for instance, board certification or years of experience), organizations (for instance, staffing patterns or types of equipment available), and patients (for instance, type of insurance or severity of illness).
- *Process measures* include the ways in which clinicians and patients interact and the appropriateness of medical treatment for a specific patient.
- *Outcomes measures* include changes in patients' current and future health status, including health-related quality of life and satisfaction with care.

The indicators included in the QA Tools system are primarily process indicators. We deliberately chose such indicators because the system was designed to assess care for which we can hold providers responsible. However, we collect data on a number of intermediate outcomes measures (for example, glycosylated hemoglobin, blood pressure, and cholesterol) that could be used to construct intermediate clinical outcomes indicators.

In many instances, the measures included in the QA Tools system are used to determine whether interventions have been provided in response to poor performance on such measures (for instance, whether persons who fail to control their blood sugar on dietary therapy are offered oral hypoglycemic therapy).

The Expert Panel Process

We convened expert panels to evaluate the indicators and to make final selections using the RAND/UCLA Appropriateness Method, a modified Delphi method developed at RAND and UCLA (Brook 1994). In general, the method quantitatively assesses the expert judgment of a group of clinicians regarding the indicators by using a scale with values ranging from 1 to 9.

The method is iterative with two rounds of anonymous ratings of the indicators by the panel and a face-to-face group discussion between rounds. Each panelist has equal weight in determining the final result: the quality indicators that will be included in the QA Tools system.

The RAND/UCLA Appropriateness Method has been shown to have a reproducibility consistent with that of well accepted diagnostic tests such as the interpretation of coronary angiography and screening mammography (Shekelle et al., 1998a). It has also been shown to have content, construct, and predictive validity in other applications (Brook, 1994; Shekelle et al., 1998b; Kravitz et al., 1995; Selby et al., 1996).

Approximately six weeks before the panel meeting, we sent panelists the reviews of the literature, the staff-proposed quality indicators, and separate rating sheets for each clinical area. We asked the panelists to examine the literature review and rate each indicator on a nine-point scale on each of two dimensions: validity and feasibility.

A quality indicator is defined as valid if:

1. Adequate scientific evidence or professional consensus exists supporting the indicator.

2. There are identifiable health benefits to patients who receive care specified by the indicator.

3. Based on the panelists' professional experience, health professionals with significantly higher rates of adherence to an indicator would be considered higher quality providers

4. The majority of factors that determine adherence to an indicator are under the control of the health professional (or are subject to influence by the health professional—for example, smoking cessation).

Ratings of 1-3 mean that the indicator is not a valid criterion for evaluating quality. Ratings of 4-6 mean that the indicator is an uncertain or equivocal criterion for evaluating quality. Ratings of 7-9 mean that the indicator is clearly a valid criterion for evaluating quality.

A quality indicator is defined as feasible if:

1. The information necessary to determine adherence is likely to be found in a typical medical record.

2. Estimates of adherence to the indicator based on medical record data are likely to be reliable and unbiased.

3. Failure to document relevant information about the indicator is itself a marker for poor quality.

Ratings of 1-3 mean that it is not feasible to use the indicator for evaluating quality. Ratings of 4-6 mean that there will be considerable variability in the feasibility of using the indicator to evaluate quality. Ratings of 7-9 mean that it is clearly feasible to use the indicator for evaluating quality.

The first round of indicators was rated by the panelists individually in their own offices. The indicators were returned to RAND staff and the results of the first round were summarized. We encouraged panelists to comment on the literature reviews, the definitions of key terms, and the indicators. We also encouraged them to suggest additions or deletions to the indicators.

At the panel meeting, participants discussed each clinical area in turn, focusing on the evidence, or lack thereof, that supports or refutes each indicator and the panelists' prior validity rankings. Panelists had before them the summary of the panel's first round ratings and a confidential reminder of their own ratings.

The summary consisted of a printout of the rating sheet with the distribution of ratings by panelists displayed above the rating line (without revealing the identity of the panelists) and a caret (^) marking the individual panelist's own rating in the first round displayed below the line. An example of the printout received by panelists is shown in Figure I.1.

panelist _; round 1; page 1   **September 14, 1997**

Chapter 1
ASTHMA   Validity   Feasibility

DIAGNOSIS

3. Spirometry should be measured in patients   1   1 2 3 1 1   3 4 2
with chronic asthma at least every 2 years.   1 2 3 4 5 6 7 8 9   1 2 3 4 5 6 7 8 9   (1- 2)
                                                              ^   ^

TREATMENT

7. Patients requiring chronic treatment with
systemic corticosteroids during any 12 month
period should have been prescribed inhaled
corticosteroids during the same 12 month   1 6   2   2 3 4
period.   1 2 3 4 5 6 7 8 9   1 2 3 4 5 6 7 8 9   (3- 4)
                                                              ^   ^

10. All patients seen for an acute asthma
exacerbation should be evaluated with a
complete history including all of the
following:
                                                    2 2 2   3   2 2   1 1 3
    a. time of onset   1 2 3 4 5 6 7 8 9   1 2 3 4 5 6 7 8 9   (5- 6)
                                                              ^   ^

                                                        4 1 4   3 1 5
    b. all current medications   1 2 3 4 5 6 7 8 9   1 2 3 4 5 6 7 8 9   (7- 8)
                                                              ^   ^

    c. prior hospitalizations and emergency   5 1 3   5 1 3
       department visits for asthma   1 2 3 4 5 6 7 8 9   1 2 3 4 5 6 7 8 9   (9-10)
                                                              ^   ^

    d. prior episodes of respiratory   1 1 3 2 2   1   2   3 1 2
       insufficiency due to asthma   1 2 3 4 5 6 7 8 9   1 2 3 4 5 6 7 8 9   (11-12)
                                                              ^   ^

Scales: 1 = low validity or feasibility; 9 = high validity or feasibility

Figure I.1 - Sample Panelist Summary Rating Sheet

Panelists were encouraged to bring to the discussion any relevant published information that the literature reviews had omitted. In a few cases, they supplied this information which was, in turn, discussed. In several cases, the indicators were reworded or otherwise clarified to better fit clinical judgment.

After further discussion, all indicators in each clinical area were re-ranked for validity. These final round rankings were analyzed in a manner similar to past applications of the RAND/UCLA Appropriateness Method (Park et al., 1986; Brook, 1994). The median panel rating and measure of dispersion were used to categorize indicators on validity.

We regarded panel members as being in *disagreement* when at least three members of the panel judged an indicator as being in the highest tertile of validity (that is, having a rating of 7, 8, or 9) and three members rated it as being in the lowest tertile of validity (1, 2, or 3) (Brook, 1994). Indicators with a median validity rating of 7 or higher without disagreement were included in the system.

We also obtained ratings from the panelists about the feasibility of obtaining the data necessary to score the indicators from medical. This was done to make explicit that failure to document key variables required to score an indicator would be treated as though the recommended care was not provided.

Although we do not intend for quality assessment to impose significant additional documentation burdens, we wanted the panel to acknowledge that documentation itself is an element of quality particularly when patients are treated by a team of health professionals. Because of the variability in documentation patterns and the opportunity to empirically evaluate feasibility, indicators with a median feasibility rating of 4 and higher were accepted into the system. Indicators had to satisfy both the validity and feasibility criteria.

Five expert panels were convened on the topics of children's care, care for women 18-50, general medicine for adults, oncologic conditions and HIV, and cardiopulmonary conditions.

The dates on which the panels were conducted are shown in Table I.2.

Table I.2

Dates Expert Panels Convened

Children	October 1995
Women	November 1995
Cardiopulmonary	September 1997
Oncology/HIV	October 1997
General Medicine	November 1997

Tables I.3 through I.6 summarize the distribution of indicators by level of evidence, type of care (preventive, acute, chronic), function of medicine (screening, diagnosis, treatment, follow-up, continuity), and modality (for example, history, physical examination, laboratory test, medication) (Malin et al., 2000; Schuster et al., 1997).

The categories were selected by the research team and reflect terminology commonly used by health services researchers to describe different aspects of health service delivery. The categories also reflect the areas in which we intend to develop aggregate quality of care scores. However, a significant benefit of the QA Tools system is its adaptability to other frameworks.

Note: In the following tables, the figures in some columns may not total exactly 100 percent due to the rounding of fractional numbers.

Table I.3

Distribution of Indicators (%) by Level of Evidence

Level Of Evidence	Children	Women	Cancer/HIV	Cardio-pulmonary	General Medicine
Randomized trials	11	22	22	18	23
Nonrandomized trials	6	16	37	4	17
Descriptive studies	72	59	26	71	57
Added by panel	12	4	15	7	4
Total	101	101	100	100	101

Table I.4

Distribution of Indicators (%) by Type of Care

Type Of Care	Children	Women	Cancer/HIV	Cardio-pulmonary	General Medicine
Preventive	30	11	20	3	18
Acute	36	49	7	26	38
Chronic	34	41	74	71	44
Total	100	101	101	100	100

Table I.5

Distribution of Indicators (%) by Function of Medicine

Function Of Medicine	Children	Women	Cancer/HIV	Cardio-pulmonary	General Medicine
Screening	23	18	9	3	12
Diagnosis	31	30	27	54	41
Treatment	36	43	53	36	41
Follow-up	10	12	10	8	6
Total	100	103	99	101	100

Table I.6

Distribution of Indicators (%) by Modality

Modality	Children	Women	Cancer/HIV	Cardio-pulmonary	General Medicine
History	19	18	4	11	23
Physical	19	10	5	21	15
Lab/Radiology	21	23	24	23	18
Medication	25	29	25	25	26
Other	17	19	42	20	17
Total	101	99	100	100	99

DEVELOPING QUALITY INDICATORS FOR WOMEN

We now describe in more detail the process by which we developed quality indicators for women, ages 18-50.

Selecting Clinical Areas

We began by examining national data sources to identify the leading causes of mortality, morbidity, and functional limitation among women. The principal data sources for this review were Vital Statistics, the National Health Interview Survey (NHIS), the National Ambulatory Medical Care Survey (NAMCS), and the National Hospital Discharge Survey (NHDS). From the leading causes of morbidity and mortality, we selected areas that would be representative of primary, secondary, and tertiary care.

We completed literature reviews and proposed quality of care criteria for the following clinical areas for women (in alphabetical order):

- Acne
- Alcohol use
- Allergic rhinitis
- Asthma
- Breast mass
- Cesarean delivery (prior cesarean, failure to progress in labor, fetal distress and other fetal status problems, prophylactic antibiotic use)
- Cigarette use
- Corticosteroids for fetal maturation
- Depression
- Diabetes mellitus
- Family planning/contraception
- Headache
- Hypertension
- Low back pain (acute)
- Prenatal care
- Preventive care (immunizations, sexually transmitted diseases and HIV, prevention, obesity counseling, seat belt use, breast examination, hyperlipidemia, hypertension, cervical cancer)
- Upper respiratory infections (acute pharyngitis, acute bronchitis, influenza, nasal congestion and rhinorrhea, acute sinusitis, chronic sinusitis)
- Urinary tract infections

- Vaginitis and sexually transmitted diseases (vulvovaginitis, diseases characterized by cervicitis, pelvic inflammatory disease, diseases characterized by genital ulcers)

The system is designed to evaluate services for a substantial portion of the ambulatory care received by the population. In order to determine the percentage of ambulatory care visits the indicator system would cover, we classified the 1993 NAMCS data ICD-9 codes for women 18 to 50 years of age into the 20 conditions for which we will develop quality indicators. This information is presented in Table I.7, which takes a fairly broad approach to categorizing an area as "included" in the quality indicators. In addition, cesarean section is an inpatient procedure and is underrepresented by visits captured in the NAMCS data.

As indicated in the table, by developing indicators for the 20 women's clinical areas listed above, we will capture over one-half (52 percent) of all the diagnoses in the 1993 NAMCS data. The diagnoses with the highest frequency include upper respiratory infections (8.3 percent), prenatal care (6.6 percent), and allergic rhinitis (6.0 percent).

Table I.7

Proportion of Ambulatory Care Estimated to be Evaluated in the QA Tool Indicator System, Based on 1993 NAMCS Data for Women 18-50 Years of Age

Clinical Area	Frequency of Visits (in thousands)	Percent of Total
Acne	219	2.4
Alcohol Dependence	4	0.0
Allergic Rhinitis	553	6.0
Asthma	367	4.0
Breast Mass	448	4.9
Cesarean Delivery	31	0.3
Cigarette Use Counseling	3	0.0
Depression	497	5.4
Diabetes Mellitus	34	0.4
Family Planning/Contraception	52	0.6
Headache	225	2.4
Hypertension	94	1.0
Low Back Pain (Acute)	151	1.6
Prenatal Care	607	6.6
Preterm Labor	2	0.0
Preventive Care	354	3.9
Upper Respiratory Infections	758	8.3
Urinary Tract Infections	100	1.1
Vaginitis and STDs	208	2.3
Medications	0	0.0
Visits with codes applicable to more than one clinical area	95	1.0
Total Included	4,802	52.2
Overall Total	9,187	

Conducting Literature Reviews

The literature reviews were conducted as described earlier in this Introduction by a team of 14 physician investigators, many of whom have clinical expertise in the conditions selected for this project. Each investigator drafted a review of the literature for his or her topic area, focusing on important areas for quality measurement (as opposed to a clinical review of the literature, which would focus on clinical management) and drafted potential indicators.

Every indicator table was reviewed by Dr. Kerr for content, consistency, and the likely availability of information necessary to score adherence to the indicator from the medical record. On a few occasions, when questions remained even after detailed literature review, we requested that a clinical leader in the field read and comment on the draft review and indicators.

Because of the breadth of topics that we were trying to address in this project, many of the literature reviews relied exclusively on textbooks and review articles. Nonetheless, we believe that for the purposes of this project, the reviews represent a reasonable summary of current clinical opinion and key research in each of the areas.

Developing Indicators

In each clinical area, we developed indicators to define the explicit criteria by which quality of care would be evaluated. Indicators were developed, where appropriate, for screening, diagnosis, treatment, and follow-up.

Our approach makes a strong distinction between indicators of quality of care and practice guidelines (see Table I.8). Whereas guidelines are intended to be comprehensive in scope, indicators are meant to apply to specific clinical circumstances where there is believed to be a strong link between a measurable health care process and patient outcomes. Indicators are not intended to measure all possible care for a condition. Furthermore, guidelines are intended to be applied prospectively at the individual patient level, whereas indicators are applied retrospectively and scored at an aggregate level. Finally, indicators must be written precisely in order to be *operationalized* (that is, to form useful measures of quality based on medical record or administrative data).

Table I.8

Clinical Guidelines versus Quality Indicators

Guidelines	Indicators
Comprehensive: Cover virtually all aspects of care for a condition.	**Targeted**: Apply to specific clinical circumstances in which there is evidence of a process-outcome link.
Prescriptive: Intended to influence provider behavior prospectively at the individual patient level.	**Observational:** Measure past provider behavior at an aggregate level.
Flexible: Intentionally allow room for clinical judgment and interpretation.	**Operational:** Precise language that can be applied systematically to medical records or administrative data.

The indicator tables at the end of each chapter of this book
- identify the population to whom the indicators apply
- state the indicator itself
- provide a "grade" for the quality of the scientific evidence that supports the indicator
- list the specific literature used to support the indicator
- provide a statement of the health benefits of complying with the indicator
- give comments to further explain the purpose or reasoning behind the indicator.

Selecting Panel Participants

We requested nominations for potential participants in the expert panel process from the American College of Physicians, the American Academy of Family Practice, and the American College of Obstetricians and Gynecologists. A few supplemental recommendations were made by research staff. We received a total of 81 nominations from the professional societies.

Each nominee was sent a letter summarizing the purpose of the project and indicating which group recommended them. Interested candidates were asked to return a curriculum vitae and calendar with available dates for a two-day panel meeting. We received positive responses from 156 potential panelists. The quality of the recommended panelists was excellent.

We sought to assemble a panel that was diverse with respect to type of practice (academic, community practice, managed care practice), geographic location, and specialty. Because of the wide variety of conditions that would be considered by the panel, we decided on a specialty distribution of four family practitioners, three internists, and two OB/GYNs. The panel was chaired by an internist (Dr. Ambrosini). (See the Acknowledgements at the front of this book for the list of panelists.)

Selecting the Final Indicators

The panel process was conducted as described above. The summary ratings sheets for women are shown in Appendix B. Figure I.2 provides an example of a final summary rating sheet. The chapter number and clinical condition are shown in the top left margin. The rating bar is numbered from 1 to 9, indicating the range of possible responses. The number shown above each of the responses in the rating bar indicates how many panelists provided that particular rating for the indicator. Below the score distribution, in parentheses, the median and the mean absolute deviation from the median are listed. Each dimension is assigned an A for "Agreement", D for "Disagreement", and I for "Indeterminate" based on the score distribution.

5. Initial laboratory tests should include the following:

	Validity	Feasibility
a. Urinalysis.	1 1 1 1 1 4 1 2 3 4 5 6 7 8 9 (7.0, 1.8, I)	1 2 6 1 2 3 4 5 6 7 8 9 (8.0, 0.9, A)
b. Glucose.	1 1 2 4 1 1 2 3 4 5 6 7 8 9 (7.0, 1.3, I)	1 1 4 3 1 2 3 4 5 6 7 8 9 (7.0, 1.2, A)
c. Potassium.	2 4 3 1 2 3 4 5 6 7 8 9 (7.0, 0.6, A)	1 4 4 1 2 3 4 5 6 7 8 9 (7.0, 0.6, A)
d. Calcium.	4 4 1 1 2 3 4 5 6 7 8 9 (6.0, 0.6, A)	2 3 4 1 2 3 4 5 6 7 8 9 (7.0, 0.9, A)
e. Creatinine.	4 5 1 2 3 4 5 6 7 8 9 (8.0, 0.4, A)	1 8 1 2 3 4 5 6 7 8 9 (8.0, 0.1, A)
f. Uric acid.	1 1 2 3 2 1 2 3 4 5 6 7 8 9 (5.0, 1.0, A)	1 1 3 4 1 2 3 4 5 6 7 8 9 (7.0, 1.2, A)
g. Cholesterol.	8 1 1 2 3 4 5 6 7 8 9 (7.0, 0.1, A)	4 5 1 2 3 4 5 6 7 8 9 (8.0, 0.4, A)
h. Triglycerides.	1 2 1 5 1 2 3 4 5 6 7 8 9 (7.0, 1.1, I)	1 5 3 1 2 3 4 5 6 7 8 9 (7.0, 0.8, A)
i. Electrocardiogram.	1 2 1 3 2 1 2 3 4 5 6 7 8 9 (7.0, 2.0, D)	1 2 6 1 2 3 4 5 6 7 8 9 (8.0, 0.9, I)
j. Echocardiogram.	1 2 5 1 1 2 3 4 5 6 7 8 9 (3.0, 0.6, A)	1 3 2 1 2 1 2 3 4 5 6 7 8 9 (5.0, 1.9, D)

(TREATMENT)
6. First-line treatment for [Stage 1-2] hypertension is
lifestyle modification. The medical record should indicate
counseling for at least one of the following interventions
prior to pharmacotherapy:
- weight reduction,
- increased physical activity,
- low sodium diet, or
- alcohol intake reduction.

	Validity	Feasibility
	3 5 1 1 2 3 4 5 6 7 8 9 (8.0, 0.4, A)	1 3 3 2 1 2 3 4 5 6 7 8 9 (7.0, 1.0, I)

Scales: 1 = low validity or feasibility; 9 = high validity or feasibility.

Figure I.2 - Sample Rating Results Sheet

We recommend caution when reviewing the ratings for each indicator. The overall median does not tell us anything about the extent to which these indicators occur in clinical practice. To determine that, actual clinical data to assess the indicators must be collected and analyzed.

Analyzing The Final Indicators

Of the 373 indicators initially proposed by staff, 15 were deleted or merged with other indicators and 33 were added or split into separate indicators. Of the 33 indicators added or split, 15 of these were added during the panel meeting discussions. Therefore, a total of 391 indicators were available for final rating at the panel meeting. A total of 340 (87%) were retained. Of the 51 dropped, 48 were dropped because of low validity scores, 1 for substantial disagreement on validity, and 2 by consensus.

A crosswalk table including the original indicators proposed by staff, the modified indicators (based on panel input), and comments explaining any changes (additions, deletions, or modifications) to the indicators is provided in Appendix C. This table is useful for tracking the progress of indicator development and selection.

Because the quality indicators are designed to produce aggregate scores, it is useful to examine the distribution of indicators by type of care (preventive, acute and chronic), function of medical care (screening, diagnosis, treatment, and follow-up), and modality of care delivered (such as history, physical examination, laboratory study, medication; other interventions such as counseling, education, procedure, psychotherapy, surgery; and other contact such as general follow-up, referral to subspecialist, or hospitalization. Indicators are assigned to one type of care, but can have up to two functions or three modalities.

As indicated in Table I.9, of the final set of 340 indicators, 11 percent are preventive care, 49 percent acute care, and 41 percent chronic care. When categorized by function, almost three-fourths of the indicators fell into the diagnosis and treatment categories. Finally, there was a fairly even distribution of indicators by modality, with almost one-half falling into the laboratory or radiologic study (23 percent) and medication (29 percent) categories.

Table I.9

Distribution of Final Set of Women's Indicators by Type of Care, Function, and Modality

Category	Adult Women Indicators, % of Each Category
Type of Care	
Preventive	11
Acute	49
Chronic	41
Function	
Screening	18
Diagnosis	30
Treatment	43
Follow-up	12
Modality	
History	18
Physical Examination	10
Laboratory or Radiologic Study	23
Medication	29
Other Intervention	12
Other Contact	7

Note: Percentages do not always add to 100% due to rounding.

As discussed earlier in this Introduction, each indicator was assigned a strength of evidence code of I (randomized controlled trial [RCT]), II (nonrandomized controlled trial, cohort or case-control study, multiple time series), or III (expert opinion or descriptive study). Table I.10 shows the distribution of the indicators by strength of evidence for the original indicators proposed by staff, the indicators that were voted on by panelists, and the final set of indicators. The majority (57 percent) of the final set of 340 indicators was based on expert opinion or descriptive studies. Twenty-two percent were based on randomized clinical trials and 18 percent on other rigorous studies. Panelists were more likely to retain indicators based on experimental or observational trials than those based only on expert opinion.

4 -

Table I.10

Distribution of Women's Indicators by Strength of Evidence

Strength of Evidence*	Original % (n)	Voted On % (n)	After Vote % (n)
I	20 (75)	21 (84)	22 (74)
II	17 (64)	16 (62)	18 (61)
III	63 (234)	59 (229)	57 (193)
N/A		4 (16)	4 (12)
Total**	100 (373)	100 (391)	100 (340)

* I = randomized controlled trial; II=nonrandomized controlled trial, cohort or case-control study, multiple time series; III=expert opinion or descriptive study; NA=indicator for which strength of evidence is not available because it was added after literature reviews were completetd.
** Percentages do not always add up to 100% due to rounding.

Conclusion

We have demonstrated that it is possible to develop a comprehensive set of quality indicators for women. These indicators cover 20 clinical conditions, span a range of clinical functions and modalities, and are supported by the literature.

The comprehensive nature of this system is evident upon examination of the type and nature of the indicators. Out of a total of 391 indicators available for rating at the panel meeting, 340 (87 percent) were retained by the panel. Although the majority of health care visits for this population is generally for acute care purposes, one-half of the indicators cover preventive and chronic care, with the remaining half covering acute care. Unlike other quality assessment tools, this system covers all four functions of medicine including, screening, diagnosis, treatment, and follow-up. Moreover, the indicators cover a variety of modes of care provision including history, physical examination, laboratory study, medication, and other interventions and contacts.

There are many advantages to a comprehensive quality assessment system such as this one. Not only does it cover the broadest possible range of health conditions experienced by the target population, but it designed to target populations vulnerable to underutilization. In addition, because of the extent of the system (340 indicators) it is difficult for health care organizations to focus on a few indicators to increase their quality scores.

Finally, it is a system that can be effective for both internal and external quality reviews. Health plans can use the system in order to improve the overall quality of the care provided. And, because of the simple summary scores that will be produced, it will be an important tool for purchasers who are making choices about health plans.

ORGANIZATION OF THIS DOCUMENT

The rest of this volume is organized as follows:

- Each chapter summarizes
    - results of the literature review for one condition
    - provides a table of the staff recommended indicators based on that review
    - lists the cited studies.
- Appendix A provides definitions of terms used in the indicator tables.
- Appendix B contains the panel rating sheets for each condition.
- Appendix C shows the original proposed definition of each indicator, notes any modifications resulting from the panel process, and provides additional comments, including whether the panel adopted or rejected the indicator.

REFERENCES

Asch, S. M., E. A. Kerr, E. G. Hamilton, J. L. Reifel, E. A. McGlynn (eds.), *Quality of Care for Oncologic Conditions and HIV: A Review of the Literature and Quality Indicators*, Santa Monica, CA: RAND, MR-1281-AHRQ, 2000.

Brook, R. H., "The RAND/UCLA Appropriateness Method," *Clinical Practice Guideline Development: methodology perspectives*, AHCPR Pub. No. 95-0009, Rockville, MD: Public Health Service, 1994.

Kerr E. A., S. M. Asch, E. G. Hamilton, E. A. McGlynn (eds.), *Quality of Care for Cardiopulmonary Conditions: A Review of the Literature and Quality Indicators*, Santa Monica, CA: RAND, MR-1282-AHRQ, 2000a.

Kerr E. A., S. M. Asch, E. G. Hamilton, E. A. McGlynn (eds.), *Quality of Care for General Medical Conditions: A Review of the Literature and Quality Indicators*, Santa Monica, CA: RAND, MR-1280-AHRQ, 2000b.

Kravitz R. L., M. Laouri, J. P. Kahan, P. Guzy, et al., "Validity of Criteria Used for Detecting Underuse of Coronary Revascularization," *JAMA* 274(8):632-638, 1995.

Malin, J. L., S. M. Asch, E. A. Kerr, E. A. McGlynn. "Evaluating the Quality of Cancer Care: Development of Cancer Quality Indicators for a Global Quality Assessment Tool," *Cancer*, 88:701-7, 2000.

McGlynn E. A., C. Damberg, E. A. Kerr, M. Schuster (eds.), *Quality of Care for Children and Adolescents: A Review of Selected Clinical Conditions and Quality Indicators*, Santa Monica, CA: RAND, MR-1283-HCFA, 2000.

Park R. A., Fink A., Brook R. H., Chassin M. R., et al., "Physician Ratings of Appropriate Indications for Six Medical and Surgical Procedures," *AJPH* 76(7):766-772, 1986.

Schuster M. A., S. M. Asch, E. A. McGlynn, et al., "Development of a Quality of Care Measurement System for Children and Adolescents: Methodological Considerations and Comparisons With a System for Adult Women," *Archives of Pediatrics and Adolescent Medicine*, 151:1085-1092, 1997.

Selby J. V., B. H. Fireman, R. J. Lundstrom, et al., "Variation among Hospitals in Coronary-Angiography Practices and Outcomes after Myocardial Infarction in a Large Health Maintenance Organization," *N Engl J Med*, 335:1888-96, 1996.

Shekelle P. G., J. P. Kahan, S. J. Bernstein, et al., "The Reproducibility of a Method to Identify the Overuse and Underuse of Medical Procedures," *N Engl J Med*, 338:1888-1895, 1998b.

Shekelle P. G., M. R. Chassin, R. E. Park, "Assessing the Predictive Validity of the RAND/UCLA Appropriateness Method Criteria for Performing Carotid Endarterectomy," *Int J Technol Assess Health Care*, 14(4):707-727, 1998a.

1. ACNE

Lisa Schmidt, M.P.H., and Eve A. Kerr, M.D.

Approach

The general approach to summarizing the key literature on acne in adolescents and adult women was to review two adolescent health text books (Vernon and Lane, 1992; Paller et al., 1992) and two articles chosen from a MEDLINE search of all English language articles published between the years of 1990 and 1995 on the treatment of acne.

IMPORTANCE

Acne is the most common skin disorder seen during adolescence. Forty percent of children between the ages of 8 and 10 develop early acne lesions, and eventually 85 percent of adolescents develop some degree of acne (Vernon and Lane, 1992; Paller et al., 1992). Acne can persist into mid-adulthood in some persons, and can also present initially in adulthood. It is estimated that 40 to 50 percent of adult women are affected by a low-grade persistent form of acne (Nguyen et al., 1994). Overall, acne affects approximately 10 percent of the U.S. population (Glassman et al., 1993). Acne was the most common reason for visits to dermatologists over the two-year period from 1989 to 1990, accounting for 16.6 percent of all visits (Nelson, 1994). Although acne is not associated with severe morbidity, mortality, or disability it can produce psychological effects. For instance, it has been reported that some adolescents with acne avoid social situations or athletic activities (Brook et al., 1980). Furthermore, in severe cases, acne can lead to physical scarring which may exacerbate the emotional effects of the disease.

EFFICACY AND/OR EFFECTIVENESS OF INTERVENTIONS

Screening

There is no role for screening for acne.

Diagnosis

Common acne is a disorder of the pilosebaceous glands and is characterized by follicular occlusion and inflammation (Paller et al., 1992). Acne occurs primarily on the face, but it can occur on the back, chest, and shoulders. Four factors contribute to the development of acne: 1) the sebum excretion rate, 2) sebaceous lipid composition, 3) bacteriology of the pilosebaceous duct, and 4) obstruction of the pilosebaceous duct. The anaerobic bacterium *Propionibacterium acnes* appears to play an important role in the pathogenesis of acne (Paller et al., 1992). *P. acnes* is capable of releasing lipolytic enzymes that convert the triglycerides in sebum into irritating fatty acids and glycerol, which may contribute to inflammation (Paller et al., 1992).

There are six types of acne lesions: comedones, papules, pustules, nodules, cysts, and scars. Individual patients may have one or more predominant type of lesion or a mixture of many lesions (Paller et al., 1992).

Vernon and Lane (1992) and Glassman et al. (1993) recommend the following in diagnosing acne:

Documentation of the acne history including:

- age at onset of acne;
- location (face, back, neck, chest);
- aggravating factors (stress, seasons, cosmetics, cremes);
- menstrual history and premenstrual worsening of acne;
- previous treatments;
- family history of acne; and
- medications and drug use.

The physical examination should include:

- location of acne;
- types of lesions present;
- severity of disease (numbers of each type of lesion and intensity of inflammation); and
- complications (extent and severity of hyperpigmentation and scarring).

Treatment

Medical treatment of acne is determined by the extent and severity of disease, prior treatments, and therapeutic goals. Each regimen must be followed for a minimum of 4 to 6 weeks before determining whether it is effective (Vernon and Lane, 1992). Table 1.1 lists guidelines to be used in the treatment of acne.

Table 1.1

Guidelines for the Treatment of Acne

Clinical Appearance	Treatment
Comedonal Acne - no inflammatory lesions	Topical tretinoin *or* benzoyl peroxide
Mild to Moderate Inflammatory Acne - red papules, few pustules	Topical tretinoin *and* benzoyl peroxide *and/or* topical antibiotic If acne is resistant to above therapy, add oral antibiotic.
Moderate to Severe Inflammatory Acne - red papules, many pustules	Topical tretinoin; topical antibiotic *or* benzoyl peroxide; *and* oral antibiotics
Severe Nodulocystic Acne - red papules, pustules, cysts and nodules	Topical tretinoin; benzoyl peroxide *or* topical antibiotic; oral antibiotics; *and* consider isotretinoin

Adapted from: Weston and Lane, 1991; Vernon and Lane 1992; Nguyen, 1994; Taylor, 1991.

Tretinoin and Benzoyl Peroxide

Topical keratolytic therapy is recommended as the primary treatment for comedonal acne to prevent new acne lesions as well as to treat preexisting ones (Paller et al., 1992). Two classes of keratolytics, tretinoin (retin A) and benzoyl peroxide, can be used alone or in combination with each other and will control 80 to 85 percent of acne (Taylor, 1991; Weston and Lane, 1991; Nguyen, 1994). Cream preparations of both tretinoin and benzoyl peroxide should be used because they are less irritating to the skin than gel forms. Tretinoin has a propensity to severely irritate the skin if used incorrectly. To avoid irritation, a low strength (0.025 percent) cream should be applied every other night for one week and then nightly. In addition, because skin treated with tretinoin is more sensitive to sun exposure, sunscreen should be used.

Tretinoin should be avoided during pregnancy because of the potential of photoisomerization to isotretinoin (a teratogen) (Weston and Lane, 1991; Vernon and Lane, 1992). Improvement of acne after treatment of tretinoin can take six to twelve weeks and flare-ups of acne can occur during the first few weeks due to surfacing of the lesions onto the skin (Nguyen, 1994). Benzoyl peroxide is available over-the-counter in various strengths and applications (gels, creams, lotions, or soaps). All concentrations seem to be therapeutically equivalent (Nguyen, 1994). Mild redness and scaling of the skin may occur during the first week of use.

Topical Antibiotics

Topical antibiotics decrease the quantity of *P. acnes* in the hair follicles. However, they are less effective than oral antibiotics because of their low solubility and consequent difficulty in penetrating sebum-filled follicules (Nguyen, 1994). Topical erythromycin and clindamycin are similar in efficacy and can be used once or twice a day (Weston, and Lane, 1991; Nguyen, 1994). Some percutaneous absorption may rarely occur with clindamycin, resulting in diarrhea and colitis (Weston and Lane, 1991; Nguyen, 1994). Topical antibiotics are frequently used in combination with keratolytics and are most useful for maintenance therapy if improvement after 1 to 2 months of oral antibiotics is observed (Weston and Lane, 1991).

Oral Antibiotics

Patients with moderate to severe inflammatory acne will require oral antibiotics in addition to topical therapy. Tetracycline and erythromycin are the most commonly used systemic antibiotics. Because tetracycline can cause enamel hyperplasia and tooth discoloration it should not be used in pregnant women or in children under 12 years of age (Nguyen, 1994). Minocycline is very effective for many adolescents who have used tetracycline without success (Weston and Lane, 1991). The cost of minocycline, however, limits its use to those patients with severe or recalcitrant acne. When tetracycline is prescribed for female patients, pregnancy status must be monitored since tetracycline is teratogenic (Glassman et al., 1993). There is the potential for broad-spectrum antibiotics to alter the absorption of oral contraceptives

(OCs); therefore, it may be prudent for women on OCs to use an alternate method of birth control when possible.

Isotretinoin

The oral retinoid isotretinoin has been very efficacious in nodulocystic acne resistant to standard therapeutic regimens. In appropriate regimens, isotretinoin has resulted in long-term remission of acne in approximately 60 percent of patients treated (Weston and Lane, 1991). However, it is not recommended as the drug of first choice because of its severe teratogenicity. Current recommendations for women of child-bearing age are: to obtain informed consent; to perform pregnancy tests throughout treatment; to postpone initiating therapy until the menstrual cycle begins; and, to use two effective birth control methods from the month before treatment to one month after discontinuing treatment (Weston and Lane, 1991). Side effects of isotretinoin include dryness and scaliness of the skin, dry lips and occasionally dry eyes and nose. It can also cause decreased night vision, hypertriglyceridemia, abnormal liver function, electrolyte imbalance, and elevated platelet count. Glassman et al. (1993) recommend monthly liver function tests to monitor potential for liver toxicity. Up to 10 percent of patients experience mild hair loss, but the effect is reversible (Weston and Lane, 1991).

Follow-up

Follow-up visits for acne should be scheduled initially every 4 to 6 weeks. Ideal control is defined as no more than a few new lesions every two weeks (Weston and Lane, 1991).

RECOMMENDED QUALITY INDICATORS FOR ACNE

The following criteria apply to women under 50 years of age.

Diagnosis

	Indicator	Quality of evidence	Literature	Benefits	Comments
1.	For patients presenting with acne, the following history should be documented in their chart: a. location of lesions (back, face, neck, chest); b. aggravating factors (stress, seasons, cosmetics, creams); c. menstrual history and premenstrual worsening of acne; d. previous treatments; and e. medications and drug use	III	Glassman, et al., 1992 and Vernon and Lane, 1992	Improve acne; decrease psychological effects of acne; and, decrease potential physical scarring.	An adequate history is necessary to determine any potential causes or exacerbating factors of the acne and to document severity and response to treatments.

Treatment

	Indicator	Quality of evidence	Literature	Benefits	Comments
2.	If oral antibiotics are prescribed, there must be documentation of moderate to severe acne (papules and pustules).	III	Vernon and Lane, 1992; Glassman et al., 1993; Weston and Lane, 1991	Improve acne; decrease psychological effects of acne; and, decrease potential physical scarring.	If only comedones are present, antibiotics should not be prescribed since they are not effective for comedones and have potential toxicities.
3.	If tetracycline is prescribed, there must be documentation of the last menstrual period or a negative pregnancy test for women of child-bearing age.	III	Vernon and Lane, 1992	Prevent birth defects.	Tetracycline is a known teratogen.
4.	If isotretinoin is prescribed, there must be documentation of severe acne (papules, pustules, cysts and nodules) and a failure of previous therapy.	III	Vernon and Lane, 1992; Glassman et al., 1993; Weston and Lane, 1991; Nguyen, 1994	Improve acne; decrease psychological effects of acne; and, decrease potential physical scarring.	Isotretinoin has severe teratogenic effects and potential for liver toxicity. Its use should be restricted to those with severe, recalcitrant nodulocystic acne.
5.	If isotretinoin is prescribed, a negative pregnancy test should be obtained within two weeks of start of therapy.	III	Vernon and Lane, 1992; Glassman et al., 1993; Weston and Lane, 1991	Prevent teratogenic effects to fetus.	Isotretinoin has severe teratogenic effects. Serum or urine tests for pregnancy are acceptable.

Indicator	Quality of evidence	Literature	Benefits	Comments
6.	If isotretinoin is prescribed, there should be documentation that counseling regarding use of an effective means of contraception (including abstinence) was provided.	III	Weston and Lane, 1991	Prevent teratogenic effects to fetus.	Isotretinoin has severe teratogenic effects.

Follow-up

	Indicator	Quality of evidence	Literature	Benefits	Comments
7.	If isotretinoin is prescribed, monthly pregnancy tests should be be performed.	III	Vernon and Lane, 1992; Glassman et al., 1993; Weston and Lane, 1991	Prevent teratogenic effects to fetus.	Isotretinoin has severe teratogenic effects. Serum or urine tests may be used to screen for pregnancy.
8.	If isotretinoin is prescribed, monthly liver function tests should be performed.	III	Glassman et al., 1993	Prevent liver disease.	Isotretinoin has the potential effects on the liver such as toxicity or failure.

Quality of Evidence Codes:

I: RCT
II-1:   Nonrandomized controlled trials
II-2:   Cohort or case analysis
II-3:   Multiple time series
III: Opinions or descriptive studies

REFERENCES - ACNE

Brook, RH, KN Lohr, GA Goldberg, et al. 1980. *Conceptualization and Measurement of Physiologic Health for Adults: Acne*. RAND, Santa Monica, CA.

Glassman, PA, D Garcia, and JP Delafield. 1993. *Outpatient Care Handbook*. Philadelphia, PA: Hanley and Belfus, Inc.

Nelson, C. 10 March 1994. Office visits to dermatologists: National Ambulatory Medical Care Survey, United States, 1989-90. *Advance Data*. National Center for Health Statistics. U.S. Department of Health and Human Services, Hyattsville, MD.

Nguyen QH, YA Kim, RA Schwartz, et al. July 1994. Management of acne vulgaris. *American Family Physician* 50 (1): 89-96.

Paller AS, EA Abel, and IJ Frieden. 1992. Dermatologic problems. In *Comprehensive Adolescent Health Care*. Editors Friedman SB, M Fisher, and SK Schonberg, 584-64. St. Louis, MO: Quality Medical Publishing, Inc.

Taylor MB. June 1991. Treatment of acne vulgaris. *Postgraduate Medicine* 89 (8): 40-7.

Vernon HJ, and AT Lane. 1992. Skin disorders. In *Textbook of Adolescent Medicine*. Editors McAnarney ER, RE Kreipe, DP Orr, et al., 272-82. Philadelphia, PA: W.B. Saunders Company.

Weston WL, and AT Lane. 1991. Acne. In *Color Textbook of Pediatric Dermatology*. 15-25. St. Louis, MO: Mosby-Year Book, Inc.

2. ALCOHOL DEPENDENCE
Steven Asch, M.D., M.P.H.

We relied on four main sources to construct quality indicators for alcohol abuse among adult women. Three are the reports of federally sponsored task forces (United States Preventive Services Task Force [USPSTF], 1989; Committee of the Institute of Medicine [IOM], 1990; National Institutes of Health [NIH], 1993) and one is a review article (Fleming, 1993). When these core references cited studies to support individual indicators, we have referenced the original source. When the core references were unclear in their support for a particular indicator, we performed a narrow MEDLINE search of English-language articles addressing that topic from January 1966 to 1995.

IMPORTANCE

Alcohol is consumed by over half of all American adults, and about 10 percent of users meet criteria for dependence (see below). It has been estimated that alcohol accounts for 69,000 deaths annually, including those resulting from alcohol-related motor vehicle deaths, homicides, and suicides, as well as the clinical sequelae of chronic use like cirrhosis, pancreatitis, gastrointestinal bleeding, and cardiomyopathy (USPSTF, 1989). Annual societal costs exceed $115 billion in medical treatment, lost productivity, and property damage (Kamerow et al., 1986). The lifetime prevalence rate of alcohol dependence among all individuals in the U.S. aged 18 years and older has been estimated at 13 percent (Regier et al., 1988). The one-month prevalence rate of alcohol dependence in women between the ages of 25 and 44 is about 1 percent, somewhat higher than in older women and considerably lower than among men (Regier et al., 1988), although the gap between men and women is probably smaller than reported because alcohol abuse by women tends to be hidden (Halliday and Bush, 1987, in Barnes et al., 1987; Cyr and Moulton, 1990). In addition, evidence has accumulated that women are more susceptible to cirrhotic, traumatic and cardiomyopathic complications of heavy alcohol use (Bigby and Cyr, 1995, in Carlson et al., 1995; Gearhart et al., 1991; Urbano-Marquez et al., 1995), perhaps as a result of lower levels of gastric alcohol dehydrogenase (Frezza et al., 1990); however, similar to men, light to moderate alcohol use by women may actually decrease overall mortality (Fuchs et al., 1995).

Table 2.1

Standardized One-Month Prevalence Rates of Alcohol Dependence By Sex and Age

Age	One-Month Prevalence (percent)	
	Women	Men
18-24	2.3	6.0
25-44	1.1	6.2
45-64	0.3	4.0
65+	0.3	1.8
All ages	0.9	5.0

Source: Regier et al., 1988
NOTE: The rates are standardized to the age, sex, and race distribution of the 1980 noninstitutionalized population.

EFFICACY AND/OR EFFECTIVENESS OF INTERVENTIONS

Screening

Common definitions of *alcohol dependence* require several basic elements (American Psychiatric Association [APA], 1994):

(1) regular or binge use,

(2) tolerance of the psychoactive effects,

(3) physical dependence, and/or

(4) interference with social function.

The APA defines *alcohol abuse* as a social disorder distinct from dependence in that the patient continues to drink despite the knowledge of recurrent social, occupational, psychological, physical or legal problems. Routine measures of biochemical markers like gamma-glutamyl transferase (GGT) are probably less sensitive and certainly less specific than clinical history in detecting dependence and abuse (Hoeksema and de Bock, 1993; USPSTF, 1989). Screening questionnaires have reasonable sensitivity and specificity in detecting dependence (see below), but can be unwieldy to apply *en bloc* to an unselected population. For that reason, many authors recommend instead that primary care providers at least ask patients about the first basic element, regular or binge use. Regular or binge use of alcohol is usually defined as more than 2 drinks/day, 11 drinks/week, or 5 drinks in any one day in the last month. (A drink is generally defined in ethanol equivalents with 1 ounce representing 1-2 drinks.) Though estimates of the sensitivity of patients' responses to such questions are lower than the estimated sensitivity of questionnaires (perhaps 50 percent), it can serve as a screen for further evaluation (Fleming, 1993; Cyr and Wartman, 1988; NIH, 1993).

Initial Evaluation

If patients show evidence of regular or binge use, there are many questionnaires that can assist in determining if the patient meets the other criteria for alcohol dependence. The lengthy Michigan Alcoholism Screening Test (MAST) has a reported sensitivity between 84 and 100 percent and a reported specificity of between 87 and 95 percent. The much shorter and more popular CAGE has only 4 items and an estimated sensitivity and specificity of 49-89 percent and 79-95 percent, respectively. Other questionnaires include the Self-Administered Alcoholism Screening Test (SAAST) (Swenson and Morse, 1975), Alcohol Use Disorder Identification Test (AUDIT) (Babor and Grant, 1989), the Short MAST (SMAST) (Selzer et al., 1975), and Health Screening Survey (HSS) (Fleming and Barry, 1991). If the patient reports regular or binge drinking, we propose that the chart should indicate some assessment of the three other criteria for alcohol dependence or the administration of one of the above-mentioned questionnaires.

Treatment

Treatment of alcohol dependence is usually divided into three phases:

1) detoxification,

2) active treatment and rehabilitation, and

3) relapse prevention.

The Institute of Medicine (IOM) reviewed more than 60 controlled trials evaluating specific treatments for one of these three phases, including inpatient and outpatient rehabilitation, mutual help groups, supportive psychotherapy, disulfuram, benzodiazapines, and aversion therapy. While various treatment modalities have clinical trial support when compared with no treatment, the IOM concluded that there was insufficient evidence to recommend any one modality over another. The Secretary's Eighth Special Report to Congress on Alcohol and Health (NIH, 1993) came to a similar conclusion, though the authors emphasized the need to tailor the treatment to the individual patient. In particular, they note one randomized controlled trial of 200 women assigned to a single gender vs. a mixed gender treatment group (Dahlgren and Willander, 1989). In this trial, the women assigned to the single gender group remained in treatment longer and had higher rates of program completion. However, the authors were reluctant to base recommendations on this single trial because treatment conditions varied in more aspects than gender segregation. We propose simply that the medical record should indicate referral for one of the above treatment modalities for alcohol dependent patients.

Regular or binge drinkers who do not meet criteria for dependence can still benefit from medical intervention. Two recent randomized trials have shown that primary care providers can reduce alcohol use among regular or binge drinkers. A British study of 47 medical practices and 909 patients who reported they drank more than 35 drinks per week found that a brief intervention decreased alcohol use, episodes of binge drinking, and GGT levels (Wallace et al., 1988). The intervention in this study consisted of physician advice, a self-help booklet, a weekly diary of alcohol use, and a written contract in the form of a prescription. A U.S. study of 72 women and 54 men who reported drinking between 21 and 70 drinks per week found that a brief intervention reduced alcohol use in men but not in women (Scott and

Anderson, 1990). The intervention in this trial consisted of a 10-minute brief advice session with the patient's primary care provider. Two other randomized trials have also found brief advice to be equally effective in reducing alcohol use as inpatient treatment (Edwards et al., 1977; Drummond et al., 1990). Given the low cost of such an intervention, many experts have recommended its widespread adoption (NIH, 1993; Fleming and Barry, 1991).

Follow-up

The core references agree that the third phase of treatment, relapse prevention, is the most difficult and least well evaluated. Most of the predictors of relapse (psychosocial stressors, mood state, concomitant psychiatric diagnoses) are difficult to modify. Two randomized trials comparing aftercare protocols have only shown that those patients who adhere to the assigned protocol relapse less often, regardless of the type of protocol used (Gilbert, 1988; McLatchie and Lomp, 1988; NIH, 1993). These trials compared different aftercare protocols head-to-head and found no difference in relapse rates by protocol, but did find that those who did not drop out relapsed less often. The outcome could be a result of self-selection of compliant or motivated patients. Observational trials of perhaps the best known aftercare program of all, Alcoholics Anonymous (AA), can be interpreted in the same way. Patients who subscribe to the 12-step AA philosophy or who maintain affiliation relapse less often (Gilbert, 1991; Cross, 1990), but the results could be due to patient self-selection. A trial of randomized court mandated attendance of AA meetings vs. no treatment showed no long-term difference in the likelihood of relapse (Brandsma et al., 1980). Given this weak evidence, we cannot recommend any particular aftercare program. Instead, we follow Fleming's recommendation that providers review all regular or binge drinkers' alcohol consumption at all subsequent visits (Fleming, 1993).

RECOMMENDED QUALITY INDICATORS FOR ALCOHOL DEPENDENCE

The following criteria apply to women age 18-50.

Diagnosis

	Indicator	Quality of evidence	Literature	Benefits	Comments
	Screening				
1.	New patients should be screened for problem drinking. This should include an assessment of at least one of the following: a. Quantity (e.g., drinks per day) b. Binge drinking (e.g., more than 5 drinks in a day in the last month)	II-III	Fleming, 1993	Reduce alcohol-associated pathology.*	Diagnosis of alcohol dependence requires regular or binge use. Sensitivity of history probably about 50 percent. Increased detection of problem drinkers may lead to counseling and detoxification and ultimately cessation of alcohol intake.
	Initial Assessment				
2.	The record should indicate more detailed screening for dependence, tolerance of psychoactive effects, loss of control and consequences of use (examples include but are not confined to the following questionnaires: CAGE, MAST, HSS, AUDIT, SAAST, and SMAST), if the medical record indicates any of the following: a. Patient drinks more than 2 drinks each day. b. Patient drinks more than 11 drinks per week. c. Patient drinks more than 5 drinks in a day in the last month.	II	Fleming, 1993; Babor and Grant, 1989; Swenson and Morse, 1975; Selzer et al., 1975	Reduce alcohol-associated pathology.*	Diagnosis of alcohol dependence requires evidence of dependence, loss of control and consequences. Sensitivity and specificity of questionnaires are 49-100 percent and 75-95 percent, respectively. Increased detection of alcohol dependence may lead to detoxification, treatment, and cessation.

Treatment

	Indicator	Quality of evidence	Literature	Benefits	Comments
3.	Patients diagnosed with alcohol dependence should be referred for further treatment to at least one of the following: a. Inpatient rehabilitation program b. Outpatient rehabilitation program c. Mutual help group (e.g., AA) d. Supportive psychotherapy e. Aversion therapy	I	NIH, 1993	Reduce alchohol-associated pathology.*	Multiple clinical trials show effectiveness of various treatment modalities, though no one treatment has consistently been demonstrated to be most effective.

Follow-up

	Indicator	Quality of evidence	Literature	Benefits	Comments
4.	Regular or binge drinkers (as defined above) should be advised to decrease their drinking.	I	Wallace et al., 1988; Scott and Anderson, 1990	Reduce alchohol-associated pathology.*	Two randomized trials have shown effectiveness of a brief intervention to reduce alcohol use in regular or binge drinkers, though one found no effect among women.
5.	Providers should reassess the alcohol intake of patients who report regular or binge drinking at every visit.	III	Fleming, 1993	Reduce alchohol-associated pathology.*	Prevention of relapse is the most difficult phase of treatment. Experts recommend frequent reassessment to evaluate success of intervention.

* Alcohol associated pathology includes: cirrhosis, pancreatitis, gastrointestinal bleeding, cardiomyopathy, assault, suicide and motor vehicle accidents. Cirrhosis, cardiomyopathy and pancreatitis may cause chronic decreases in health-related quality of life due to vomiting, ascites, abdominal pain, bleeding, shortness of breath and may eventually result in mortality. Gastrointestinal bleeding has a short-term mortality risk as well as a chronic impact on health-related quality of life due to anemia and other complications. Motor vehicle accidents and assaults may result in chronic disability from injuries and death. The health-related quality of life of persons other than the patient may also be affected. Liver disease and alcohol-related trauma are more common in women.

Quality of Evidence Codes:

I:	RCT
II-1:	Nonrandomized controlled trials
II-2:	Cohort or case analysis
II-3:	Multiple time series
III:	Opinions or descriptive studies

REFERENCES - ALCOHOL DEPENDENCE

American Psychiatric Association. 1994. Substance-related disorders. In *Diagnostic and Statistical Manual of Mental Disorders: DSM-IV*, Fourth ed. 175-205. Washington, DC: American Psychiatric Association.

Babor TF, and M Grant. 1989. From clinical research to secondary prevention: International collaboration in the development of the alcohol use disorders identification test (AUDIT). *International Perspectives* 13 (4): 371-4.

Bigby J, and MG Cyr. 1995. Alcohol and drug abuse. In *Primary Care of Women*. Editors Carlson KJ, and SA Eisenstat, 427-30. St. Louis, MO: Mosby-Year Book, Inc.

Brandsma, JM. 1980. Outpatient treatment of alcoholism: a review and comparative study. Baltimore: University Park Press.

Committee of the Institute of Medicine, Division of Mental Health and Behavioral Medicine. 1990. *Broadening the Base of Treatment for Alcohol Problems*. Washington, DC: National Academy Press.

Cross GM, CW Morgan, AJ Mooney, et al. March 1990. Alcoholism treatment: A ten-year follow-up study. *Alcoholism: Clinical and Experimental Research* 14 (2): 169-73.

Cyr MG, and AW Moulton. December 1990. Substance abuse in women. *Obstetrics and Gynecology Clinics of North America* 17 (4): 905-25.

Cyr MG, and SA Wartman. 1 January 1988. The effectiveness of routine screening questions in the detection of alcoholism. *Journal of the American Medical Association* 259 (1): 51-4.

Dahlgren L, and A Willander. July 1989. Are special treatment facilities for female alcoholics needed? A controlled 2-year follow-up study from a specialized female unit (EWA) versus a mixed male/female treatment facility. *Alcoholism: Clinical and Experimental Research* 13 (4): 499-504.

Drummond DC, B Thom, C Brown, et al. 1990. Clinical practice: Specialist versus general practitioner treatment of problem drinkers. *Lancet* 336: 915-8.

Edwards G, J Orford, S Egert, et al. 1977. Alcoholism: A controlled trial of "treatment" and "advice". *Journal of Studies on Alcohol* 38 (5): 1004-31.

Fleming MF. 1993. Screening and brief intervention for alcohol disorders. *Journal of Family Practice* 37 (3): 231-4.

Fleming MF, and KL Barry. 1991. The effectiveness of alcoholism screening in an ambulatory care setting. *Journal of Studies on Alcohol* 52 (1): 33-6.

Frezza M, C di Padova, G Pozzato, et al. 11 January 1990. High blood alcohol levels in women: The role of decreased gastric alcohol dehydrogenase activity and first-pass metabolism. *New England Journal of Medicine* 322 (2): 95-9.

Fuchs CS, MJ Stampfer, GA Colditz, et al. 11 May 1995. Alcohol consumption and mortality among women. *New England Journal of Medicine* 332 (19): 1245-50.

Gearhart JG, DK Beebe, HT Milhorn, et al. September 1991. Alcoholism in women. *American Family Physician* 44 (3): 907-13.

Gilbert FS. 1991. Development of a "steps questionnaire". *Journal of Studies on Alcohol* 52 (4): 353-60.

Gilbert FS. 1988. The effect of type of aftercare follow-up on treatment outcome among alcoholics. *Journal of Studies on Alcoholism* 49: 149-59.

Halliday A, and B Bush. 1987. Women and alcohol abuse. In *Alcoholism: A Guide for the Primary Care Physician*. Editors Barnes HN, MD Aronson, and TL Delbanco, 176-80. New York, NY: Springer-Verlag, Inc.

Hoeksema HL, and GH de Bock. 1993. The value of laboratory tests for the screening and recognition of alcohol abuse in primary care patients. *Journal of Family Practice* 37 (3): 268-76.

Kamerow DB, HA Pincus, and DI Macdonald. 18 April 1986. Alcohol abuse, other drug abuse, and mental disorders in medical practice. *Journal of the American Medical Association* 255 (15): 2054-7.

McLatchie BH, and KGE Lomp. 1988. An experimental investigation of the influence of aftercare on alcoholic relapse. *British Journal of Addiction* 83: 1045-54.

National Institutes of Health. September 1993. *Eighth Special Report to the U.S. Congress on Alcohol and Health--from the Secretary of Health and Human Services*. U.S. Department of Health and Human Services, Washington, DC.

Regier DA, JH Boyd, JD Burke, et al. 1988. One-month prevalence of mental disorders in the United States. *Archives of General Psychiatry* 45:977-986.

Scott E, and P Anderson. 1990. Randomized controlled trial of general practitioner intervention in women with excessive alcohol consumption. *Drug and Alcohol Review* 10: 313-21.

- 46 -

Selzer ML, A Vinokur, and L van Rooijen. 1975. A self-administered short Michigan alcoholism screening test (SMAST). *Journal of Studies on Alcoholism* 36 (1): 117-26.

Swenson WM, and RM Morse. April 1975. The use of a self-administered alcoholism screening test (SAAST) in a medical center. *Mayo Clinic Proceedings* 50: 204-8.

U.S. Preventive Services Task Force. 1989. *Guide to Clinical Preventive Services: An Assessment of the Effectiveness of 169 Interventions*. Baltimore, MD: Williams and Wilkins.

Urbano-Marquez A, R Estruch, J Fernandez-Sola, et al. 12 July 1995. The greater risk of alcoholic cardiomyopathy and myopathy in women compared with men. *Journal of the American Medical Association* 274 (2): 149-54.

Wallace P, S Cutler, and A Haines. 10 September 1988. Randomised controlled trial of general practitioner intervention in patients with excessive alcohol consumption. *British Medical Journal* 297: 663-8.

3. ALLERGIC RHINITIS
Eve A. Kerr, M.D., M.P.H.

We conducted a MEDLINE search of review articles on rhinitis between the years of 1990-1995 and selected articles pertaining to allergic rhinitis. We also performed a MEDLINE search of randomized controlled trials on allergic rhinitis patients between January 1990 and May 1995. Identified studies tended to use investigative therapies or compare new formulations of nasal steroids or antihistamines to previously used formulations. Since the general approach to treatment of allergic rhinitis is currently not controversial, these were not separately reviewed.

IMPORTANCE

Allergic rhinitis ranks thirteenth among the principal diagnoses rendered by physicians, based on the 1991 National Ambulatory Medical Care Survey (National Center for Health Statistics [NCHS], 1994c), accounting for over 11 million visits to the physician in that year. In fact, allergic rhinitis affects about 20 percent of the American population (Bernstein, 1993). Allergic rhinitis results in limitation of daily activities, and time lost from school and work (Bernstein, 1993). Complications of allergic rhinitis include serous otitis media (especially in children) and bacterial sinusitis (Kaliner and Lemanske, 1992).

EFFICACY/EFFECTIVENESS OF INTERVENTIONS

Diagnosis

The history is the fundamental diagnostic tool in allergic rhinitis. Symptoms include sneezing, itching of the nose, eyes, palate or pharynx, nasal stuffiness, rhinorrhea and post-nasal drip (Kaliner and Lemanske, 1992). A careful history of allergen exposure may reveal exacerbating allergies. In addition, one should inquire as to use of medications, especially nose drops or sprays. On physical exam, pale, edematous nasal turbinates and clear secretions are characteristic.

Temperature elevation, purulent nasal discharge, or cervical adenopathy should indicate the possibility of sinusitis, otitis, pharyngitis, or bronchitis (Kaliner and Lemanske, 1992).

Selected skin testing with appropriate allergens is the least time-consuming and expensive diagnostic modality, when confirmation of allergen sensitivity is necessary. Specific serum IgE determinations, although more expensive, may also be employed. Results need to be interpreted in the context of the patient's history. Total IgE levels and peripheral eosinophil counts are neither sensitive nor specific. Nasal smears for eosinophils are not specific for allergic rhinitis (Kaliner and Lemanske, 1992).

Treatment

Treatment rests with allergen avoidance, use of pharmaceutical agents and, when indicated, immunotherapy. Careful counseling regarding allergen avoidance is the mainstay of treatment (Naclerio, 1991). If it is unclear which allergen causes moderate to severe symptoms, skin testing should be performed (Naclerio, 1991). In addition, oral antihistamines (first- or second-generation H1-antagonistic drugs) are appropriate first-line agents, and decrease local and systemic symptoms of allergic rhinitis (Kaliner and Lemanske, 1992; Bernstein, 1993). Antihistamines may also be used in combination with decongestants for symptomatic relief. Topical nasal decongestants should be used for a maximum of four days. Nasal cromolyn sodium can be useful as a single agent, but requires regular, frequent dosing for optimal benefit (Bernstein, 1993). Topical nasal corticosteroids are effective in treating allergic rhinitis, but have no effect on ocular symptoms. Local burning, irritation, epistaxis and, very rarely, nasal septal perforation, are the reported side effects. Currently, both antihistamines and topical steroids have been advocated as first-line agents (Kaliner and Lemanske, 1992).

Immunotherapy should be considered if symptoms are present more than a few weeks of the year and medication and avoidance measures are ineffective (Naclerio, 1991). Allergy injections are reported to reduce symptoms in more than 90 percent of patients (Bernstein, 1993).

Reported toxicities, although uncommon, include hives, asthma and hypotension. The duration of treatment for optimal effect and maintenance of benefits after treatment cessation are unclear (Creticos, 1992).

RECOMMENDED QUALITY INDICATORS FOR ALLERGIC RHINITIS

The following criteria apply to women age 18-50.

Diagnosis

Indicator	Quality of evidence	Literature	Benefits	Comments
1. If a diagnosis of allergic rhinitis is made, the search for a specific allergen by history should be documented in the chart (for initial history).	III	Kaliner and Lemanske, 1992; Naclerio, 1990	Decrease nasal congestion, rhinorrhea, and itching.	Allergen avoidance is the mainstay of treatment
2. If a diagnosis of allergic rhinitis is made, history should include whether the patient uses any topical nasal decongestants.	III	Bernstein, 1993	Decrease nasal congestion, rhinorrhea, and itching.	Chronic use of topical nasal decongestants can cause rhinitis medicamentosa and may mimic allergic rhinitis

Treatment

Indicator	Quality of evidence	Literature	Benefits	Comments
3. Treatment for allergic rhinitis should include at least one of the following: antihistamine, nasal steroids, nasal cromolyn.	I-III	Naclerio, 1991; Kaliner and Lemanske, 1992	Decrease nasal congestion, rhinorrhea, and itching.	These have proven efficacy in allergic rhinitis
4. If topical or systemic nasal decongestants are prescribed, duration of treatment should be for no longer than 4 days.	II	Stanford et al., 1992; Barker, 1991	Decrease nasal congestion, rhinorrhea, and itching.	Longer treatment may cause rebound congestion.

Quality of Evidence Codes:

I: RCT
II-1:   Nonrandomized controlled trials
II-2:   Cohort or case analysis
II-3:   Multiple time series
III: Opinions or descriptive studies

50

REFERENCES - ALLERGIC RHINITIS

Bernstein JA. 1 May 1993. Allergic rhinitis: Helping patients lead an unrestricted life. *Postgraduate Medicine* 93 (6): 124-32.

Creticos PS. 25 November 1992. Immunotherapy with allergens. *Journal of the American Medical Association* 268 (20): 2834-9.

Kaliner M, and R Lemanske. 25 November 1992. Rhinitis and asthma. *Journal of the American Medical Association* 268 (20): 2807-29.

Naclerio RM. 19 September 1991. Allergic rhinitis. *New England Journal of Medicine* 325 (12): 860-9.

National Center for Health Statistics. 1994. *National Ambulatory Medical Care Survey: 1991 summary*. U.S. Department of Health and Human Services, Hyattsville, MD.

4. ASTHMA

Eve A. Kerr, M.D., M.P.H.

The general approach to developing quality indicators for asthma
diagnosis and treatment was based on *Guidelines for the Diagnosis and
Management of Asthma* (National Asthma Education Program [NAEP], 1991).
These guidelines, issued by the National Heart, Lung, and Blood
Institute (NHLBI), are based on expert consensus and scientific
literature review.[1] The expert panel was convened by the Coordinating
Committee of the National Asthma Education Program (NAEP). These
guidelines were reproduced in the September 1991 issue of the *Journal of
Allergy and Clinical Immunology*. We also reviewed the standards issued
by the American Thoracic Society for the diagnosis and care of patients
with chronic obstructive pulmonary disease and asthma.[2] Further, we
conducted a MEDLINE literature search to identify randomized controlled
trials (RCTs) related to asthma and its treatment or the prevention and
control of asthma exacerbations published in English between January 1,
1991 and April 1, 1995. We reviewed select articles dealing with areas
where management controversy exists.

IMPORTANCE

NHLBI defines asthma as "..a lung disease with the following
characteristics: (1) airway obstruction that is reversible (but not
completely so in some patients) either spontaneously or with treatment;
(2) airway inflammation; and (3) increased airway responsiveness to a
variety of stimuli." Approximately 10 million persons (adults and
children) in the US have asthma (NAEP, 1991), with an increase in
prevalence of 29 percent from 1980 to 1987. During the same period, the
death rate from asthma increased 31 percent. In 1990, total asthma-
related health care expenditures exceeded $6 billion in the United
States (Barach, 1994; Weiss et al., 1992).

---

[1]The material reviewed is current to January 1, 1991.
[2]The American Thoracic Society adopted the standards in November,
1986.

Diagnosis

The diagnosis of asthma is based on the patient's medical history, physical examination, and laboratory test results. Symptoms include cough, wheezing, shortness of breath, chest tightness, and sputum production. Precipitating and/or aggravating factors may include viral respiratory infections, exposure to environmental or occupational allergens, irritants, cold air, and drugs (e.g., aspirin), exercise, and endocrine factors. Severity of disease ranges widely, with some patients having rare symptoms and others having severe limitation of daily activity with frequent exacerbations. Consequently, the use of health care services and the impact of asthma on an individual's quality of life also vary widely.

Spirometry to document severity of airflow obstruction and to establish acute bronchodilator responsiveness should be performed for all patients in whom the diagnosis of asthma is being considered (NAEP, 1991). The results of spirometry should demonstrate an obstructive process. Additional laboratory testing, such as chest x-rays, complete blood count, sputum examination, complete pulmonary function studies, and determination of specific IgE antibodies to common allergens should be considered, but need only be performed when appropriate for the clinical situation (NAEP, 1991).

Peak expiratory flow rate (PEFR) is the greatest flow velocity that can be obtained during a forced expiration starting with fully inflated lungs. PEFR correlates well with forced expiratory volume at 1 second (FEV_1) measured by spirometry (NAEP, 1991). Measurement of PEFR is useful both in the medical and home setting. NHLBI suggests the following as guidelines for adult patients.

Measure PEFR in the Clinician's Office/Emergency Department

Chronic Asthma

1. Measure PEFR in all patients at each office visit for therapeutic judgments. This will help judge the need for increases or decreases in medication.

2. Measure PEFR to confirm exercise-induced asthma as a diagnostic tool.

Acute Exacerbations

1. Measure PEFR during all acute exacerbations as a means to judge how far the patient is from baseline measurements and to make decisions regarding management.

2. Measure PEFR after $beta_2$-agonist inhalation to judge response.

3. Measure PEFR just prior to discharge from emergency department. This will help determine need for a steroid taper.

Hospital

1. Measure PEFR two to four times per day to follow course of asthma therapy.

Home

1. Consider measuring PEFR in all patients with moderate or severe asthma to monitor course of asthma.

2. Measure PEFR diagnostically before and after exposure.

3. Measure PEFR during acute exacerbations to monitor course of exacerbation and response to therapy.

When using PEFR measurements to judge response to treatment or severity of exacerbation, it is useful to compare the measurement to patient "baseline." This baseline is usually regarded as the norm or personal best PEFR for the individual patient. Alternately, one can use standard PEFR measurements that are based on age and height (see Table 4.1).

Table 4.1

Predicted Average Peak Expiratory Flow for Normal Males and Females

	Height							
	60"		65"		70"		75"	
Age	M	F	M	F	M	F	M	F
20	554	423	602	460	649	496	693	529
25	543	418	590	454	636	490	679	523
30	532	413	577	448	622	483	664	516
35	521	408	565	442	609	476	651	509
40	509	402	552	436	596	470	636	502
45	498	397	540	430	583	464	622	495
50	486	391	527	424	569	457	607	488
55	475	386	515	418	556	451	593	482
60	463	380	502	412	542	445	578	475
65	452	375	490	406	529	439	564	468
70	440	369	477	400	515	432	550	461

Source: Excerpted from NAEP, 1991.

EFFICACY AND/OR EFFECTIVENESS OF INTERVENTIONS

According to the NHLBI, asthma therapy has several components: patient education, environmental control, and pharmacologic therapy, as well as the use of objective measures to monitor the severity of disease and the course of therapy (NAEP, 1991).

Patient Education

Patient education is one of the most important modalities in asthma control (NAEP, 1991). Asthma education programs have led to improved patient outcomes, including reduced hospitalizations and emergency room visits (Lawrence, 1995), fewer asthma symptoms and physician visits, and improvement in asthma management skills (Kotses et al., 1995). However, the performance and adequacy of education is not easily assessed through medical record review. Therefore, the review and the indicators that follow will not focus on the patient-education component of care.

Pharmacologic Therapy

Corticosteroids

The duration and severity of an acute asthma exacerbation can be reduced by therapy with corticosteroids; their use decreases the need for emergency department visits and hospitalizations (NAEP, 1991). Inhaled corticosteroids, at currently approved doses, are safe and effective for the treatment of asthma and are being utilized more frequently as primary therapy for patients with moderate and severe asthma. Some investigators feel that inhaled corticosteroids are also appropriate as first line therapy in mild asthma (Haahtela et al., 1991). In any patient requiring chronic treatment with oral corticosteroids (i.e., exceeding one month in duration), a trial of inhaled corticosteroids should be attempted in an effort to reduce or eliminate oral steroids. High doses of inhaled steroids should be used if conventional doses fail to permit oral steroid tapering. Pulmonary functions (PEFR or FEV_1) should be monitored during tapering. Prolonged daily use of oral corticosteroids is reserved for patients with severe asthma despite use of high-dose inhaled corticosteroids. In patients on long-term oral corticosteroids, pulmonary function tests should be used to objectively assess efficacy.

Cromolyn sodium

Cromolyn sodium is a nonsteroidal anti-inflammatory drug that is used prophylactically with few toxicities. According to the NHLBI, there is no way to reliably predict who will respond to cromolyn sodium therapy. Therefore, NHLBI advocates a 4- to 6-week trial to determine efficacy in individual patients.

Beta₂-agonists

Inhaled beta$_2$-agonists are the medication of choice for immediate treatment of asthma exacerbations and for the prevention of exercise-induced asthma. Regular use of beta$_2$-agonists may be a marker for severity. However, there appears to be some consensus in the medical community that regular (i.e., 4 times daily) use of beta$_2$-agonists should be discouraged in favor of anti-inflammatory treatment (Executive Committee of the American Academy of Allergy and Immunology, 1993). Although inhaled beta$_2$-agonists are often used chronically, this use of beta$_2$-agonists has recently been associated with worsening of asthma control in some patients (NAEP, 1991). Correct use of metered-dose inhalers is critical.

Theophylline

Theophylline, which is used in some patients primarily for its bronchodilator effects, has the major disadvantages of variable clearance from the body and potential for multiple toxicities. Monitoring serum theophylline concentrations at initiation of therapy and subsequently at least yearly is therefore useful (NAEP, 1991). Theophylline levels should also be checked for patients who do not exhibit the expected bronchodilator effect or who develop an exacerbation while on their usual dose (NAEP, 1991). The use of theophylline may be particularly useful for nocturnal asthma.

Diagnosis and Treatment of Allergic Asthma

Allergy may have a significant role in the symptoms of asthma for some persons. A determination of an allergic component may be made in persons whose asthma worsens when they are exposed to allergens (e.g., dust mites, animal allergens) or who have seasonal worsening of symptoms. A careful history plays the most critical role in patients suspected of having allergic asthma. In such patients, determination of specific IgE antibodies, skin testing, and/or a referral to an immunologist, may be useful (NAEP, 1991).

Once it is determined (through history and/or ancillary testing) that allergy plays a role in the person's asthma, allergen avoidance should be the first recommendation (NAEP, 1991). However, when avoidance is not possible and appropriate medication fails to control symptoms of allergic asthma, immunotherapy should be considered (NAEP, 1991). Randomized controlled studies, reviewed in the NHLBI guidelines, demonstrate a reduction of symptoms through the use of immunotherapy to a number of allergens (NAEP, 1991). Immunotherapy should only be administered in a physician's office where facilities and trained personnel are available to treat potential life-threatening reactions.

GENERAL MANAGEMENT PRINCIPLES

The NHLBI guidelines state that therapeutic agents to prevent or reverse airway hyperresponsiveness are considered first-line therapy. Specific asthma therapy must be selected to fit the needs of individual patients. Treatment recommendations are based on severity of disease. However, it must be recognized that grading severity is not straightforward. For example, in some severity measures, need for certain medications, such a steroids, indicates "severe" asthma. Yet this definition complicates interpreting recommendations that state that patients who have "severe" asthma should be using inhaled steroids. Criteria for determining the severity of asthma are summarized below and are based on NHLBI guidelines.

Chronic Mild Asthma

According to NHLBI, persons with mild asthma:
1) have intermittent, brief (<1 hour) wheezing, coughing, or dyspnea up to 2 times weekly;
2) are asymptomatic between exacerbations;
3) have brief (<1/2 hour) wheezing/coughing/dyspnea with activity; and,
4) have infrequent (<2 times a month) nocturnal coughing/wheezing.

For these patients, asthma symptoms often occur following exercise, exposure to irritants or allergens, or respiratory infections. For patients with mild asthma, the use of inhaled $beta_2$-agonists on an as-needed-basis usually suffices. However, if patients are using inhaled $beta_2$-agonists more than 3 to 4 times per day (NAEP, 1991), have more than 8 inhalations per day (Practice parameters), or use inhaled $beta_2$-agonists on a daily basis, additional daily therapy may be indicated.

Chronic Moderate Asthma

Patients who have symptoms that are poorly regulated by episodic administration of $beta_2$-agonists may need more continuous treatment.

Included in this category are persons who have symptomatic exacerbations more than twice per week, including at night; exacerbations that last several days; and, occasional emergency care. Since it may be inadvisable to prescribe prolonged administration of regularly scheduled beta$_2$-agonists, patients with moderate asthma may need longer-acting bronchodilators (e.g., theophylline) and/or anti-inflammatory agents (e.g., inhaled corticosteroids, cromolyn). A patient who was previously controlled with only as-needed beta$_2$-agonists and who exhibits a deterioration in clinical status probably needs the addition of an inhaled anti-inflammatory agent. Patients who require frequent bursts of prednisone (two or three five-day courses in a six-month period) who are not already taking inhaled corticosteroids should be started on them; the dose should be increased for those already on inhaled corticosteroids.

Chronic Severe Asthma

Patients who are not controlled on maximal doses of bronchodilators and inhaled anti-inflammatory agents may need systemic corticosteroids on a routine basis. The lowest possible dose must be sought and should be administered under the supervision of an asthma specialist (NAEP, 1991).

Other Management Measures

The U.S. Preventive Services Task Force recommends pneumococcal vaccination and regular influenza vaccination for those with chronic cardiac or pulmonary disease (U.S. Preventive Services Task Force [USPSTF], 1989). The NHLBI guidelines state that "influenza vaccinations and pneumococcal vaccine should be considered for patients with moderate or severe asthma in order to avoid aggravation of asthma."

Care of an Acute Asthma Exacerbation

The NHLBI has outlined four general principles of treatment of asthma exacerbations:

* early recognition;
* prompt communication between patient and health care provider;

- appropriate intensification of anti-asthma medications (treatment can begin at home); and
- removal of the allergen or irritant, if one or the other triggered the exacerbation.

Patients at high risk of death from exacerbations should be counseled to seek immediate medical care rather than initiate home therapy. Patients at high risk include those with a history of:

- prior intubation;
- two or more hospitalizations for asthma in past year;
- three or more emergency care visits for asthma in the past year;
- hospitalization or emergency care visit within the past month;
- current use of systemic corticosteroids or recent withdrawal from systemic corticosteroids;
- past history of syncope/hypoxic seizure due to asthma;
- prior admission for asthma to hospital-based intensive care unit; or
- serious psychiatric or psychosocial problems.

In general, patients who do not have a good response to home inhaled beta$_2$-agonist treatment should contact their health care provider. Severe symptoms at rest, such as breathlessness, speech fragmented by rapid breathing and inability to walk 100 feet without stopping to rest, that are unimproved within 30 minutes, indicate a visit to the emergency department.

All patients seen in the emergency department or other urgent care setting should be evaluated with a complete history including:

- length of current exacerbation;
- severity of symptoms;
- all current medications, including use of systemic corticosteroids;
- prior hospitalizations and emergency department visits for asthma;
- prior episodes of respiratory intubation due to asthma; and

- significant prior cardiopulmonary disease.

All patients presenting to the emergency department with an asthma exacerbation should be evaluated with at least one measurement of airflow obstruction:
- peak expiratory flow rate measured with a peak flow meter; or
- one-second forced expired volume (FEV_1) determined by spirometry.

In general, all patients should receive initial treatment with inhaled beta$_2$-agonists (McFadden and Hejal, 1995). Patients should be re-evaluated at least three times within 90 minutes of treatment.

Patients who have persistent symptoms, diffuse wheezes audible on chest auscultation, and a PEFR or $FEV_1 \leq 40$ percent of predicted or baseline should be admitted to the hospital.

Patients with a good response to inhaled beta$_2$-agonist treatment should be observed for 30 to 60 minutes after the last treatment to ensure stability prior to discharge.

The following are recommended steps for follow-up care once a patient has been stabilized following an acute exacerbation:

1) Treatment regimen should be given for at least three days.
2) Treatment regimen should include oral corticosteroids for all patients with an FEV_1 or PEFR ≤ 70 percent of baseline (or predicted) at discharge, and for all patients at increased risk for potential life-threatening deterioration.
3) A follow-up medical appointment should occur within 48 to 72 hours of discharge.

Care of Patients Hospitalized for Asthma

Patients whose airflow obstruction does not respond to intensive bronchodilator treatment require close attention in the hospital. These patients should be followed with lung function measurement (PEFR or spirometry) at least twice per day before and after bronchodilator therapy (NAEP, 1991). Patients who are admitted to the intensive care unit or who have had multiple hospital admissions should have a consultation with an asthma specialist.

All patients with asthma who are admitted to the hospital should receive systemic corticosteroids (preferably via intravenous route) and beta$_2$-agonists. The NHLBI guidelines also recommend that all hospitalized patients be administered oral or intravenous methylxanthines (e.g., theophylline or aminophylline). Oxygen should be given to all patients with an oxygen saturation less than 90 to 92 percent. Measurement of oxygen saturation by oximetry is recommended. Chest physical therapy has not been found to be helpful for most patients. Use of mucolytics (e.g., acetylcysteine, potassium iodide) and sedation (i.e., with anxiolytics and hypnotic drugs) should be strictly avoided. Since bacterial and mycoplasmal respiratory infections are thought to contribute only infrequently to severe exacerbations of asthma, use of antibiotics should be reserved for those patients with purulent sputum and/or fever.

Patients with PEFR or FEV$_1$ of less than 25 percent of baseline or predicted should receive an arterial blood gas measurement to evaluate pCO$_2$. If pCO$_2$ is greater than 40 mm Hg, the patient will require repeated arterial blood gas measurement to evaluate their response to treatment, preferably in an intensive care setting.

The NHLBI recommends close medical follow-up during the tapering period, but does not specify a follow-up interval. Since most patients' taper will be finished within 14 days, a follow-up visit within 14 days seems reasonable.

RECOMMENDED QUALITY INDICATORS FOR ADULT ASTHMA

The following apply to women age 18-50 who have chronic asthma and excludes patients with only exercise-induced asthma.

Diagnosis

	Indicator	Quality of evidence	Literature	Benefits	Comments
1.	Patients with the diagnosis of asthma should have had some historical evaluation of asthma precipitants (environmental exposures, exercise, allergens) within six months (before or after) of diagnosis.	III	NAEP, 1991	Decrease baseline shortness of breath. Improve exercise tolerance. Decrease steroid toxicity.* Decrease number of exacerbations.**	This may result in improved control of asthma and less need for medications such as steroids, which have undesirable toxicities.*
2.	Patients with the diagnosis of asthma should have baseline spirometry performed within six months of diagnosis.	III	NAEP, 1991	Decrease baseline shortness of breath.	By documenting the diagnosis with spirometry, one can initiate the appropriate therapy, minimize inappropriate use of medications, and assess future worsening or improvement.
3.	Peak expiratory flow rate (PEFR) or FEV_1 should be measured in patients with chronic asthma at least annually.	III	NAEP, 1991	Decrease shortness of breath. Improve exercise tolerance.	Sequential measurement of PEFR are useful for therapeutic decisions. Knowing the person's baseline is useful for treatment of exacerbations. However, no randomized trial has been done to demonstrate improved outcomes among patients who received routine PEFR measurements in the office.

Therapy

	Indicator	Quality of evidence	Literature	Benefits	Comments
4.	Patients with the diagnosis of asthma should have been prescribed a beta$_2$-agonist inhaler for symptomatic relief of exacerbations to use as needed.	III	NAEP, 1991	Decrease shortness of breath. Prevent need for emergency room treatment.	Beta$_2$-agonists are first-line therapy for asthma exacerbations. Asthmatics should have ready access to this therapy.
5.	Patients who report using a beta$_2$-agonist inhaler more than 3 times per day on a daily basis (not only during an exacerbation) should be prescribed a longer acting bronchodilator (theophylline) and/or an anti-inflammatory agent (inhaled corticosteroids, cromolyn).	II, III	NAEP, 1991; Executive Committee of the American Academy of Allergy and Immunology, 1993	Decrease baseline shortness of breath. Improve exercise tolerance.	This is somewhat controversial since some clinicians are still advocating chronic treatment with beta$_2$-agonists. However, chronic treatment with beta$_2$-agonists appears to increase bronchial reactivity and may contribute to asthma mortality.
6.	Patients with asthma should not receive beta-blocker medications (e.g., atenolol, propanalol).	III	NAEP, 1991	Prevent worsening of shortness of breath.	Beta-blockade promotes airway reactivity.
7.	Asthmatic patients who require systemic steroids in the past should have documented current or past inhaled steroid use.	III	NAEP, 1991	Decrease steroid toxicity.*	Inhaled steroids have lower toxicities than oral steroids. It is unclear if it would be useful to attempt a trial every year or so, or if a single attempt is sufficient. This may be difficult to operationalize.
8.	Patients on theophylline should have at least one serum theophylline level determination per year.	III	NAEP, 1991	Decrease shortness of breath. Improve exercise tolerance. Prevent theophylline toxicity.	Clearance of theophylline can vary even within the same individual. Patients may therefore become subtherapeutic or toxic on doses that were previously therapeutic. Toxicities include tremulousness and agitation, nausea, vomiting, and cardiac arrhythmias.
9.	Patients with the diagnosis of asthma should have a documented flu vaccination in the fall/winter of the previous year (September - January).	III	NAEP, 1991; CDC, 1993	Prevent pneumonia secondary to influenza infection. Prevent asthma exacerbation.**	Influenza can precipitate exacerbations and lead to secondary pneumonia in patients with asthma.
10.	Patients with the diagnosis of asthma should have a pneumococcal vaccination documented in the chart.	III	USPSTF, 1989	Prevent pneumonia.	Pneumonia is more life-threatening in persons with asthma.

65

Treatment of exacerbations

	Indicator	Quality of evidence	Literature	Benefits	Comments
11.	Patients presenting to the physician's office with an asthma exacerbation or historical worsening of asthma symptoms should be evaluated with PEFR or forced expiratory volume at 1 second (FEV_1).	III	NAEP, 1991	Decrease shortness of breath.	Objective measurements are useful for treatment decisions. They help inititate appropriate level of theraputic intervention, whether that be with beta$_2$-agonists, steroids, or hospitalization.
12.	At the time of an exacerbation, patients on theophylline should have theophylline level measured.	III	NAEP, 1991	Decrease shortness of breath.	Theophylline clearance may vary to a great degree. Subtherapeutic levels in persons on chronic treatment may add to an exacerbation.
13.	A physical exam of the chest should be performed in patients presenting with an asthma exacerbation.	III	NAEP, 1991; McFadden and Hejal, 1995	Prevent mortality due to asthma.	A silent chest may predict more severe asthma. A physical exam helps guide therapy by evaluating severity.
14.	Patients presenting to the physician's office or ER with an FEV_1 or PEFR≤70% of baseline (or predicted) should be treated with beta$_2$-agonists before discharge.	III	NAEP, 1991; McFadden and Hejal, 1995	Decrease shortness of breath.	The percentage cut-off for this and the next three indicators are achieved through expert opinion; 70% is generally felt to be a cut-off for moderately severe exacerbations. It is generally agreed, however, that beta$_2$-agonists are first-line drugs in an exacerbation. Lack of improvement indicates the need for additional therapy. If baseline is not available, predicted will be used.
15.	Patients who receive treatment with beta$_2$-agonists in the physician's office or ER for FEV_1<70% of baseline (or predicted) should have an FEV_1 or PEFR repeated prior to discharge.	III	NAEP, 1991	Decrease shortness of breath.	Repeat measures assess response (or lack thereof) to therapy.
16.	Patients with an FEV_1 or PEFR≤70% of baseline (or predicted) after treatment for asthma exacerbation in the physician's office should be placed on an oral corticosteroid taper.	III	NAEP, 1991; McFadden and Hejal, 1995	Decrease shortness of breath.	Steroids have been shown to improve recovery, but little objective data exists to back up the appropriate cut-off. If patients do not improve significantly with beta$_2$-agonists alone, then the severity of the exacerbation warrants steroid treatment.
17.	Patients who have a PEFR or FEV_1≤40% of baseline (or predicted) after treatment with beta$_2$-agonists should be admitted to the hospital.	III	NAEP, 1991; McFadden and Hejal, 1995	Prevent mortality from asthma	The cut-off, though arbitrary, reflects severe asthma exacerbation. These patients require close supervision to prevent mortality.

Hospital Treatment

Indicator	Quality of evidence	Literature	Benefits	Comments
18. Patients admitted to the hospital for asthma exacerbation should have oxygen saturation measured.	III	NAEP, 1991	Prevent mortality. Prevent cardiac ischemia. Decrease shortness of breath.	Oxygen saturation identifies patients who are hypoxemic and for whom oxygen therapy should be initiated.
19. Hospitalized patients with PEFR or FEV_1 less than 25 percent of predicted or personal best should receive arterial blood gas measurement.	III	NAEP, 1991	Prevent mortality.	Arterial blood gases identify acidosis and hypercarbia, which indicate potential need for intubation.
20. Hospitalized patients should receive systemic steroids (either PO or IV).	III	NAEP, 1991	Prevent mortality. Decrease shortness of breath.	Steroids improve recovery from severe asthma exacerbation. There is a debate regarding the preference of IV versus PO steroids.
21. Hospitalized patients should receive treatment with beta$_2$-agonists.	III	NAEP, 1991	Prevent mortality. Decrease shortness of breath.	These are first-line agents for treatment of bronchoconstriction
22. Hospitalized patients should receive treatment with methylxanthines.	III	NAEP, 1991	Prevent mortality. Decrease shortness of breath.	This is an area of controversy, and not well backed up by RCTs, but is indicated by the NHLBI.
23. Hospitalized patients with oxygen saturation less than 90 percent should receive supplemental oxygen.	III	NAEP, 1991	Prevent mortality. Prevent cardiac ischemia. Decrease shortness of breath.	90% is a conservative cut-off.
24. Hospitalized patients with pCO_2 of greater than 40 should receive at least one additional blood gas measurement to evaluate response to treatment.	III	NAEP, 1991	Decrease shortness of breath. Prevent mortality.	CO_2 retention indicates poor gas exchange and fatigue, and these patients should be monitored closely for treatment response.
25. Hospitalized patients with pCO_2 of greater than 40 should be monitored in an intensive care setting.	III	NAEP, 1991	Prevent mortality.	CO_2 retention indicates poor gas exchange and fatigue, and these patients should be monitored closely for treatment response.
26. Patients with 2 or more hospitalizations for asthma exacerbation in the previous year should receive (or should have received) consultation with an asthma specialist.	III	NAEP, 1991	Improve quality of life by decreasing future hospitalizations. Decrease shortness of breath.	Hospitalization is a marker for severity and poor control. Patients with frequent hospitalizations may benefit from evaluation by an expert.
27. Hospitalized patients should not receive sedative drugs (e.g., anxiolytics).	III	NAEP, 1991	Prevent worsening of shortness of breath.	Sedation may worsen exacerbation.

Follow-up

	Indicator	Quality of evidence	Literature	Benefits	Comments
28.	Patients with the diagnosis of asthma should have at least 2 visits within a calendar year.	III	NAEP, 1991; Starfield et al., 1994	Decrease baseline shortness of breath.	Minimum visit intervals have not been well specified or studied. However, follow-up visits should serve to optimize treatment regimen.
29.	Patients whose asthma medication requires changes (new medication added, current medication dose decreased or increased) during one visit should have a follow-up visit within 4 weeks.	III	NAEP, 1991	Decrease shortness of breath. Minimize medication toxicity.	If medication regimen is altered, a change in symptoms is expected. Follow-up should indicate if new medication regimen is working appropriately. However, the time interval is arbitrary and this may not take into account telephone follow-up.
30.	Patients on chronic oral corticosteroids (three or more corticosteroid tapers for exacerbations in the past year; or continuous treatment with any dose prednisone; or three or more administrations of intramuscular corticosteroids in the past year) should have follow-up visits at least 4 times in a calendar year.	III	NAEP, 1991	Decrease toxicities of oral steroids.** Prevent exacerbations.	Minimum follow-up intervals have not been defined. Patients on chronic oral steroids have severe asthma and should be monitored more closely.
31.	Patients seen in the emergency department with an asthma exacerbation should have a follow-up re-assessment within 72 hours.	III	NAEP, 1991	Prevent exacerbation recurrence.	NHLBI recommends that treatment be given for 3 days and then patient be reassessed. Worsening of an exacerbation usually occurs in this time period. The guidelines do not specify whether telephone follow-up is adequate.
32.	Patients with a hospitalization for asthma exacerbation should receive outpatient follow-up within 14 days.	III	NAEP, 1991	Prevent exacerbation recurrence.	NHLBI recommends follow-up but does not state a time interval. Two weeks seems reasonable since a taper off steroids is usually for approximately 2 weeks. Four weeks would be the outside range.

*Toxicites of glucocorticoid therapy include fluid/electrolyte disturbances, peptic ulcer disease, ulcerative esophagitis, diabetes mellitus, glaucoma, psychosis, myopathy, osteoporosis, pancreatitis, impaired wound healing, adrenal atrophy, cataracts, and increased susceptibility to infections. (Barker et al., 1991).

**An asthma exacerbation is characterized by acute obstruction to airflow. Exacerbations may be initiated through exposure to allergens and irritants, influenza, pneumonia, as well as other unidentified factors. Patients become acutely short of breath, tachycardic, and if severe, use accessory muscles of respiration. Exacerbation could lead to death if improperly treated. Treatment for an exacerbation should begin at home with beta2-agonists. Physicians need to evaluate the severity of the exacerbation in order to initiate appropriate treatment.

Quality of Evidence Codes:

I: RCT
II-1:   Nonrandomized controlled trials
II-2:   Cohort or case analysis
II-3:   Multiple time series
III: Opinions or descriptive studies

68

REFERENCES - ADULT ASTHMA

Barker LR, JR Burton, and PD Zieve, Editors. 1991. *Principles of Ambulatory Medicine*, Third ed.Baltimore, MD: Williams and Wilkins.

Executive Committee of the American Academy of Allergy and Immunology. 1993. Inhaled beta-2-adrenergic agonists in asthma. *Journal of Allergy and Clinical Immunology* 91: 1234-7.

Haahtela T, M Jarvinen, T Kava, et al. 8 August 1991. Comparison of a beta-2-agonist, terbutaline, with an inhaled corticosteroid, budesonide, in newly detected asthma. *New England Journal of Medicine* 325 (6): 388-92.

Kotses H., IL Bernstein, DI Bernstein, et al. February 1995. A self-management program for adult asthma. Part I: Development and evaluation. *Journal of Allergy and Clinical Immunology* 95 (2): 529-40.

Lawrence G. January 1995. Asthma self-management programs can reduce the need for hospital-based asthma care. *Respiratory Care* 40 (1): 39-43.

McFadden ER, and R Hejal. 13 May 1995. Asthma. *Lancet* 345: 1215-20.

Nathan RA. 1992. Beta 2 Agonist therapy: Oral versus ihnaled delivery. *Journal of Asthma* 29 (1): 49-54.

National Asthma Education Program. August 1991. *Guidelines for the diagnosis and management of asthma*. U.S. Department of Health and Human Services, Hyattsville, MD.

U.S. Preventive Services Task Force. 1989. *Guide to Clinical Preventive Services: An Assessment of the Effectiveness of 169 Interventions*. Baltimore, MD: Williams and Wilkins.

Weiss KB, PJ Gergen, and TA Hodgson. 26 March 1992. An economic evaluation of asthma in the United States. *New England Journal of Medicine* 326 (13): 862-6.

5. BREAST MASS

Lisa Schmidt, M.P.H., and Eve A. Kerr, M.D.

The general approach to breast mass work-ups was obtained from opinions of the Committee of Gynecologic Practice of the American College of Obstetrics and Gynecology (ACOG) (ACOG, 1994 and ACOG, 1991). In addition, review articles were selected from a MEDLINE search that identified all English language review articles on breast mass work-ups between the years of 1990 and 1995.

IMPORTANCE

Breast cancer is the most commonly diagnosed cancer and the second leading cause of cancer deaths among women (CDC, 1992b). It accounts for 32 percent of all cancers in women and 18 percent of female cancer deaths (ACOG, 1991). Survival after diagnosis and treatment is directly related to the stage at diagnosis; the earlier the breast cancer is diagnosed, the better the survival rates (Austoker, 1994). Should a breast mass be detected by clinical breast examination (CBE) during screening, immediate follow-up is essential. This chapter focuses on CBE as the screening technique for women less than 50 years of age--see discussion in CBE section of chapter 16.

EFFICACY AND/OR EFFECTIVENESS OF INTERVENTIONS

Clinical examination of the breast can detect a mass, but it is not useful to distinguish a benign from a malignant process (Donegan, 1992). Although there are some characteristics of breast cancer that may distinguish it from a benign breast mass (e.g., indistinct borders, skin dimpling or nipple retraction), these cannot reliably differentiate a malignant tumor from a benign mass. In addition, a clinical exam cannot distinguish a cystic from a solid breast mass (Donegan, 1992).

ACOG (1991) recommends that all positive findings of a CBE be documented in writing or with an appropriate drawing in the patient's chart. In addition, a comprehensive history, including age, menstrual status, parity, previous history of breast-feeding, family medical history, and drug usage should be noted (Bland and Love, 1992).

Some type of follow-up should be provided for all women with a breast mass detected on physical examination. Bland and Love (1992) and Dixon and Mansel (1994) recommend fine needle aspiration for any palpable breast mass. Fine needle aspiration and cytologic examination have been shown to be efficacious, cost-effective, and highly reliable when cytologic preparation and cellular sampling are properly done (Bland and Love, 1992). Aspiration is also effective for differentiating a cyst from a solid mass (Donegan, 1992). If the fine needle aspiration cannot rule out cancer of the breast, an open biopsy should be performed (ACOG, 1994). In addition, ACOG (1991) suggests that any of the following findings require an open biopsy following fine needle aspiration:

- bloody cyst fluid on aspiration;
- failure of mass to disappear completely upon fluid aspiration;
- recurrence of cyst after one or two aspirations;
- solid dominant mass not diagnosed as fibroadenoma;
- bloody nipple discharge;
- nipple ulceration or persistent crusting; or
- skin edema and erythema suspicious of inflammatory breast carcinoma.

Mammography is an essential part of the examination of a woman with a palpable breast mass (ACOG, 1994 and Donegan, 1992). Significant mammographic findings consist of alterations in density of breast tissue, calcifications, thickening of skin, fibrous streaks, and nipple discharge (ACOG, 1991). However, mammography alone may not be sufficient to rule out malignant pathology. Ultrasonography or magnified mammographic imaging of the breast containing the mass may provide additional information and may identify cysts or variations in normal breast architecture that account for the palpable abnormality (ACOG, 1994). Sonograms, however, cannot distinguish benign from malignant masses, although they can accurately identify masses as cystic or solid (Donegan, 1992). Sonograms are most helpful when a mass cannot be felt, when the patient will not permit aspiration, or when a mass is too small and deep to offer a reliable target for aspiration (Donegan, 1992).

The combination of physical examination, mammography, and fine-needle aspiration is highly accurate when all the tests give the same results (Donegan, 1992). Layfield et al., found cancer in only 3 of 457 cases in which all three evaluations indicated that a mass was benign (Donegan, 1992).

RECOMMENDED QUALITY INDICATORS FOR BREAST MASS

The following criteria apply to women under 50 years of age.

Diagnosis

Indicator	Quality of evidence	Literature	Benefits	Comments
1. If a palpable breast mass has been detected, at least one of the following procedures should be completed within 6 months: • Fine needle aspiration • Mammography • Ultrasound • Biopsy • Follow-up visit	III	ACOG, 1991; ACOG, 1994; Bland & Love, 1992; Dixon & Mansel, 1994	Reduce late-stage breast cancer. Decrease mortality from breast cancer.	Any breast mass may be an indicator of cancer and needs to be followed closely and/or investigated further. The six-month time period is not specified in the literature but is probably generous. The modality of follow-up may differ depending on the patient and mass characteristics.
2. If a breast mass has been detected on two separate occasions, then either a biopsy or FNA should be performed within 6 months of the second visit.	III	ACOG, 1991; ACOG, 1994; Bland & Love, 1992; Dixon & Mansel, 1994	Reduce late-stage breast cancer. Decrease mortality from breast cancer.	A definite mass (as opposed to fibrocystic changes) needs further work-up. While a follow-up visit to determine change in nature or size with menstrual cycle may be appropriate one time, if a definite mass is palpated twice, then biopsy or FNA for diagnosis needs to occur. The timeframe is debatable.

Quality of Evidence Codes:

I:	RCT
II-1:	Nonrandomized controlled trials
II-2:	Cohort or case analysis
II-3:	Multiple time series
III:	Opinions or descriptive studies

REFERENCES - BREAST MASS

American College of Obstetricians and Gynecologists. June 1991. Nonmalignant conditions of the breast. *ACOG Technical Bulletin* 156: 1-6.

American College of Obstetricians and Gynecologists. June 1994. The role of the obstetrician-gynecologist in the diagnosis and treatment of breast disease. *ACOG Committee Opinion* 140: 1-2.

Austoker J. 16 July 1994. Cancer prevention in primary care: Screening and self examination for breast cancer. *British Medical Journal* 309: 168-74.

Bland KI, and N Love. October 1992. Evaluation of common breast masses. *Postgraduate Medicine* 92 (5): 95-112.

Centers for Disease Control. 24 April 1992. Cancer screening behaviors among U.S. women: Breast cancer, 1987-1989, and cervical cancer, 1988-1989. *Morbidity and Mortality Weekly Report* 41 (SS-2): 17-34.

Dixon JM, and RE Mansel. 17 September 1994. Symptoms assessment and guidelines for referral. *British Medical Journal* 309: 722-6.

Donegan WL. 24 September 1992. Evaluation of a palpable breast mass. *New England Journal of Medicine* 327 (13): 937-42.

6. CESAREAN DELIVERY
Deidre Gifford, M.D.

Prior cesarean, failure to progress in labor, and fetal distress are three of the most common indications for cesarean delivery in the United States, accounting for 35 percent, 30 percent, and 8 percent of cesareans, respectively (Shearer, 1993). Because the majority of cesareans performed will be for at least one of these three indications, we chose to develop quality indicators involving each, where sufficient data were available. The development of the specific indicators was based on four main sources of data. We used these resources to establish quality indicators that were clinically important, and that were based on evidence in the literature:

1) The document published by the American College of Obstetricians and Gynecologists (ACOG) in 1994, "Quality Assessment and Improvement in Obstetrics and Gynecology." This document contains several "criteria sets" whose purpose is to "...identify a threshold below which most physicians would agree that the care may be substandard and above which there may be several levels of acceptable care." Although these criteria represent a generally agreed upon standard, the process by which they were arrived at is not explicitly discussed.

2) Technical Bulletins and Committee opinions, periodically published by ACOG as educational aids to the practicing physician. These are "prepared by an expert or panel of experts, based on both scientific literature and personal expertise. Each document is reviewed and approved by the committee responsible for its development. Second, an oversight committee within ACOG performs a thorough review. Third, the ACOG executive board which represents all regions of the nation reviews it and grants final approval."

3) Since these ACOG publications are developed through an informal consensus process, we performed a literature search using MEDLINE to review each of the included topics.

4) The text, *Effective Care in Pregnancy and Childbirth* (Crowther et al., 1989; Enkin, 1989; Enkin et al., 1989; Grant, 1989; and Keirse, 1989; in Chalmers et al., 1989). This text contains meta-analyses of most known randomized trials in the field of obstetrics.

IMPORTANCE

The rate of cesarean delivery has increased from 5.5 percent in 1970, to 23.5 percent in 1991. Cesareans account for nearly one million of the four million births that occur annually in the United States, making it the most commonly performed major surgical procedure (Center for Disease Control [CDC], 1993). While the cesarean delivery rate has leveled since 1988 (CDC, 1993), questions remain about the appropriate use of cesarean delivery for many indications. These questions are motivated by several observations. First, the United States has higher rates of infant mortality than many developed countries in which cesarean rates are less than half of those in the U.S. (Notzon et al., 1987; CDC, 1993). Second, there is considerable variation in the use of cesareans between regions of the United States (CDC, 1993), and from hospital to hospital (Shiono et al., 1987). This variation does not appear to be explained by differences in clinical risk factors, since nonclinical factors such as hospital ownership, hospital teaching status, payment source, and volume of deliveries have also been shown to influence the rate of cesarean births (Stafford, 1991; King and Lahiri, 1994). All of these observations suggest that factors other than the health benefit to mother or infant may influence the decision to perform cesarean delivery.

Physician and hospital charges for cesarean delivery in 1991 were $7286, 66 percent higher than the charges of $4720 for vaginal delivery. The additional charge for cesarean delivery includes $611 for physician fees and $2495 for hospital charges (CDC, 1993). The CDC has estimated that a savings of one billion dollars would have occurred in 1991 if the cesarean delivery rate had been 15 per 100 births (U.S. Department of Health and Human Services [DHHS], 1990), rather than the actual 23.5 per 100 (CDC, 1993). With 3.9 million births annually in the United States, a 1 percent drop in the cesarean rate could reduce annual medical charges by an estimated $170 million (Keeler and Brodie, 1993).

Cesarean births require on average two additional days of hospitalization when compared to vaginal deliveries, and in some states women are given two weeks' extra disability payment following cesarean delivery (Keeler and Brodie, 1993). In addition, cesarean birth poses increased risks of morbidity for the mother when compared to vaginal birth. The most common complications following cesarean delivery are infectious (endometritis and urinary tract infection), but more serious complications such as excessive blood loss, venous thrombosis, damage to internal organs, anesthetic complications and death are also more common following cesarean birth (VanTuinen and Wolfe, 1992).

The decision to perform a cesarean involves calculating the trade-offs between risk and benefit to both mother and fetus simultaneously. While cesarean delivery may be more morbid for the mother, it is often perceived as being the safest route of delivery for the infant (Feldman and Freiman, 1985). Ideally, information about risks and benefits to both mother and infant, at least in the most common clinical situations, would be available to assist decisionmaking. However, in many cases such information does not exist (Gifford, 1995).

PRIOR CESAREAN DELIVERY

IMPORTANCE

Traditional obstetric practice dictated that women who had one cesarean should have all subsequent births by cesarean. This was due to the perceived risk of uterine rupture during labor, with subsequent maternal hemorrhage and possible fetal death. Repeat cesarean deliveries have accounted for 48 percent of the rise in cesareans between 1980 and 1985 (Taffel et al., 1987), and are currently the leading indication for cesarean delivery. In 1980, a NIH Consensus Development Conference on Cesarean Childbirth reviewed the topic and concluded that "...a proper selection of cases should permit a safe trial of labor and vaginal delivery for women who have had a previous low-segment transverse cesarean delivery" (NIH Consensus Statement, 1981). ACOG has subsequently published a committee opinion (1994) stating that "... in the absence of a contraindication, a woman with one previous cesarean delivery with a lower uterine segment incision should be counseled and encouraged to undergo a trial of labor in her current pregnancy." Despite these recommendations in 1991, less than 25 percent of women with prior cesareans currently have vaginal births (CDC, 1993).

EFFICACY AND/OR EFFECTIVENESS OF INTERVENTIONS

Treatment with Repeat Cesarean vs. Trial of Labor

There have been no randomized trials of a trial of labor vs. elective cesarean delivery for women with prior cesareans. However, a summary of seven cohort studies (Enkin, 1989, in Chalmers et al., 1989) showed that 80 percent (range 60 to 85 percent) of women who attempt a vaginal birth after cesarean will be successful. The same summary found that the maternal morbidity following elective cesarean *exceeds* that which follows a trial of labor. The incidence of uterine rupture or dehiscence in the review ranged from 0.5-3.3 percent in the trial of labor groups, and from 0.5-2.0 percent in the elective repeat cesarean groups. Overall, dehiscences or ruptures occurred in 1.5 percent of the women who had elective cesareans, and in 0.8 percent of the women with a trial of labor. Febrile morbidity was more common in the women who had elective cesarean delivery than in those who had a trial of labor. There are no data to suggest a benefit in infant outcomes following elective repeat cesarean delivery. Iatrogenic prematurity and respiratory distress can be the result of cesarean delivery scheduled and performed prior to term (because of inaccurate estimates of gestational age). No estimate of the frequency with which this currently occurs is available.

Data from managed care settings are sparser, but also raise the question about the utility of elective repeat cesareans. One recently-

published prospective cohort study of 7229 patients in a Health
Maintenance Organization examined outcomes following a trial of labor
(n=5022) vs. elective cesarean delivery (n=2207) (Flamm et al., 1994).
The success rate of a trial of labor ranged from 70 to 82 percent among
ten hospitals. The rate of uterine rupture was 0.8 percent in the trial
of labor group, and was not reported in the elective cesarean group.
There were no maternal or infant deaths related to uterine rupture in
either group. The elective cesarean groups had significantly longer
hospital stays (85 hours vs. 57 hours, p=.0001), more transfusions (1.72
percent vs. 0.72 percent, p=.0001), more postpartum fever (16.4 percent
vs. 12.7 percent, p=.0001). Hysterectomy was rare and not significantly
different between the two groups (0.27 percent vs. 0.12 percent, p=.21).
The trial of labor group had more infants with five minute Apgar scores
<7 (1.48 percent vs. 0.68 percent, p=.004). There were no perinatal or
maternal deaths related to uterine rupture in either group. One
maternal death occurred in the trial of labor group, as the result of an
anesthetic complication during emergency cesarean delivery.

It is important to note that the risk of uterine rupture during or
prior to labor following a prior cesarean depends on the type of uterine
scar which is present. For women with a prior transverse lower segment
incision, the risk of uterine rupture during a trial of labor appears to
be much less than the risk with a vertical uterine incision (Enkin,
1989, in Chalmers et al., 1989). The decision about whether or not to
undergo a trial of labor is therefore dependent on knowledge of the
previous type of uterine scar. The vast majority of women in the U.S.
are eligible to have a trial of labor because vertical incisions are
used so infrequently (Flamm et al., 1994).

In summary, both NIH and ACOG have endorsed the safety and efficacy
of a trial of labor following one prior transverse lower segment
cesarean section. No randomized trials on the topic exist, but multiple
observational studies have given consistent results showing:

1) The majority of women who attempt a vaginal birth after
   cesarean will be successful.
2) There is excessive maternal morbidity and no improvement in
   infant health with elective repeat cesarean delivery.

3) When the type of uterine scar is a classical or vertical scar, the rate of uterine rupture is higher, and elective repeat cesarean should be done.

4) The cost of routine elective repeat cesarean exceeds that of a trial of labor, both because of higher physician fees and longer hospital stays, and because of the increased maternal morbidity of cesarean delivery.

RECOMMENDED QUALITY INDICATORS FOR PRIOR CESAREAN DELIVERY

The following criteria apply to all women admitted for labor and delivery.

Treatment

	Indicator	Quality of evidence	Literature	Benefits	Comments
1.	For women who have delivered by cesarean, the type of uterine incision used (transverse lower segment or vertical) should be noted in the medical record.	III	Enkin, 1989, in Chalmers et al., 1989	Prevent uterine rupture in future pregnancies.	Decisions about future method of delivery are dependent on the availability of this information. This indicator is indirectly suggested by data on differential rupture rates in previous vertical versus transverse cesareans. Documentation of the type of incision at the time of delivery will provide the most accurate measure of the risk associated with a future trial of labor, reducing the risk of adverse outcomes.
2.	For women with a cesarean delivery in a prior pregnancy, the number and type of previous uterine scar(s) should be noted in the current delivery medical record. (If this information is not available, an attempt to locate it should be documented in the chart.)	II-2	Enkin, 1989, in Chalmers et al., 1989	Prevent uterine rupture during labor. Reduce morbidity by avoiding cesarean delivery.*	Allows for the most appropriate mode of delivery in the current pregnancy to be chosen, reducing the risk of adverse outcomes.
3.	Women with one prior transverse lower segment cesarean should undergo a trial of labor unless another indication for cesarean delivery is present.	II-2	Enkin, 1989, in Chalmers et al., 1989; Flamm et al., 1994	Reduce morbidity by avoiding cesarean delivery.*	A trial of labor means that the subject should have regular painful uterine contractions that result in cervical dilation or descent of the fetal presenting part. No difference in fetal outcomes has been shown for repeat cesarean versus trial of labor, but maternal morbidity is reduced with a trial of labor. Approximately 70% of women who attempt a trial of labor after cesarean will deliver vaginally.
4.	Women with a prior vertical cesarean should have a scheduled repeat cesarean delivery.	II-2	Enkin, 1989, in Chalmers et al., 1989	Prevent uterine rupture.	The percentage of women with a vertical incision is low, but in these women there will be a decreased risk of catastrophic uterine rupture with a planned cesarean. Risks are minimal with a small number of women receiving unnecessary cesareans. Although spontaneous labor may unexpectedly ensue prior to the date of the planned cesarean, a cesarean should be carried out as soon as the woman presents in labor. No trial of vaginal delivery should occur.

*Morbidity is primarily for the mother, with increased risk of transfusion, fever, infection and prolonged recovery time.

83

Quality of Evidence Codes:

I:	RCT
II-1:	Nonrandomized controlled trials
II-2:	Cohort or case analysis
II-3:	Multiple time series
III:	Opinions or descriptive studies

CESAREAN DELIVERY FOR FAILURE TO PROGRESS IN LABOR

IMPORTANCE

Disorders of the progress of labor, or "failure to progress in labor" can be caused by disproportion in the size of the fetal head and the maternal pelvis or ineffective uterine contractions. These disorders sometimes fall under the heading of "dystocia," a broad term used to describe a heterogeneous group of labor abnormalities. Some authors have suggested that the diagnosis of dystocia in first pregnancies is primarily responsible for the increase in cesareans seen in the United States, since primary cesareans for dystocia have usually been followed by repeat cesareans for "prior cesarean" (Boylan and Frankowski, 1986). Three times as many women are diagnosed with dystocia now than were so diagnosed in 1970 (VanTuinen and Wolfe, 1992), but the reasons for the increased use of this diagnosis are unknown. Both the NIH Consensus Development Conference on Cesarean Childbirth (1981) and the Canadian National Consensus Conference on Aspects of Cesarean Birth (1986) pointed to the increasing use of this diagnosis as an area for concern, and formulated recommendations regarding the diagnosis. Subsequently, ACOG developed a "criteria set" involving the diagnosis of failure to progress in labor which specifies criteria to be met before assigning the diagnosis and actions to be taken prior to carrying out a cesarean delivery (ACOG, 1994).

EFFICACY AND/OR EFFECTIVENESS OF INTERVENTIONS

Diagnosis

The diagnosis of dystocia can be made in either the first or second stage of labor. The course of labor is generally described by three stages (Figure 6.1). The first stage begins with the onset of labor and continues until complete cervical dilatation (10 cm) is reached. The second stage of labor begins at the time of complete dilatation and ends with complete expulsion of the fetus. The third stage of labor lasts from the delivery of the fetus until expulsion of the placenta. The

first stage of labor is divided into two phases, the latent phase and
the active phase. During the latent phase, contractions are often less
strong and more irregular than during the active phase, and the rate of
cervical dilatation is much slower.

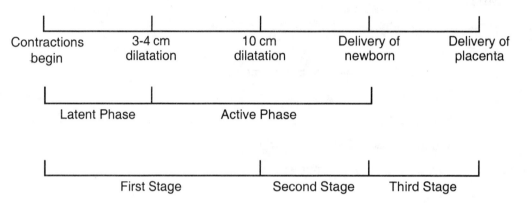

Figure 6.1 - Standard Terminology Describing the Course of Labor

During the latent phase of labor, change in cervical dilatation is
slow with a mean of 7 hours to reach a dilatation of 2.0 to 2.5 cm. At
3 to 4 cm of cervical dilatation, the active phase of labor is entered,
and the rate of cervical dilatation increases to 1.0 to 3.0 cm per hour
(Crowther et al., 1989, in Chalmers et al., 1989). The second stage of
labor begins when the laboring woman has reached 10 cm of cervical
dilatation, and ends with delivery of the infant. Controversy remains
regarding the definition of abnormal progress in labor, and its effects
on the mother and infant. According to ACOG, the rate of cervical
dilatation in the active phase below which progress should be considered
"abnormal" is 1.5 cm per hour for multiparas or 1.2 cm per hour for
nulliparas, based on the observations by Friedman (ACOG Technical
Bulletin, No. 137, 1989). The Canadian consensus panel (1989) has
suggested that progress of less than 0.5 cm per hour warrants a
diagnosis of dystocia. The protocol of the "active management of labor"
(O'Driscoll et al., 1984; Lopez-Zeno et al., 1992) uses a threshold of 1
cm per hour. These commonly used definitions for abnormal labor
progress have been based on means and standard deviations derived from
observing large numbers of labors (Friedman, 1989), and not necessarily
on the outcomes of such labors. It is implicit in all of these

definitions of abnormal progress that a series (at least two) of cervical exams is necessary in order to establish a lack of progress.

Although there is no consensus about the specific definition of poor progress in labor, there is one aspect of this diagnosis on which there is no disagreement in the literature. Both the ACOG (1994) and the Canadian consensus panel (1986) agree and have specified in their recommendations that before the diagnosis of "dystocia" can be entertained, a woman should have entered the active phase of labor (defined as a cervical dilatation of at least 3 cm in a nullipara and 4 cm in a multipara). This criterion is also used by those who advocate the active management of labor approach (O'Driscoll et al., 1984; Lopez-Zeno et al., 1992). Because the rate of cervical dilatation in the latent phase is known to be much slower than that in the active phase of labor, the same rate of progress is not to be expected. Although a prolonged latent phase may be associated with later labor abnormalities (Chelmow et al., 1993), there is no evidence and no consensus that cesarean delivery for lack of progress in the latent phase, no matter how slow the progress, is of any benefit to the mother or infant in the absence of another indication for cesarean. Despite this, there is evidence from both Canada and the United States that the diagnosis of dystocia is used frequently prior to the establishment of active labor (Stewart et al., 1990).

Treatment

Treatment options once the diagnosis of dystocia is made include continued observation, oxytocin, amniotomy, ambulation or cesarean delivery. The most effective of these treatments for poor progress in labor has not been well-established (ACOG, 1994; Canadian Consensus Conference Report, 1986; Keirse, 1989, in Chalmers et al., 1989). Amniotomy has been shown to shorten the length of labor in nulliparous women and to decrease the incidence of subsequent dystocia (Fraser et al., 1993), but there are no trials of the efficacy of amniotomy alone as a treatment for pre-existing dystocia. A randomized trial of the so-called "active management of labor," which involves early amniotomy, frequent cervical exams and oxytocin treatment when the rate of cervical

dilatation in active labor is less than 1 cm per hour, was published in
1992 (Lopez-Zeno et al., 1992). After controlling for confounding
variables, this therapy resulted in a decrease in cesarean delivery (OR
0.57, 95 percent CI 0.36-0.95) which was statistically significant.
Labors were also shorter in the treatment than in the control group. It
is not clear which element or combination of elements in the active
management protocol contributes to the reduction in cesarean use.
Keirse (1989, in Chalmers et al., 1989) summarizes the results of four
studies of oxytocin treatment for poor progress in labor, only one of
which showed an increase in the rate of cervical dilatation in treatment
vs. control women. In two of the four trials, ambulation resulted in
the same increase in cervical dilatation as treatment with oxytocin.

ACOG (1994) has stated that cesarean delivery should be used to
treat these disorders only when "...there has been no change in either
dilatation of the cervix or descent of the presenting part after at
least 2 hours of active labor following completion of the latent phase"
(the two hour time period appears to be derived from consensus and not
from outcomes data). This recommendation is based on the observation
that "...95 percent of women will have three to five contractions every
10 minutes that are each greater than 25 mm Hg above baseline." Thus,
they suggest that it is reasonable to proceed to cesarean delivery when
a laboring woman has met this norm and still has had no change in
cervical dilatation or descent of the presenting part over a period of
two hours. The Canadian consensus panel (1986) did not make a specific
time recommendation about when to proceed to cesarean delivery. Both
groups specify that other therapeutic interventions such as amniotomy or
oxytocin should be used in an attempt to correct the problem before
resorting to cesarean delivery.

RECOMMENDED QUALITY INDICATORS FOR CESAREAN DELIVERY FOR FAILURE TO PROGRESS IN LABOR

The following criteria apply to all women admitted for labor and delivery.

Diagnosis

	Indicator	Quality of evidence	Literature	Benefits	Comments
1.	When the diagnosis of failure to progress in labor is made, a woman should be in the active phase of labor.	III	AGOG, 1994; Canadian Consensus Conference Report, 1986	Reduce morbidity by avoiding cesarean section delivery.*	Reduces the number of unnecessary cesarean deliveries because the diagnosis of failure to progress in labor is not applicable in the latent phase. Unlike the active phase, there are no accepted standards for dilatation during the latent phase. Risks are minimal. Other terms for failure to progress are: "cephalopelvic disproportion," "protracted or prolonged active phase," "protracted or prolonged first stage," "feto-pelvic disproportion," and "arrest of dilatation." The active phase of labor is defined as a cervical dilatation of 3 cm for nulliparas and 4 cm for multiparas.
2.	When the diagnosis of failure to progress in labor is made, at least two exams of cervical dilatation separated in time by at least 2 hours should have been done and recorded in the medical record.	III	ACOG, 1994; Canadian Consensus Conference Report, 1986	Reduce morbidity by avoiding cesarean section delivery.*	This is implicit in recommendations that the observation of progress over time is necessary to establish the diagnosis. Repeat exams increase the accuracy of diagnosis since the lack of a change over time is necessary to assess the progression of labor and helps reduce the likelihood of an unnecessary cesarean delivery. Risks are minimal.

89

Treatment

	Indicator	Quality of evidence	Literature	Benefits	Comments
3.	Before a cesarean delivery is used to treat failure to progress in labor, at least one of the following therapeutic interventions should have been tried after the time of the diagnosis of FTP: 1) Amniotomy 2) Oxytocin 3) Ambulation	III	ACOG, 1994; Canadian Consensus Conference Report, 1986	Reduce morbidity by avoiding cesarean section delivery.*	There is no clear evidence that any one of these interventions is more effective than the others in treating failure to progress in labor. These measures should result in a shorter length of labor. May lead to a decrease in the cesarean delivery rate with certain protocols. Risk is minimal.

*Morbidity is mainly for the mother, with increased risk of transfusion, fever, infection and prolonged recovery time.

Quality of Evidence Codes:

I: RCT
II-1:   Nonrandomized controlled trials
II-2:   Cohort or case analysis
II-3:   Multiple time series
III: Opinions or descriptive studies

FETAL DISTRESS/NON-REASSURING FETAL STATUS AND INTRAPARTUM FETAL HEART RATE MONITORING

IMPORTANCE

Cesarean deliveries for "fetal distress" account for about 10 percent of all cesareans. The incidence of this diagnosis increased dramatically during the 1980s, from 1.2 percent of all deliveries in 1980 to 6.3 percent in 1989 (VanTuinen and Wolfe, 1992). This increase coincided with the increase in use of electronic fetal monitoring (EFM), a technology which was adopted and enjoyed widespread use prior to extensive study in randomized trials. The goal of electronic fetal heart rate monitoring is to detect changes in the fetal heart rate that are indicative of fetal hypoxia (commonly known as "fetal distress" or "non-reassuring fetal status"), and that might eventually lead to either permanent neurologic injury or death.

EFFICACY AND/OR EFFECTIVENESS OF INTERVENTIONS

Diagnosis

The development of procedures such as EFM to screen for fetal distress, has been made difficult by the lack of a "gold standard" against which they can be assessed. Initially, Apgar scores were used to determine the presence or absence of "true" distress, but they have been shown to correlate poorly with other morbidity measures and with long-term outcomes (Sykes et al., 1982). Measurement of fetal acid-base status, either intrapartum with scalp blood sampling, or after birth with cord blood, gives a better idea of the metabolic status of the infant, but is still not a highly reliable predictor of long-term infant morbidity or mortality (Clark and Paul, 1985). Inter- and intra-observer reliability of EFM interpretation is poor. In one study, four obstetricians were asked to read 50 different EFM tracings. Only 11 of the 50 tracings were assessed in the same way ("need for immediate delivery") by all four physicians. Twenty-one percent of the tracings were interpreted differently by individual obstetricians when reassessed two months later (Nielsen et al., 1987).

At least 10 randomized controlled trials have been published comparing routine electronic fetal monitoring in labor to either selective monitoring of high-risk pregnancies (Leveno et al., 1986) or to intermittent auscultation of the fetal heart rate (periodically listening to the fetal heart rate with either a stethoscope or Doppler device) by a nurse or midwife (Haverkamp, 1976; Renou, 1976; Kelso et al., 1978; Wood et al., 1981; Neldam, 1986; MacDonald et al., 1985; Luthy et al., 1987; Vintzileos, 1993). Meta-analysis revealed that routine electronic fetal heart rate monitoring increased the risk of cesarean delivery for "fetal distress," maternal infection and general anesthesia (Grant, 1989, in Chalmers et al., 1989). EFM did not decrease perinatal deaths, but did decrease the incidence of neonatal seizures, though the long-term benefits of this reduction in neonatal seizures are unclear (MacDonald et al., 1985). EFM may be more effective in certain subgroups.

The Dublin randomized trial of intrapartum fetal heart rate monitoring randomized over 12,000 women to either continuous EFM or intermittent auscultation. This study, which used fetal scalp sampling to document the presence or absence of fetal acidemia in conjunction with EFM, found no overall increase in cesarean deliveries with EFM (OR 1.10, 95 percent CI 0.88-1.38), but a significant increase in cesareans for fetal distress (OR 2.37, 95 percent CI 1.22-4.6). In this study, perinatal deaths were not different between the two groups, but the incidence of neonatal seizures was lower in the EFM group (OR 0.46, 95 percent CI 0.25-0.87). Retrospective re-analysis of the data from this trial showed the increase in neonatal seizures to be only among those infants where labor was induced, augmented or prolonged (Grant, 1989, in Chalmers et al., 1989). A randomized trial of 34,995 pregnancies in Dallas, Texas, compared routine EFM to EFM only in high-risk pregnancies. In this trial, there was no difference in neonatal seizures (OR 1.16, 95 percent CI 0.78-1.73) or perinatal death (OR 0.87, 95 percent CI 0.73-1.02) between the two groups. These findings have led to the suggestion that EFM is effective in preventing adverse infant outcomes in high-risk pregnancies, but has no beneficial fetal effects in pregnancies not at high risk for intrapartum distress.

The ACOG considers continuous electronic monitoring and intermittent auscultation to be equivalent methods for monitoring a fetus in labor (ACOG Technical Bulletin, No. 132, 1989), but notes that staffing limitations may limit the option for auscultation in many institutions. They do not make a distinction as to the type of monitoring that should be used for high-risk vs. low-risk pregnancies, nor do they suggest criteria for differentiating between those two subgroups. The auscultation regimen used in the randomized trials is every 15 minutes in the first stage and every 5 minutes in the second stage, requiring 1:1 nursing care. ACOG suggests that in low-risk pregnancies the heart rate should be monitored every 30 minutes in the first stage, and every 15 minutes in the second stage, although they acknowledge there are no data supporting this as the optimal time interval. In contrast to the ACOG recommendations, the U.S. Preventive Services Task Force (1989) recommends that "fetal heart rate should be measured by auscultation on all women in labor to detect signs of fetal distress. Electronic fetal monitoring should not be performed routinely on all women in labor. It should be reserved for pregnancies at increased risk for fetal distress." The Canadian Task Force on the periodic health exam has advised against routine electronic fetal monitoring in normal pregnancies, and states that the data are currently insufficient to recommend universal electronic monitoring in high-risk pregnancies (Anderson and Allison, 1990, in Goldbloom and Lawrence, 1990).

RECOMMENDED QUALITY INDICATORS FOR CESAREAN DELIVERY FOR FETAL DISTRESS

The following criteria apply to all women admitted for labor and delivery.

Diagnosis

	Indicator	Quality of evidence	Literature	Benefits	Comments
1.	Fetuses should be monitored during active labor. The forms of monitoring are: 1) intermittent auscultation with a stethoscope or doppler device; or 2) continuous electronic fetal monitoring (EFM).	III	Grant, 1989, in Chalmers et al., 1989	Decrease fetal morbidity and mortality.*	There are no trials comparing absence of fetal monitoring to monitoring during labor since there is general consensus that some form of monitoring is necessary. Active labor begins at 4 cm of cervical dilatation.

*Morbidity includes anoxia, seizures, and long-term neurologic damage.

Quality of Evidence Codes:

I: RCT
II-1:   Nonrandomized controlled trials
II-2:   Cohort or case analysis
II-3:   Multiple time series
III: Opinions or descriptive studies

PROPHYLACTIC ANTIBIOTICS FOR CESAREAN DELIVERY

IMPORTANCE

Post-partum infection is a common complication of cesarean delivery (Gibbs, 1985). Fever, endometritis, and more serious infections such as wound infection, sepsis and septic pelvic thrombophlebitis are all more likely to occur after cesarean delivery than after vaginal delivery (Enkin et al., 1989, in Chalmers et al., 1989). The prevalence of specific types of infection is not well understood because of varying definitions applied in the literature (Enkin et al., 1989, in Chalmers et al., 1989); however, estimates of endometritis range from 12 to 95 percent following cesarean delivery, depending on the patient population under study. Other infections may occur in as many as 25 percent of women delivered by cesarean (Gibbs, 1985).

EFFICACY AND/OR EFFECTIVENESS OF INTERVENTIONS

Prevention

Prophylactic antibiotics for the prevention of post-cesarean infectious morbidity have been extensively studied. Enkin et al. (1989, in Chalmers et al., 1989) summarized the results of over 90 controlled trials that examined the effect of prophylactic antibiotics in cesarean delivery (Table 6.1). A meta-analysis of 43 controlled trials showed that the odds ratio of serious infection (defined as septicemia, pelvic abscess, general peritonitis or serious wound infection) was 0.24 (95 percent CI 0.18-0.32) when use of prophylactic antibiotics was compared to no treatment. A similar effect was seen with post-partum endometritis, where an analysis of 44 studies gave an odds ratio of 0.25 (95 percent CI 0.22-0.29) when prophylactic antibiotics were compared to no treatment. A summary of 42 studies of the effects of prophylactic antibiotics on wound infection showed an odds ratio of 0.35 (95 percent CI 0.28-0.44).

While the risk of post-operative infection following cesarean is greater for emergency deliveries than for elective ones, prophylactic antibiotics have also been shown in a meta-analysis of a subset of the above studies to reduce both endometritis (OR 0.23; 95 percent CI 0.13-0.42) and wound infection (OR 0.10; 95 percent CI 0.03-0.36) following elective cesarean delivery (Enkin et al., 1989, in Chalmers et al., 1989).

Table 6.1
Effect of Prophylactic Antibiotics on Post-Cesarean Infection

| | Type of Infection | | |
	Wound infection	Endometritis	Other serious infection*
All cesareans			
OR	0.35	0.25	0.24
95% CI	0.28-0.44	0.22-0.29	0.18-0.32
No. studies	42	44	43
N	5372	5661	5777
Experi/Control	3036/2441	3235/2545	3323/2605
Elective cesareans			
OR	0.10	0.23	NA
95% CI	0.03-0.36	0.13-0.42	NA
No. studies	5	11	NA
N	164	425	NA
Experi/Control	86/78	241/214	NA

*This includes septicemia, pelvic abscess, general peritonitis or cases specified by the authors as serious wound infections. NA=not available, expt=experimental (antibiotic) group.
Source: Enkin et al., 1989, in Chalmers et al., 1989.

Penicillins, cephalosporins, metronidazole, and combinations of clindamycin plus gentamycin have all been studied for use in prophylaxis. There does not appear to be a clear advantage of any one of these antibiotics over the others (Gibbs, 1985; Enkin et al., 1995). There is some evidence that the combination of penicillin plus aminoglycoside may reduce febrile morbidity to a greater extent than penicillin alone, however the increased risk of nephrotoxicity and ototoxicity with aminoglycosides should be considered. Shorter courses of antibiotic prophylaxis appear to be less effective than longer courses in reducing febrile morbidity, but there is no agreed upon duration of prophylaxis that maximizes benefits in reducing infection and minimizes antibiotic toxicity and cost. Even single-dose therapy results in significant reductions in infectious outcomes (Enkin et al., 1995).

Potential adverse consequences of routine antibiotic prophylaxis include diarrhea, development of resistant strains, and allergic and/or toxic reactions to the antibiotic administration. The prevalence of such reactions is not well known, although there have been no reports of serious maternal side effects of antibiotic prophylaxis for cesarean delivery. The reported prevalence of mild drug reactions such as rash is less than 1 percent; however, this may be an underestimation due to under-reporting in the studies cited above (Enkin et al., 1989, in Chalmers et al., 1989). Antibiotics administered to the mother prior to the delivery of the infant can result in transfer of the medication to the fetus. This can lead to diagnostic interventions to rule out sepsis in the newborn which are costly and distressing to parents and infant. The available evidence suggests that antibiotics administered after cord clamping are just as effective as those administered pre-operatively in preventing post-operative infection (Enkin et al., 1989, in Chalmers et al., 1989).

Risk factors for infection following cesarean delivery include prolonged labor, prolonged rupture of membranes, internal monitoring, multiple vaginal exams during labor, obesity and low socioeconomic status (Gibbs, 1985; Enkin et al., 1989, in Chalmers et al., 1989). The data reviewed by Enkin (1989) suggest that prophylactic administration of antibiotics should be routine policy, except in the rare case where the prevalence of post-operative infection in an institution is low without the use of prophylaxis.

RECOMMENDED QUALITY INDICATORS FOR ANTIBIOTIC PROPHYLAXIS FOR CESAREAN DELIVERY

The following criteria apply to all women who deliver by cesarean.

Prophylactic Antibiotics for Cesarean Delivery

Indicator	Quality of evidence	Literature	Benefits	Comments
1. Women who give birth by cesarean should receive at least one dose of antibiotic prophylaxis.	I	Enkin et al., 1989, in Chalmers et al., 1989	Reduce endometritis. Reduce wound infection.	Routine prophylaxis with antibiotics results in reduction in endometritis (OR=0.23) and wound infection (OR=0.10). Side effects of antibiotics include rash and GI upset as well as a small risk of anaphylaxis.
2. Prophylactic antibiotic regimens should include one of the following: broad spectrum penicillins, broad spectrum cephalosporins, or metronidazole.	I	Enkin et al., 1989, in Chalmers et al., 1989; Enkin et al., 1995	Reduce endometritis. Reduce wound infection.	These drugs have been shown to be effective in lowering febrile morbidity and the incidence of wound infection in cesarean delivery. Categories of antibiotics other than these have not been studied and should not be used for prophylaxis.
3. Aminoglycosides should not be used, alone or in combination, for antibiotic prophylaxis.	III	Enkin et al., 1989, in Chalmers et al., 1989; Gibbs, 1985	Prevent oto- and nephro-toxicity.	There is no evidence that any additional benefit confirmed by adding aminoglycosides to the prophylactic regimen outweighs the added risk of oto- and nephro-toxicity.
4. Prophylactic antibiotics should be administered after the umbilical cord is clamped.	II	Enkin et al., 1989, in Chalmers et al., 1989; Gibbs, 1985	Prevent unnecessary transfer of medication to fetus.	Administering antibiotics after cord clamping avoids transfer of medication to the fetus and interventions to rule out sepsis in an infant "treated" with antibiotics prior to delivery are avoided. Antiobiotic effectiveness is still maintained. When chorioamnionitis is present prior to delivery, antibiotic therapy is therapeutic as opposed to prophylactic. Institution of antibiotics prior to delivery of the infant in these cases may be appropriate.

Quality of Evidence Codes:

I: RCT
II-1: Nonrandomized controlled trials
II-2: Cohort or case analysis
II-3: Multiple time series
III: Opinions or descriptive studies

98

REFERENCES - CESAREAN DELIVERY

American College of Obstetricians and Gynecologists. December 1989. Dystocia. *ACOG Technical Bulletin* 137: 1-6.

American College of Obstetricians and Gynecologists. September 1989. Intrapartum fetal heart rate monitoring. *ACOG Technical Bulletin* 132: 1-6.

American College of Obstetricians and Gynecologists. 1994. *Quality Assessment and Improvement in Obstetrics and Gynecology*. Washington, DC: ACOG.

Anderson GM, and DJ Allison. 1990. Intrapartum electronic fetal heart rate monitoring: A review of current status for the task force on the periodic health examination. In *Preventing Disease: Beyond the Rhetoric*. Editors Goldbloom RB, and RS Lawrence, 19-26. New York, NY: Springer-Verlag.

Boylan PC, and R Frankowski. August 1986. Dystocia, parity, and the cesarean problem. *American Journal of Obstetrics and Gynecology* 155 (2): 455-6.

Canadian Consensus Conference Report. 15 June 1986. Indications for cesarean section: Final statement of the panel of the National Consensus Conference on Aspects of Cesarean Birth. *Canadian Medical Association Journal* 134: 1348-52.

Centers for Disease Control. 23 April 1993. Rates of cesarean delivery--United States, 1991. *Morbidity and Mortality Weekly Report* 42 (15): 285-9.

Chelmow D, SJ Kilpatrick, and RK Laros. April 1993. Maternal and neonatal outcomes after prolonged latent phase. *Obstetrics and Gynecology* 81 (4): 486-91.

Clark SL, and RH Paul. 1 December 1985. Intrapartum fetal surveillance: The role of fetal scalp blood sampling. *American Journal of Obstetrics and Gynecology* 153 (7): 717-20.

Cohen WR, and S Yeh. March 1986. The abnormal fetal heart rate baseline. *Clinical Obstetrics and Gynecology* 29 (1): 73-82.

Crowther C, M Enkin, MJN Keirse, et al. 1989. Monitoring the progress of labour. In *Effective Care in Pregnancy and Childbirth. Volume 2: Childbirth. Parts VI-X and Index*. Editors Chalmers I, M Enkin, and MJN Keirse, 833-45. New York, NY: Oxford University Press.

Enkin M. 1989. Labour and delivery following previous caesarean section. In *EffeItive Care in Pregnancy and Childbirth. Volume 2:*

Childbirth. Parts VI-X and Index. Editors Chalmers I, M Enkin, and MJN Keirse, 1196-1215. New York, Ny: Oxford University Press.

Enkin M, E Enkin, I Chalmers, et al. 1989. Prophylactic antibiotics in association with caesarean section. In *Effecitive Care in Pregnancy and Childbirth. Volume 2: Childbirth. Parts VI-X and Index.* Editors Chalmers I, M Enkin, and MJN Keirse, 1246-69. New York, Ny: Oxford University Press.

Enkin M, MJN Keirse, M Renfrew, et al. 1995. Labour and delivery after previous caesarean section. In *A Guide to Effective Care in Pregnancy and Childbirth*, Second ed. 284-327. New York, NY: Oxford University Press.

Feldman GB, and JA Freiman. 9 May 1985. Occasional notes: Prophylactic cesarean section at term? *New England Journal of Medicine* 312 (19): 1264-7.

Flamm BL, JR Goings, Y Liu, et al. June 1994. Elective repeat cesarean delivery versus trial of labor: A prospective multicenter study. *Obstetrics and Gynecology* 83 (6): 927-32.

Fraser WD, S Marcoux, J Moutquin, et al. 22 April 1993. Effect of early amniotomy on the risk of dystocia in nulliparous women. *New England Journal of Medicine* 328 (16): 1145-49.

Friedman EA. 1989. Normal and dysfunctional labor. In *Management of Labor*, Second ed. Editors Cohen WR, DB Acker, and EA Friedman, 1-18. Rockville, MD: Aspen Publishers, Inc.

Gibbs RS. December 1985. Infection after cesarean section. *Clinical Obstetrics and Gynecology* 28 (4): 697-710.

Gifford DS, E Keeler, and KL Kahn. June 1995. Reductions in cost and cesarean rate by routine use of external cephalic version: A decision analysis. *Obstetrics and Gynecology* 85 (6): 930-6.

Grant A. 1989. Monitoring the fetus during labour. In *Effective Care in Pregnancy and Childbirth. Volume 2: Childbirth. Parts VI-X and Index.* Editors Chalmers I, M Enkin, and MJN Keirse, 846-82. New York, NY: Oxford University Press.

Haverkamp AD, HE Thompson, JG McFee, et al. 1 June 1976. The evaluation of continuous fetal heart rate monitoring in high-risk pregnancy. *American Journal of Obstetrics and Gynecology* 125 (3): 310-20.

Keeler EB, and M Brodie. 1993. Economic incentives in the choice between vaginal delivery and cesarean section. *The Milbank Quarterly* 71 (3): 365-404.

Keirse MJN. 1989. Augmentation of labour. In *Effective Care in Pregnancy and Childbirth. Volume 2: Childbirth. Parts VI-X and*

Index. Editors Chalmers I, M Enkin, and MJN Keirse, 951-66. New York, NY: Oxford University Press.

Kelso IM, RJ Parsons, GF Lawrence, et al. 1978. An assessment of continuous fetal heart rate monitoring in labor. *American Journal of Obstetrics and Gynecology* 131 (5): 526-32.

King DE, and K Lahiri. 17 August 1994. Socioeconomic factors and the odds of vaginal birth after cesarean delivery. *Journal of the American Medical Association* 272 (7): 524-9.

Leveno KJ, FG Cunningham, S Nelson, et al. 1986. A prospective comparison of selective and universal electronic fetal monitoring in 34,995 pregnancies. *New England Journal of Medicine* 315 (10): 615-9.

Lopez-Zeno JA, AM Peaceman, JA Adashek, et al. 13 February 1992. A controlled trial of a program for the active management of labor. *New England Journal of Medicine* 326 (7): 450-4.

Luthy DA, KK Shy, G van Belle, et al. May 1987. A randomized trial of electronic fetal monitoring in preterm labor. *Obstetrics and Gynecology* 69 (5): 687-95.

MacDonald D, A Grant, M Sheridan-Pereira, et al. 1 July 1985. The Dublin randomized controlled trial of intrapartum fetal heart rate monitoring. *American Journal of Obstetrics and Gynecology* 152 (5): 524-39.

National Institutes of Health Consensus Statement, Summary. 16 May 1981. Caesarean childbirth. *British Medical Journal* 282: 1600-4.

Neldam S, M Osler, PK Hansen, et al. 1986. Intrapartum fetal heart rate monitoring in a combined low- and high-risk population: A controlled clinical trial. *European Journal of Obstetrics, Gynecology, and Reproductive Biology* 23: 1-11.

Nielsen PV, B Stigsby, C Nickelsen, et al. 1987. Intra- and inter-observer variability in the assessment of intrapartum cardiotocograms. *Acta Obstetricia et Gynecologica Scandinavica* 66 (5): 421-4.

Notzon FC, PJ Placek, and SM Taffel. 12 February 1987. Comparisons of national cesarean-section rates. *New England Journal of Medicine* 316 (7): 386-89.

O'Driscoll K, M Foley, and D MacDonald. April 1984. Active management of labor as an alternative to cesarean section for dystocia. *Obstetrics and Gynecology* 63 (4): 485-90.

Renou P, A Chang, I Anderson, et al. 15 October 1976. Controlled trial of fetal intensive care. *American Journal of Obstetrics and Gynecology* 126 (4): 470-6.

Shearer EL. 1993. Cesarean section: Medical benefits and costs. *Social Science and Medicine* 37 (10): 1223-31.

Shiono PH, JG Fielden, D McNellis, et al. January 1987. Recent trends in cesarean birth and trial of labor rates in the United States. *Journal of the American Medical Association* 257 (4): 494-7.

Stafford RS. 2 January 1991. The impact of nonclinical factors on repeat cesarean section. *Journal of the American Medical Association* 265 (1): 59-63.

Stewart PJ, C Dulberg, AC Arnill, et al. 1990. Diagnosis of dystocia and management with cesarean section among primiparous women in Ottawa-Carleton. *Canadian Medical Association Journal* 142 (5): 459-63.

Sykes GS, PM Molloy, P Johnson, et al. 27 February 1982. Do Apgar scores indicate asphyxia? *Lancet* 1 (8270): 494-6.

Taffel SM, PJ Placek, and T Liss. 1987. Trends in the United States cesarean section rate and reasons for the 1980-85 rise. *American Journal of Public Health* 77 (8): 955-9.

U.S. Department of Health and Human Services. 1991. *Healthy People 2000: National Health Promotion and Disease Prevention Objectives*. U.S. Government Printing Office, Washington, DC.

U.S. Preventive Services Task Force. 1989. *Guide to Clinical Preventive Services: An Assessment of the Effectiveness of 169 Interventions*. Baltimore, MD: Williams and Wilkins.

VanTuinen, I, and SM Wolfe. 1992. *Unnecessary Cesarean Sections: Halting a National Epidemic*. Washington, DC: Public Citizen's Health Research Group.

Vintzileos AM, A Antsaklis, I Varvarigos, et al. June 1993. A randomized trial of intrapartum electronic fetal heart rate monitoring versus intermittent auscultation. *Obstetrics and Gynecology* 81 (6): 899-907.

Wood C, P Renou, J Oats, et al. 1 November 1981. A controlled trial of fetal heart rate monitoring in a low-risk obstetric population. *American Journal of Obstetrics and Gynecology* 141 (3): 527-34.

7. CIGARETTE USE COUNSELING
Steven Asch, M.D., M.P.H.

We relied on Chapter 48 of the Guide to Clinical Preventive
Services published by the U.S. Preventive Services Task Force (USPSTF,
1989) to construct quality indicators for the prevention of smoking and
the screening and treatment of cigarette use. When this core reference
cited studies to support individual indicators, we have referenced the
original source. We also performed narrow MEDLINE literature searches
for articles from 1990 to 1995 to update the literature support for the
proposed indicators.

IMPORTANCE

About one-third of all Americans smoke tobacco. Even higher
proportions of African Americans and low-income patients smoke.
Although smoking in women decreased from 28 percent to 25 percent
between 1974 and 1992, the rate of decline has been slower among women
than men (American Cancer Society [ACS], 1995; United States Department
of Health and Human Services [USDHHS], 1989). In 1993, there were
approximately 22 million female smokers and 73 percent wanted to quit
smoking, but only 2.5 percent of all smokers are able to successfully
quit each year (Centers for Disease Control [CDC], 1993; CDC, 1994).
Tobacco abuse has been strongly associated with carcinoma of the lung,
trachea, bronchus, esophagus, kidney, bladder, pancreas and stomach.
Smoking also plays a large role in causing coronary heart disease,
cerebrovascular disease, and obstetrical complications. As a result,
tobacco abuse is the most important modifiable cause of death in the
United States. Smoking is related to about 400,000 deaths annually and
the total direct and indirect costs may exceed $200 billion (USDHHS,
1989; Fiore et al., 1989; ACS, 1995). Patients who stop smoking return
to baseline risk profiles for coronary artery disease within three to
five years (USDHHS, 1989; Rich-Edwards et al., 1995).

EFFICACY AND/OR EFFECTIVENESS OF INTERVENTIONS

Screening and Initial Evaluation

Many specialty societies and governmental organizations recommend asking patients if they smoke, including the American College of Physicians (ACP), American College of Obstetricians and Gynecologists (ACOG), American Academy of Pediatrics (AAP), and the National Cancer Institute (NCI), though there is little agreement as to the optimal interval for screening (ACP, 1986; Health and Public Policy Committee, 1986; ACOG, 1986; Committee on Adolescence, 1987; Glynn and Marley, 1993; USPSTF, 1989). For our quality indicator, we propose that intake history and physicals include screening for tobacco abuse. If the patient has not had an intake history and physical, at least one provider over the course of the year should ask about smoking.

Treatment and Prevention

Once a patient has been identified as a smoker, providers have modest but definite impact in helping them quit (Russell et al., 1979; Ewart et al., 1983; Wilson et al., 1982; Wilson et al., 1988). A meta-analysis of 39 controlled trials found that counseling yielded an 8.4 percent (95 percent CI 5.6-11.2) reduction in the number of smokers at six months and a 5.8 percent (95 percent CI 3.2-8.4) reduction at one year (Kottke et al., 1988). While most of the individual trials did not demonstrate an effect, the 95 percent confidence limits after pooling the subjects exclude zero for both time points (Kottke et al., 1988).

A broad-based program to stop smoking appears to be most effective. The most successful trials were more likely to employ both group and individual counseling, teams of physicians and nonphysicians, multiple reinforcement sessions, and face-to-face advice. Multivariate analysis of the attributes of successful trials showed that the number of interventions was strongly associated with the smoking cessation rate (Table 7.1) (Kottke et al., 1988).

Table 7.1

**Descriptors for Interventions (Continuous Variables) Reporting Results
12 Months After Initiation of Intervention**

Descriptors	Range	Mean ± SD	Correlation With Cessation Rate
No. of intervention modalities	1-6	2.1 ± 0.9	.48*
Participant drop-out rate	0%-51%	13.8% ± 12.0%	.05
No. of subject contacts with program	1-15	3.8 ± 4.6	.38*
Months subject in contact with program	0-12	1.1 ± 2.1	.55*
No. of participants	32-8189	608.2 ± 948.6	.20
No. of times smoking status was assessed	1-18	4.0 ± 4.5	.13
Months from first contact to last verification	0-12	7.6 ± 11.8	.16
No. of times cessation claims were validated	0-6	0.9 ± 1.2	.09
Subjective rating of study quality	0-5	3.2 ± 1.0	-.23

*$p < .01$.
Source: Kottke et al., 1988.

Adding nicotine replacement therapy may increase the success rate
of counseling alone by up to one-third, particularly in heavy smokers.
A meta-analysis of 14 randomized trials of nicotine gum compared to
placebo gum found that more patients who used nicotine gum had quit
smoking at 6 months (27 percent vs. 18 percent, n=734) and 12 months (23
percent vs. 13 percent), although this study occurred in the setting of
specialized smoking cessation clinics. The meta-analysis found lower
rates of effectiveness when the treatment occurred in general medical
clinics, however. Placebo controlled trials in general practice did not
demonstrate an effect, though uncontrolled trials show that nicotine
replacement had a modest effect at 6 months (17 percent vs. 13 percent;
n=2238) and 12 months (9 vs. 5 percent) in general practice. Given its
questionable efficacy in the setting of general practice, we propose

that nicotine replacement be prescribed as second line therapy after counseling alone has failed (Lam et al., 1987).

There are several contraindications for nicotine replacement therapy. Nicotine replacement is contraindicated in women who are pregnant or nursing because it crosses the placenta and is excreted in the breast milk. Patients with recent myocardial infarctions may have their ischemia exacerbated by nicotine replacement and patients with temporomandibular joint disease may experience symptomatic worsening. If the patient continues to smoke, the potential toxicities of nicotine replacement become much more likely. Nicotine gum may not be as effective in the absence of counseling; all the controlled studies combined gum with some form of advice (Lam et al., 1987; Oster et al., 1986; Russell et al., 1983; Benowitz, 1988; Wilson et al., 1988; Fagerström, 1984).

Follow-up

The above-mentioned meta-analysis of 39 clinical trials of smoking cessation counseling showed that one of the common attributes of successful programs is reinforcement through follow-up appointments. Both the number of subject contacts with the program and the number of months duration of the program were positively correlated with the cessation rate (see Table 7.1). We propose that the medical record should indicate a plan for such reinforcement either by adding tobacco abuse to the patient's problem list or through addressing the problem during at least one subsequent visit.

RECOMMENDED QUALITY INDICATORS FOR CIGARETTE USE COUNSELING

These indicators apply to women aged 18-50.

Screening and Initial Evaluation

	Indicator	Quality of evidence	Literature	Benefits	Comments
1.	Enrollees should have the presence or absence of tobacco use noted in the medical record at the intake history and physical or at least once during the course of a year.	III	ACP, 1986; AAP, 1987; ACOG, 1986; NIH, 1989; USPSTF, 1989	Decrease smoking-related morbidity and mortality.*	Recommended by many medical societies and governmental agencies (see text), though no consensus on optimal screening interval. No trials on screening, but cost is very low. Prerequisite to counseling. Screening increases likelihood of detection and subsequent interventions.

Treatment

	Indicator	Quality of evidence	Literature	Benefits	Comments
2.	Current smokers should receive counseling to stop smoking.**	I	Kottke et al., 1988	Decrease smoking-related morbidity and mortality.*	Meta-analysis of 39 trials of counseling showed 8% decrease in smoking rate at six months and 6% at one year.
3.	If counseling alone fails to help the patient quit smoking, the patient should be offered nicotine replacement therapy (gum or patch).	I-II	Lam et al., 1987	Decrease smoking-related morbidity and mortality.*	Meta-analysis of RCTs of nicotine replacement therapy demonstrated efficacy in setting of specialized smoking clinics; adding nicotine replacement may increase cessation rate by one third. Weaker evidence in general practice.
4.	Nicotine replacement should only be prescribed in conjunction with counseling.**	I	Lam et al., 1987	Avert potential side effects of nicotine therapy in patients who will not benefit without concomitant counseling. Decrease smoking-related morbidity and mortality.*	All controlled trials of nicotine replacement combine it with some form of counseling.
5.	Nicotine replacement should not be prescribed if the patient: a. is pregnant or nursing b. has had a myocardial infarction in past year c. has temporomandibular joint disease d. continues to smoke	I-II	Benowitz, 1988	Avert premature births, birth defects, potential harm to nursing newborns, ischemic events.	Nicotine crosses placenta and is excreted into breast milk. It can exacerbate ongoing ischemia and worsen symptoms of temporomandibular joint disease. Continuing to smoke makes side effects of nicotine replacement much more likely.

Follow-up

	Indicator	Quality of evidence	Literature	Benefits	Comments
6.	Tobacco abuse should be added to the problem list of all current smokers or addressed within one year.	I	Kottke et al., 1988; Wilson et al., 1988	Decrease smoking-related morbidity and mortality.*	One of the common characteristics of successful counseling in the Kottke meta-analysis is reinforcement at subsequent visits.

*Smoking has been associated with increased risk of cancer of the lung, trachea, bronchus, lip, oral cavity, pharynx, larynx, esophagus, kidney, bladder, stomach, and pancreas. Smoking also causes or exacerbates COPD, asthma, bronchitis, cerebrovascular accidents and coronary heart disease. Smoking while pregnant is a contributing factor in low birthweight, shortened gestation, and sudden infant death syndrome. Each of these conditions causes a wide range of morbid symptoms and most increase mortality.

***We plan a broad operationalization of counseling to include everything from from pamphlets and brief advice in the primary care setting to specialized structured programs.

Quality of Evidence Codes:

I: RCT
II-1:   Nonrandomized controlled trials
II-2:   Cohort or case analysis
II-3:   Multiple time series
III: Opinions or descriptive studies

108

REFERENCES - CIGARETTE USE COUNSELING

American Cancer Society. 1995. *Cancer Facts and Figures-1995*. Atlanta, GA: American Cancer Society.

American College of Physicians. 9 April 1986. *Cigarette Abuse Epidemic: Position Paper of the American College of Physicians*.

American College of Obstetricians and Gynecologists. November 1986. Statement on smoking. *ACOG Statement of Policy* November 1986.:

Benowitz NL. 1988. Toxicity of nicotine: Implications with regard to nicotine replacement therapy. In *Nicotine Replacement: A Critical Evaluation*. Editors Pomerleau OF, and CS Pomerleau, 187-217. New York, NY: Alan R. Liss, Inc.

Centers for Disease Control. 23 December 1994. Cigarette smoking among adults--United States, 1993. *Morbidity and Mortality Weekly Report* 43 (50): 925-30.

Centers for Disease Control. 9 July 1993. Smoking cessation during previous year among adults--United States, 1990 and 1991. *Morbidity and Mortality Weekly Report* 42 (26): 504-7.

Committee on Adolescence. March 1987. Tobacco use by children and adolescents. *Pediatrics* 79 (3): 479-81.

Ewart CK, VC Li, and TJ Coates. June 1983. Increasing physicians' antismoking influence by applying an inexpensive feedback technique. *Journal of Medical Education* 58: 468-73.

Fagerstrom K. 1984. Effects of nicotine chewing gum and follow-up appointments in physician-based smoking cessation. *Preventive Medicine* 13: 517-27.

Fiore MC, TE Novotny, JP Pierce, et al. 6 January 1989. Trends in cigarette smoking in the United States. *Journal of the American Medical Association* 261 (1): 49-55.

Glynn, TJ, and MW Manley. 1993. *How to Help Your Patients Stop Smoking: A National Cancer Institute Manual for Physicians*. U.S. Department of Health and Human Services, Hyattsville, MD.

Health and Public Policy Committee, and American College of Physicians. 1986. Methods for stopping cigarette smoking. *Annals of Internal Medicine* 105 (2): 281-91.

Kottke TE, RN Battista, GH DeFriese, et al. 20 May 1988. Attributes of successful smoking cessation interventions in medical practice: A meta-analysis of 39 controlled trials. *Journal of the American Medical Association* 259 (19): 2883-9.

Lam W, PC Sze, HS Sacks, et al. 4 July 1987. Meta-analysis of randomised controlled trials of nicotine chewing-gum. *Lancet* 2 (8549): 27-30.

Oster G, DM Huse, TE Delea, GA Colditz. 1986. Cost-effectiveness of nicotine gum as an adjunct to physician's advice against cigarette smoking. *JAMA* 256(10):1315-1318.

Rich-Edwards JW, JE Manson, CH Hennekens, et al. 29 June 1995. The primary prevention of coronary heart disease in women. *New England Journal of Medicine* 332 (26): 1758-66.

Russell MA, R Merriman, J Stapleton, et al. 10 December 1983. Effect of nicotine chewing gum as an adjunct to general practitioners' advice against smoking. *British Medical Journal* 287: 1782-5.

Russell MAH, C Wilson, C Taylor, et al. 28 July 1979. Effect of general practitioners' advice against smoking. *British Medical Journal* 2: 231-5.

U.S. Department of Health and Human Services. 1989. *Reducing the Health Consequences of Smoking; 25 Years of Progress: A Report of the Surgeon General-1989*. Rockville, MD: U.S. Department of Health and Human Services.

U.S. Preventive Services Task Force. 1989. *Guide to Clinical Preventive Services: An Assessment of the Effectiveness of 169 Interventions*. Baltimore, MD: Williams and Wilkins.

Wilson DM, W Taylor, R Gilbert, et al. 16 September 1988. A randomized trial of a family physician intervention for smoking cessation. *Journal of the American Medical Association* 260 (11): 1570-4.

Wilson D, G Wood, N Johnston, et al. 15 January 1982. Randomized clinical trial of supportive follow-up for cigarette smokers in a family practice. *Canadian Medical Association Journal* 126: 127-9.

8. DEPRESSION

Eve A. Kerr, M.D., M.P.H.

We relied on the following sources to construct quality indicators for depression in adult women: the AHCPR Clinical Practice Guideline *Depression in Primary Care (Volumes 1 and 2): Treatment of Major Depression* (Depression Guideline Panel, 1993a and 1993b), as well as selected review and journal articles. We conducted a MEDLINE search of review articles published in English between the years 1985 and 1995.

IMPORTANCE

Major depression is a common condition, affecting more than 10 percent of adults between the ages of 14 and 55 annually (Kessler, 1994). Major depressive disorder is characterized by one or more episodes of major depression without episodes of mania or hypomania. By definition, major depressive episodes last at least two weeks, and typically much longer. Up to one in eight individuals may require treatment for depression during their lifetime (Depression Guideline Panel, 1993b). The common age of onset is from 20 to 40; however, depression can start at any age.

Approximately 11 million people in the United States suffered from depression in 1990; a disproportionate share (7.7 million) were women (Greenberg et al., 1993). The point prevalence for major depressive disorder in Western industrialized nations is 2.3 to 3.2 percent for men and 4.5 to 9.3 percent for women (Depression Guideline Panel, 1993a).[3] Katon and Schulberg (1992) report that among general medical outpatients, the prevalence rate for major depression is between 5 and 9 percent and 6 percent for the less severe diagnosis of dysthymia. Consistent with these findings, Feldman et al. (1987) found that the point prevalence of major depressive disorder in primary care outpatient settings ranged from 4.8 to 8.6 percent. The lifetime risk for developing depression is between 20 and 25 percent for women.

---

[3]For a summary of the prevalence literature, refer to pg. 25, Volume 1, *Depression Guidelines*.

Depression is associated with severe deterioration of a person's ability to function in social, occupational, and interpersonal settings (Broadhead et al., 1990; Wells et al., 1989a). Broadhead et al. (1990) found that patients with major depressive disorder reported 11 disability days per 90-day interval compared to 2.2 disability days for the general population. Roughly one-quarter of all persons with major depressive disorder reported restricted activity or bed days in the past two weeks (Wells et al., 1988). The functioning of depressed patients is comparable with or worse than that of patients with other major chronic medical conditions, such as congestive heart failure (Hays et al., 1995).

The direct costs associated with treating major depressive disorder combined with the indirect costs from lost productivity account for about $16 billion per year in 1980 dollars (Depression Guideline Panel, 1993a). Greenberg et al. (1993) estimate that the total costs of affective disorders are $12.4 billion for direct treatment, $7.5 billion for mortality costs due to suicide, and $23.8 billion in morbidity costs due to reduction in productivity ($11.7 billion from excess absenteeism and $12.1 billion while at work).

Sturm and Wells (1994) recently demonstrated the cost-effectiveness of treatment for depression. They found that treatment consistent with standards/guidelines lowers the average cost per quality-adjusted life-year when compared to no treatment or ineffective treatment (e.g., subtherapeutic doses of antidepressants). To achieve this gain, however, total costs of care are higher.

EFFICACY AND/OR EFFECTIVENESS OF INTERVENTIONS

Screening/Detection

The under-diagnosis of depression seriously impedes interventional efforts. The Depression Guidelines report that only one-third to one-half of all cases of major depressive disorders are properly recognized by primary care and non-psychiatric practitioners (Depression Guideline Panel, 1993a; Wells et al., 1989b). The Medical Outcomes Study (MOS) revealed that approximately 50 percent of patients with depression were detected by general medical clinicians, and among patients in prepaid health plans the rates of detection were much lower than those observed for patients in fee-for-service plans (Wells et al., 1989b).

No definitive screening method exists to detect major depression. Patient self-report questionnaires are available but are non-specific. These questionnaires can be used to supplement the results of direct interview by a clinician (Depression Guideline Panel, 1993a). Burnam et al. (1988) used an eight-item screen in the MOS; however, no standard screen currently exists for clinical work.

A clinical interview is the most effective method for detecting depression (Depression Guideline Panel, 1993a). Clinicians should especially look for symptoms in patients who are at high risk. Risk factors for depression include (Depression Guideline Panel, 1993a):

1) Prior episodes of depression (one major depressive episode is associated with a 50 percent chance of a subsequent episode; two episodes with a 70 percent chance and three or more with a 90 percent chance of recurrent depression over a lifetime (NIMH Consensus Development Conference, 1985);

2) Family history of depressive disorder;

3) Prior suicide attempts;

4) Female gender;

5) Age of onset under 40;

6) Postpartum period;

7) Medical comorbidity;

8) Lack of social support;

9) Stressful life events; and,

10) Current alcohol or substance abuse.

Laboratory testing for depression is effective only in identifying underlying physiologic reasons for depression (e.g., hypothyroidism). No laboratory screening test exists for depression *per se* and thus, laboratory tests should be tailored to the patient, when indicated, as part of a diagnostic work-up. Laboratory testing should especially be considered as part of the general evaluation if:

1) the medical review of systems reveals signs or symptoms that are rarely encountered in depression;

2) the patient is older;

3) the depressive episode first occurs after the age of 40-45; or

4) the depression does not respond fully to routine treatment (Depression Guideline Panel, 1993a).

Diagnosis

The diagnosis of depression is based primarily on DSM-IV criteria. The criteria state that at least five of the following symptoms must be present during the same period to receive a diagnosis of major depression (American Psychiatric Association, 1994).

1) depressed mood;

2) markedly diminished interest or pleasure in almost all activities;

3) significant weight loss/gain;

4) insomnia/hypersomnia;

5) psychomotor agitation/retardation;

6) fatigue;

7) feelings of worthlessness (guilt);

8) impaired concentration; and,

9) recurrent thoughts of death or suicide.

The symptoms should be present most of the day, nearly daily, for a minimum of two weeks.

Practitioners need to consider the presence of other comorbidities prior to making a diagnosis of major depression. Other factors that may contribute to the patient's mental health and which the clinician may want to treat first include:

1) substance abuse;

2) medications;

3) general medical disorder;

4) causal, non-mood psychiatric disorder; and/or,

5) grief reaction (Depression Guideline Panel, 1993a).

The clinician should also consider alternative diagnoses by eliciting a proper patient history. Examples of alternative diagnoses include:

1) Bipolar disorder if the patient manifests prior manic episodes;

2) Dysthymic disorder if the patient has a chronic mood disturbance (sadness) present most of the time for at least two consecutive years (Depression Guideline Panel, 1993a).

Treatment

Treatment is more effective if provided earlier in the depressive episode, prior to the condition becoming chronic (Bielski and Friedel, 1976; Kupfer et al., 1989). Unless noted otherwise, the recommendations for treatment are drawn from the *Depression Guidelines* (Depression Guideline Panel, 1993b).

Use of Antidepressant Medications

Antidepressant medications are the first-line treatments for major depressive disorder. Medications have been shown to be effective in all forms of major depressive disorder (Depression Guideline Panel, 1993b). Anti-depressant medications are highly likely to be of benefit when:

1) the depression is moderate to severe;

2) there are psychotic, melancholic, or atypical symptom features;

3) the patient requests medication;

4) psychotherapy by a trained, competent psychotherapist is not available;

5) the patient has shown a prior positive response to medication; and,

6) maintenance treatment is planned.

The choice of anti-depressant is less important than use of antidepressants at appropriate dosages (Wells et al., 1994). No single antidepressant medication is clearly more effective than another and no single medication results in remission for all patients. Pharmacologic doses are recommended in the *Depression Guidelines* (1993b)

The specific choice of medication should be based on:

1) short- and long-term side effects;

2) prior positive/negative response to medication;

3) concurrent, nonpsychiatric medical illnesses that may make selected medications more or less risky; and/or,

4) the concomitant use of other nonpsychotropic medications that may alter the metabolism or increase the side effects of the antidepressant (Depression Guideline Panel, 1993b).

In general, anti-anxiety agents should not be used (with possible exception of alprazolam) (Depression Guideline Panel, 1993b).

Use of Psychotherapy

Maintenance medication clearly prevents recurrences, while, to date, maintenance psychotherapy does not (Depression Guideline Panel, 1993a). Clinicians should consider psychotherapy alone for major depression as a first-line treatment if the episode is mild to moderate AND the patient desires psychotherapy as the first-line therapy (Depression Guideline Panel, 1993b). If psychotherapy is completely ineffective by 6 weeks of treatment or if psychotherapy does not result in nearly a fully symptomatic remission within 12 weeks, then a switch to medications is appropriate due to the clear evidence of the efficacy of treatment with medications (Depression Guideline Panel, 1993b).

Medication Plus Psychotherapy

Clinicians should consider combined treatment initially with medications and psychotherapy if:

1) the depression is chronic or characterized by poor inter-episode recovery;

2) either treatment alone has been only partially effective;

3) the patient has a history of chronic psychosocial problems; or,

4) the patient has a history of treatment adherence difficulties.

However, there is little evidence that indicates that patients being seen in primary care practices who have major depression require initial psychotherapy in addition to medication. It is recommended that medication be added to (or substituted for) psychotherapy if:

1) there is no response to psychotherapy at 6 weeks;

2) there is only partial response at 12 weeks;

3) the patient worsens with psychotherapy; or,

4) the patient requests medications and symptoms are appropriate (Depression Guideline Panel, 1993b).

Clinicians may add psychotherapy to prescribed medications if:

1) residual symptoms are largely psychological (e.g., low self-esteem); or

2) patient has difficulty with adherence.

Follow-up

Most patients with major depressive disorder respond partially to medication within 2 to 3 weeks and full symptom remission is typically seen within 6 to 8 weeks (Depression Guideline Panel, 1993a). Most patients who receive time-limited psychotherapy respond partially by 5 to 6 weeks and fully by 10 to 12 weeks. Office visits or telephone contacts to manage indications should occur weekly for the first 3 to 4 weeks following initial diagnosis to ensure adherence to medication regimen, adjust dosage, and detect and manage side effects. The depression panel recommends that patients with severe depression be seen weekly for the first 6 to 8 weeks (Depression Guideline Panel, 1993a). Once the depression has resolved, visits every 4 to 12 weeks are reasonable (Depression Guideline Panel, 1993a). The Depression Guideline Panel recommended the following guidelines for evaluating patients at each subsequent visit.

Failure to Respond to Medications

If the patient shows no response to the current medication by six weeks, then the clinician should both reassess adequacy of the diagnosis and reassess adequacy of treatment. Change in diagnosis or treatment plan (e.g., change of medication, referral to mental health specialist) is indicated (Depression Guideline Panel, 1993b).

If the patient exhibits a partial response by six weeks, but cognitive symptoms remain, then the clinician should:

- continue treatment;
- reassess response to treatment in six more weeks;

- increase the dose of the current medication or change the medication entirely if reevaluation reveals only a partial response. Alternately, referral to a mental health specialist for addition of psychotherapy may be warranted;
- consult a psychiatrist if two attempts at acute-phase medication have failed to resolve symptoms (Depression Guideline Panel, 1993b).

Continuation of Treatment

Unless maintenance treatment is planned, anti-depressant medication should be discontinued at four to nine months (Depression Guideline Panel, 1993b, pg. 109). Patients should be followed for the next several months to ensure that a new depressive episode does not occur. We recommend follow-up visits at 16-week intervals; the Depression Guideline Panel recommended 12-week intervals, but did not have any evidence about optimal timing. It is unclear from the literature when the optimal time is to discontinue psychotherapy.

Maintenance

Maintenance treatment is designed to prevent new episodes of depression. Patients should be considered for maintenance treatment if they have had:

a) Three or more episodes of major depressive disorder; or

b) Two episodes of major depressive disorder and other circumstance (i.e., family history of bipolar disorder, history of recurrence within one year after previously effective medication was discontinued, family history of recurrent major depression, early onset (prior to age 20) of the first depressive episode, both episodes were severe, sudden, or life-threatening in the past three years) (Depression Guideline Panel, 1993b).

RECOMMENDED QUALITY INDICATORS FOR DEPRESSION

The following indications apply to women ages 18-50.

Diagnosis/Detection

	Indicator	Quality of evidence	Literature	Benefits	Comments
1.	Clinicians should ask about the presence or absence of depression or depressive symptoms* in any person with any of the following risk factors for depression: a. divorce in past six months, b. unemployment, c. history of depression, d. death in family in past six months, or e. alcohol or other drug abuse.	III	USPSTF, 1989	Alleviate symptoms of depression.*	Risk factors for depression have been relatively well-defined in cross-sectional studies.
2.	If the diagnosis of depression is made, specific co-morbidities should be elicited and documented in the chart: a. presence or absence of substance abuse; b. medication use; and c. general medical disorder(s).	III	Depression Guideline Panel, 1993a & 1993b	Alleviate symptoms of depression.* Prevent complications of substance abuse.**	Certain co-morbidities may contribute to or cause depression. The practitioner should be aware of these co-morbidities when making a treatment plan for depression. Documentation may have occured on previous visits.

119

Treatment

	Indicator	Quality of evidence	Literature	Benefits	Comments
3.	If co-morbidity (substance abuse, contributing medication) is present that contributes to depression, the initial treatment objective should be to remove the comorbidity or treat the medical disorder.	III	Depression Guideline Panel, 1993a & 1993b (meta-analysis)	Alleviate symptoms of depression.* Prevent complications of substance abuse.**	Depression may be treated by addressing the co-morbidity. For example, alcoholism should be treated and patients should be taken off of medications that may have CNS depressant properties.
4.	Once diagnosis of major depression has been made, treatment with anti-depressant medication and/or psychotherapy should begin within 2 weeks.	I, II-1, II-2	Depression Guideline Panel, 1993a & 1993b	Alleviate symptoms of depression.* Reduce disability days.	Randomized controlled trials cited in the guidelines (not individually reviewed) substantiate the usefulness of medication and psychotherapy for the treatment of depression. Antidepressant medication therapy is probably the more effective sole modality. The guidelines recommend "prompt" treatment, but no definition of prompt is given. We suggest two weeks are a reasonable time interval.
5.	Presence or absence of suicidal ideation should be documented during the first or second diagnostic visit.	II-2, III	Depression Guideline Panel, 1993a & 1993b	Prevent death from suicide. Prevent morbidity from suicide attempts.	Presence of suicidality is a marker for severe depression and would argue for instituting therapy with anti-depressants and against psychotherapy alone. Suicidality with psychosis, drug abuse, and/or plan of action warrants hospitalization.
6.	Medication treatment visits or telephone contacts should occur weekly for a minimum of 4 weeks.	III	Depression Guideline Panel, 1993a & 1993b	Alleviate symptoms of depression.* Reduce disability days.	Once treatment is started, the practitioner needs to document improvement. Most patients improve at least partially within 3 weeks. The guidelines advocate weekly follow-up by phone or in person for 4-6 weeks. Our indicator specifies the lower end of the recommendations.
7.	At least one of the following should occur if there is no or incomplete response to therapy for depression at 6 weeks: • Referral to psychotherapist, if not already seeing one; • Change or increase in dose of medication, if on medication; • Addition of medication, if only using psychotherapy • Change in diagnosis documented in chart	III	Depression Guideline Panel, 1993a & 1993b	Alleviate symptoms of depression.* Reduce disability days.	Almost all clinical depression responds at least partially by 6 weeks. If response is incomplete, the diagnosis needs to be re-evaluated and/or treatment plan changed/augmented.

#	Indicator		Reference	Objective	Comment
8.	Anti-depressants should be prescribed at appropriate dosages.	I	Depression Guideline Panel, 1993b; Wells, 1994	Alleviate symptoms of depression.* Reduce disability days.	Only appropriate doses of anti-depressants will be effective in treatment, yet subtherapeutic doses are often used. For example, a patient on 25 mg of amitryptilline at bedtime is not on a therapeutic antidepressant dose. Since these indicators only apply to women under age 50, we will not need to adjust for change in dose requirements in the elderly. We will exclude those with renal and hepatic dysfunction from this indicator.
9.	Anti-anxiety agents should generally NOT be used (except alprazolam).	I	Depression Guideline Panel, 1993b	Alleviate symptoms of depression.* Reduce disability days. Avoid dependence on anti-anxiety agents.	With the possible exception of alprazolam, anti-anxiety agents have not shown to be of benefit and may be of harm. Foregoing antidepressants in favor of anxiolytics deprives patients of potential benefits of antidepressant treatment.
10.	Persons who have suicidality should be asked if they have specific plans to carry out suicide.	III	Depression Guideline Panel, 1993b	Prevent death from suicide. Prevent morbidity from suicide attempts.	If a person has a plan to carry out suicide, the risk of success increases. These persons should be hospitalized.
11.	Persons who have suicidality and have any of the following risk factors should be hospitalized: • psychosis • current alcohol or drug abuse • specific plans to carry out suicide (e.g., obtaining a weapon, putting affairs in order, making a suicide note).	III	Depression Guideline Panel, 1993b	Prevent death from suicide. Prevent morbidity from suicide attempts.	Presence of risk factors for successful suicide in a person who admits to suicidality warrants hospitalization.

Follow-up

	Indicator	Quality of evidence	Literature	Benefits	Comments
12.	Once depression has resolved, follow-up visits should occur every 16 weeks at a minimum, while patient is still on medication, for the first year of treatment.	III	Depression Guideline Panel, 1993b	Alleviate symptoms of depression.* Reduce disability days. Reduce remissions.	The guidelines recommend visit intervals every 12 weeks for the duration of treatment. Occasionally, patients may be on indefinite treatment. In order to allow variation in follow-up times given patient preferences and long-term duration of treatment, we recommend 16-week interval visits during the first year of treatment. Even so, it may be difficult to penalize a practitioner whose patients are seeing a psychotherapist in addition to him/herself for not seeing a patient on a frequent basis.
13.	At each visit during which depression is discussed, degree of response/remission and side effects of medication should be assessed and documented during the first year of treatment.	III	Depression Guideline Panel, 1993b	Alleviate symptoms of depression.* Reduce toxicities of medication. Reduce remission.	Even effectively treated patients may relapse or develop toxicities to medications. While most persons will be off of medications after one year, the optimal time to remove medications is still not well established.
14.	Persons hospitalized for depression should have follow-up with a mental health specialist or their primary care doctor within two weeks of discharge.	III	Depression Guideline Panel, 1993b	Alleviate symptoms of depression.* Reduce disability days. Prevent death from suicide. Prevent morbidity from suicide attempts.	The guidelines do not specifically address time-interval between discharge and follow-up. However, given severity of disease, morre than two weeks should probably not pass before re-evaluation. If the patient is also seeing a mental health specialist, the two week interval can apply to that specialist instead of the primary care provider.

*Symptoms of depression include depressed mood, diminished interest or pleasure in activities, weight loss/gain, impaired concentration, suicidality, fatigue, feelings of worthlessness and guilt, and psychomotor agitation/retardation.

**Medical complications of substance abuse are numerous and include: for alcohol, blackouts, seizures, delerium, liver failure; for IV drugs of any kind, local infection, endocarditis, hepatitis and HIV, death from overdose; for cocaine and amphetamines, seizures, myocardial infarction, and hypertensive crises.

Quality of Evidence Codes:

I:	RCT
II-1:	Nonrandomized controlled trials
II-2:	Cohort or case analysis
II-3:	Multiple time series
III:	Opinions or descriptive studies

REFERENCES - DEPRESSION

American Psychiatric Association. 1994. Substance-related disorders. In *Diagnostic and Statistical Manual of Mental Disorders: DSM-IV*, Fourth ed. 175-205. Washington, DC: American Psychiatric Association.

Bielski RJ, and RO Friedel. December 1976. Prediction of tricyclic antidepressant response: A critical review. *Archives of General Psychiatry* 33: 1479-89.

Broadhead WE, DG Blazer, LK George, et al. 21 November 1990. Depression, disability days, and days lost from work in a prospective epidemiologic survey. *Journal of the American Medical Association* 264 (19): 2524-8.

Burnam MA, KB Wells, B Leake, et al. 1988. Development of a brief screening instrument for detecting depressive disorders. *Medical Care* 26: 775-89.

Depression Guideline Panel. April 1993. *Depression in Primary Care: Volume 1. Detection and Diagnosis. Clinical Practice Guideline, Number 5.* AHCPR Publication No. 93-0550. Rockville, MD: U.S. Department of Health and Human Services, Public Health Service, Agency for Health Care Policy and Research.

Depression Guideline Panel. April 1993. *Depression in Primary Care: Volume 2. Treatment of Major Depression. Clinical Practice Guideline, Number 5.* AHCPR Publication No. 93-0551. Rockville, MD: U.S. Department of Health and Human Services, Public Health Service, Agency for Health Care Policy and Research.

Feldman E, R Mayou, K Hawton, et al. May 1987. Psychiatric disorder in medical in-patients. *Quarterly Journal of Medicine* New Series 63 (241): 405-12.

Greenberg PE, LE Stiglin, SN Finkelstein, et al. November 1993. Depression: A neglected major illness. *Journal of Clinical Psychiatry* 54 (11): 419-24.

Hays RD, KB Wells, CD Sherbourne, et al. January 1995. Functioning and well-being outcomes of patients with depression compared with chronic general medical illness. *Archives of General Psychiatry* 52: 11-9.

Katon W, and H Schulberg. 1992. Epidemiology of depression in primary care. *General Hospital Pscyhiatry* 14: 237-47.

Kessler RC, KA McGonagle, S Zhao, et al. January 1994. Lifetime and 12-month prevalence of DSM-III-R psychiatric disorders in the United States. *Archives of General Psychiatry* 51: 8-19.

Kupfer DJ, E Frank, and JM Perel. September 1989. The advantage of early treatment intervention in recurrent depression. *Archives of General Psychiatry* 46: 771-5.

NIMH Consensus Development Conference. April 1985. Mood disorders: Pharmacologic prevention of recurrences. *American Journal of Psychiatry* 142 (4): 469-76.

Sturm, R, and KB Wells. June 1994. *Can Prepaid Care for Depression Be Improved Cost-Effectively?* RAND, Santa Monica, CA.

Wells KB, JM Golding, and MA Burnam. June 1988. Psychiatric disorder and limitations in physical functioning in a sample of the Los Angeles general population. *American Journal of Psychiatry* 145 (6): 712-7.

Wells KB, RD Hays, MA Burnam, et al. 15 December 1989. Detection of depressive disorder for patients receiving prepaid or fee-for-service care: Results from the medical outcomes study. *Journal of the American Medical Association* 262 (23): 3298-3302.

Wells KB, W Katon, B Rogers, et al. May 1994. Use of minor tranquilizers and antidepressant medications by depressed outpatients: Results from the medical outcomes study. *American Journal of Psychiatry* 151 (5): 694-700.

Wells KB, A Stewart, RD Hays, et al. 18 August 1989. The functioning and well-being of depressed patients: Results from the Medical Outcomes Study. *Journal of the American Medical Association* 262 (7): 914-9.

9. DIABETES MELLITUS

Steven Asch, M.D., M.P.H.

Several recent reviews provided the core references in developing quality indicators for diabetes (Singer et al., 1991, in Eddy, 1991; Bergenstal, 1993; Gerich, 1989; Nathan, 1993, in Rubenstein and Federman, 1993; Garnick et al., 1994). Where these core references cited studies to support individual indicators, we have included the original references. We also performed narrow MEDLINE searches of the medical literature from 1985 to 1995 to supplement these references for particular indicators. Indicators of quality of care for gestational diabetes are covered in Chapter 14.

IMPORTANCE

Diabetes is a heterogeneous, yet often serious, and common chronic condition prevalent throughout the world. In 1992, the number of diabetics in the United States alone was estimated to be 7.2 million. The prevalence was estimated at 26.1 per 1,000 population, including all ages, while the prevalence in people under 44 was 6.8. Diabetes occurs more frequently among women than men, and among nonwhites than whites (American Diabetes Association [ADA], 1993).

The complications of diabetes include visual loss and dysfunction of the heart, peripheral vasculature, peripheral nerves, and kidneys. Diabetes is the primary cause of blindness in the United States, and diabetics are at much higher risk of developing cataracts, glaucoma, and poor near vision. The deleterious effect of diabetes on the cardiovascular system contributes significantly to the risk of heart attacks, strokes, and, together with diabetic neuropathy, is the principal reason for amputations due to gangrene (Garcia et al., 1974). About half of insulin-dependent diabetics develop kidney failure (Bergenstal et al., 1993). All of these complications taken together result in much higher death rates among diabetics than the remainder of the population (Palumbo et al., 1976). Much of the benefit of high quality care will accrue years later from the prevention of morbidity and mortality from such complications. Death rates from diabetes itself increase with age ranging from 0.2 per 100,000 for those between 15 and 19 years of age to 14.6 per 100,000 for those between 50 and 54 years; older patients experience even higher rates (National Center for Health Statistics [NCHS], 1994a).

The treatment of diabetes is resource intensive, with total costs estimated at $30-40 billion annually in 1992 (ADA, 1993), or one of every seven dollars spent on health care in 1992 (Rubin et al., 1994). Diabetes was the eighth most common reason for a patient visiting a physician's office in 1992 (NCHS, 1994b).

EFFICACY AND/OR EFFECTIVENESS OF INTERVENTIONS

Screening

Indicators of the quality of screening diabetics for complications of diabetes are covered under diagnosis below. This section covers screening patients not known to be diabetic for the disease. Both the American College of Physicians (ACP) (Singer et al., 1991, in Eddy, 1991) and the Canadian Task Force (CTF) on the Periodic Health Examination (1979) recommended that asymptomatic patients need not undergo screening for diabetes. These recommendations were based on the poor evidence that treatment of patients so identified would prevent complications. Though many persons have asymptomatic hyperglycemia, most complications of diabetes occur late in the course of the disease, limiting the benefits of early identification. Since the publication of those recommendations, the Diabetes Control and Complication Trial (DCCT) (see below) has added evidence for the efficacy of tight control in known diabetics in preventing complications (DCCT, 1993a). However, we have found no subsequent studies directly evaluating the efficacy of screening asymptomatic patients in reducing morbidity or mortality from diabetes (Singer, 1988; CTF, 1979).

Diagnosis

The initial diagnosis of diabetes depends upon the measurement of a fasting blood sugar greater than 140/mg/dl or a postprandial blood sugar of greater than 200/mg/dl. If a recorded blood sugar meets the above criteria, we recommend looking for notation of the diagnosis of diabetes in the progress notes or problem list. Most experts also recommend a complete history and physical examination, dietary evaluation, urinalysis for protein, measurement of blood creatinine, and a lipid panel at the time of initial diagnosis (ADA, 1989). We do not propose any of these as quality indicators for the initial diagnosis because of the small number of incident cases in our sample and the difficulty of defining the time of initial diagnosis.

We instead concentrate on the routine diagnostic tests that known diabetics should undergo regardless of their clinical status and stage of disease. The first of these is the measurement of glycosylated hemoglobin to monitor glycemic control. A randomized controlled trial of 240 patients found that measuring hemoglobin A_{1c} every three months led to changes in diabetic treatment and improvement in metabolic control, indicated by a lowering of average hemoglobin A_{1c} values (Larsen et al., 1990). The landmark DCCT followed 1,441 insulin-dependent diabetics for 9 years and found that tight glycemic control and lower hemoglobin A_{1c} values decreased rates of diabetic complications (DCCT, 1993a). Despite recommendations from a number of specialty and generalist physician societies, there is great variation in the use of this test (ADA, 1993; Bergenstal et al., 1993; Garnick et al., 1994; Goldstein et al., 1994). We propose as a quality indicator a hemoglobin A_{1c} test be done for all diabetics at six-month intervals, the longest recommended interval.

Home blood glucose monitoring has been shown to aid glycemic control in diabetics treated with insulin. The DCCT employed home blood glucose monitoring for its population of insulin-dependent diabetics, rather than the more easily tolerated urine glucose monitoring to achieve tight control, because moderate hyperglycemia (180 mg/dl) may not cause glycosuria. At least one small randomized trial (n=23) has shown home blood glucose monitoring to improve glycemic control in obese insulin-dependent diabetics (Allen et al., 1990). The optimal frequency of monitoring has not yet been determined, though some studies have questioned patients' ability to comply with frequent measurement (Bergenstal et al., 1993; Health and Public Policy Committee, 1983;

Muchmore et al., 1994; Gordon, 1991). Observational data have failed to find any strong relationship between home blood glucose monitoring and glycemic control in noninsulin-dependent diabetics (Patrick, 1994; Allen et al., 1990). Specialty societies recommend that patients on insulin be offered training and equipment for home glucose monitoring, and we propose this as another indicator of diagnostic quality (ADA, 1993). For patients not taking insulin, randomized trials have not shown home blood glucose to be any more effective at maintaining glycemic control than urine testing (Allen et al., 1990).

Because of the frequency of vision, cardiovascular, and renal complications among diabetics, many of which may be asymptomatic, the ADA (1989) has recommended several screening tests on an annual basis: eye exam, tests of triglycerides, total cholesterol, HDL cholesterol, urinalysis, and total urinary protein excretion. An annual eye and vision exam conducted by an ophthalmologist, beginning five years after diagnosis, has also been recommended by the ACP, the ADA, and the American Academy of Ophthalmology (AAO) (ACP, ADA and AAO, 1992). Retinal examination by generalists has been shown to be much less effective in detecting retinopathy at an early treatable stage (Reenders et al., 1992). The routine evaluation of the other screening recommendations has never been tested in controlled trials, but the conditions screened for (hyperlipidemia, nephropathy, and ESRD) are both more common in diabetics and amenable to intervention (The Carter Center, 1985). Compliance with ADA screening recommendations has been estimated to vary from 20 to 50 percent (Garnick et al., 1994; Brechner et al., 1993).

Other common treatable complications of diabetes include hypertension, cellulitis, and osteomyelitis. The ADA recommends blood pressure measurement and examination of the feet at every visit to detect these complications early in their course as well as a careful history to elicit signs and symptoms of hypoglycemia and hyperglycemia. No controlled trials have examined the efficacy of a regular history and physical examination.

Treatment

Recent debate in the area of diabetic treatment hinges on the utility of tight glycemic control. The goal of tight control and prevention of long-term complications through aggressive treatment is supported by the DCCT (DCCT, 1993a). The DCCT randomized 1,441 insulin-dependent diabetics into conventional therapy or intensive therapy that included daily adjustments of insulin dosage, frequent home glucose monitoring, and nutritional advice. Under the optimal circumstances present in the DCCT trial, 44 percent of the intervention group achieved glycosolated hemoglobin values under the goal of 6.05 mg/dl percent at least once, but only 5 percent maintained average values in that range. The intervention group developed 76 percent less retinopathy, 57 percent less albuminuria, and 60 percent less clinical neuropathy, but this reduction in diabetic complications may come at the expense of quality of life (Nerenz et al., 1992). For example, the tight control group in DCCT experienced a two- to three-fold increase in hypoglycemic episodes. The efficiency of such methods in general practice has not received adequate evaluation. Nonetheless, the ADA recommends that all diabetics over the age of seven be offered similar aggressive therapy.

Treatment strategies are different for Type I diabetes (complete pancreatic deficiency of insulin) and Type II diabetes (abnormal secretion of insulin and resistance to insulin action). In Type I diabetes, emphasis is placed on avoidance of diabetic ketoacidosis and tight control of blood sugar levels through the judicious use of insulin. In Type II diabetes, the focus shifts to control of symptoms, usually with a combination of diet, exercise, and oral hypoglycemic agents. If these measures fail to maintain adequate control in Type II diabetics, then insulin therapy is warranted. We will review the evidence for quality indicators for each of these treatment modalities in turn.

Adherence to the ADA-recommended diet decreases insulin and oral hypoglycemic requirements and serum lipids (Bantle, 1988). The DCCT trial relied on dieticians and revealed that greater adherence to dietary instructions resulted in better control (DCCT, 1993b). Exercise improves glucose tolerance and may reduce or eliminate the need for drug therapy (Raz et al., 1994). The ADA and the American Board of Family Practice recommend dietary and exercise counseling at both the initial diagnosis and before starting oral hypoglycemics or insulin (ADA, 1989; Bergenstal et al., 1993). We recommend evaluating the medical record for evidence that all diabetics have received dietary and exercise counseling and that Type II diabetics have undergone a trial of this conservative therapy prior to pharmaceutical intervention.

Randomized controlled trials have shown oral hypoglycemic agents to effectively improve glycemic control and prevent hyperglycemic coma. Although the effectiveness of these agents in preventing longer-term complications of Type II diabetes has been questioned, particularly in the controversial UGDP Trial of the 1970's (Gerich, 1989; Kilo et al., 1980; Knatterud, 1978), we recommend evaluating the medical record to determine if oral hypoglycemic therapy has been offered to symptomatic Type II diabetics who have already received a trial of dietary therapy.

Insulin treatment is essential for Type I diabetics and a treatment of last resort for Type II diabetics. The literature contains varied recommendations as to the optimal timing and content of insulin injections (Gregerman, 1991, in Barker et al., 1991; Knatterud, 1978), and no single regimen has emerged as superior. However, the ADA recommends that all diabetics taking insulin receive formal instruction in the technique of injection (ADA, 1989; Bergenstal et al., 1993). We recommend evaluating the medical record for evidence that this has taken place. We also recommend that symptomatic Type II diabetics who have failed oral hypoglycemics be offered insulin.

Though quality indicators for treatment of hypertension are covered elsewhere (Chapter 12), the intersection of diabetes and hypertension poses special treatment challenges. Control of hypertension is perhaps the most crucial step in preventing diabetic nephropathy. In particular, ACE inhibitors and possibly calcium channel blockers have been shown to reduce hyperalbuminuria and delay the progression to diabetic nephropathy (Lederle, 1992; Anderson, 1990). Beta blockers on the other hand may block the symptoms of hypoglycemia, and thus may be contraindicated in treated diabetics (Hamilton, 1990). We propose that diabetics with hypertension receive ACE inhibitors or calcium channel blockers as first-line pharmacotherapy if diet has failed to control blood pressure.

Follow-up

A study of internists and family practitioners using patient vignettes found wide variation in recommended follow-up intervals for diabetics (Petitti and Grumbach, 1993). The ADA (1989) guidelines recommend that regular visits be scheduled every three months for insulin-dependent diabetics and every six months for other diabetics. As a minimum standard of care for patients with diabetes, we suggest a visit every six months.

RECOMMENDED QUALITY INDICATORS FOR DIABETES MELLITUS

The following criteria apply to nonpregnant women age 18-50.

Diagnosis

	Indicator	Quality of evidence	Literature	Benefits	Comments
1.	Patients with fasting blood sugar >140 or postprandial blood sugar >200 should have diabetes noted in progress notes or problem list.	III	ADA, 1989	Prevent diabetic complications.*	This definition of diabetes is accepted worldwide. Blood sugar tests are often ordered as part of panels; this indicator will test the timeliness of follow-up on an abnormal result.
2.	Patients with the diagnosis of diabetes should have glycosylated hemoglobin every 6 months.	I, III	ADA, 1989; Larsen et al., 1990; ACP, ADA and AAO, 1992	Prevent diabetic complications.*	Randomized controlled trial of 240 patients indicated a significant decrease in hemoglobin A_{1c} among those whose hemoglobin A_{1c} was monitored. Time interval is that used in most clinical trials.
3.	Patients with the diagnosis of diabetes should have each of the following at least once a year: a. Eye and visual exam; b. Triglycerides; c. Total cholesterol; d. HDL cholesterol; and e. Urinalysis.	I, III	ADA, 1989; Larsen et al., 1990; ACP, ADA and AAO, 1992	Prevent diabetic complications.* Prevent retinopathy, hyperlipidemia, atherosclorotic complications, and renal disease.	Eye and visual exam shown to detect retinopathy at an earlier treatable stage. Other recommendations based on expert opinion, though studies have shown conditions they screen for to be more common in diabetics and all are susceptible to treatment with improved outcomes resulting from earlier detection.
4.	Patients with the diagnosis of diabetes should have each of the following at every visit: f. examination of feet; and g. measurement of blood pressure.	I, III	ADA, 1989; Larsen et al., 1990; ACP, ADA and AAO, 1992	Prevent diabetic complications.* Prevent lower renal disease, extremity amputation, reduced morbidity from foot infections.	These are ADA recommendations. Earlier detection of treatable disease reduces probability of developing serious complications. Exam provides an opportunity for patient education.
5.	Patients taking insulin should monitor their glucose at home.	III	ADA, 1993	Prevent hypoglycemic episodes. Prevent diabetic complications.*	A small RCT found that home glucose monitoring increases glycemic control in insulin dependent diabetics. Another study found no difference in control by frequency of monitoring. Recommended by the ADA.

132

	Indicator	Quality of evidence	Literature	Benefits	Comments
6.	Diabetics should receive dietary and exercise counseling.	II	Raz et al., 1994; Delahanty and Halford, 1993; ADA, 1989; Bergenstal et al., 1993	Reduce diabetic complications.*	Adherence to ADA diet decreases insulin and oral hypoglycemic requirements and serum lipids. Exercise improves glucose tolerance and may reduce or eliminate need for drug therapy. DCCT used dieticians and found that adherence to diet improved control and the ADA and the ABFP recommend their use. No study has found that dietary counseling reduces diabetic complications.
7.	Type II diabetics who have failed dietary therapy should receive oral hypoglycemic therapy.	III	ADA, 1989; Gerich, 1989; Bergenstal et al., 1993	Reduce diabetic complications.*	Observational trials have shown oral hypoglycemics to be effective in treating hyperglycemia and improving glycemic control. No studies have shown reduction of diabetic complications. Specialty societies and review articles widely recommend their use in mild to moderate disease before starting insulin.
8.	Type II diabetics who have failed oral hypoglycemics should be offered insulin.	III	ADA, 1989; Bergenstal et al., 1993	Reduce diabetic complications.*	Recommended by the ADA and ABFP.
9.	If patient is receiving other antihypertensive therapy in the absence of ACE inhibitors or calcium channel blockers, progress note should document failure of ACE inhibitors and calcium channel blockers to control blood pressure.	I	Lederle, 1992; Anderson, 1990	Reduce rate of renal failure.	Randomized controlled trials have demonstrated a reduction in albuminuria and progression of diabetic nephropathy in hypertensive patients treated with ACE inhibitors and possibly calcium channel blockers.

133

Follow-up

	Indicator	Quality of evidence	Literature	Benefits	Comments
10.	Patients with diabetes should have a follow-up visit at least every 6 months.	III	Bergenstal et al., 1993; ADA, 1989	Reduce probability of severe diabetic complications.*	Visits for diabetic patients in control should be every 3-6 months (per ABFP). Routine monitoring facilitates early detection and treatment of complications.

*Diabetic complications include visual loss and dysfunction of the heart, peripheral vasculature, peripheral nerves, and kidneys.

Quality of Evidence Codes:

I: RCT
II-1:   Nonrandomized controlled trials
II-2:   Cohort or case analysis
II-3:   Multiple time series
III: Opinions or descriptive studies

134

REFERENCES - DIABETES

Allen BT, ER DeLong, and JR Feussner. October 1990. Impact of glucose self-monitoring on non-insulin-treated patients with type II diabetes mellitus: Randomized controlled trial comparing blood and urine testing. *Diabetes Care* 13 (10): 1044-50.

American College of Physicians, American Diabetes Association, and American Academy of Ophthalmology. 15 April 1992. Screening guidelines for diabetic retinopathy. *Annals of Internal Medicine* 116 (8): 683-5.

American Diabetes Association. 1993. *Direct and Indirect Costs of Diabetes in the United States in 1992.*Alexandria, VA: American Diabetes Association.

American Diabetes Association. May 1989. Standards of medical care for patients with diabetes mellitus. *Diabetes Care* 12 (5): 365-8.

Anderson S. 1990. Renal effects of converting enzyme inhibitors in hypertension and diabetes. *Journal of Cardiovascular Pharmacology* 15 (Suppl. 3): S11-S15.

Bantle JP. 1988. The dietary treatment of diabetes mellitus. *Medical Clinics of North America* 72 (6): 1285-99.

Bergenstal RM, WE Hall, and JA Haugen. 1993. *Diabetes Mellitus: Reference Guide*, Fourth ed.Lexington, KY: American Board of Family Practice.

Brechner RJ, CC Cowie, LJ Howie, et al. 13 October 1993. Ophthalmic examination among adults with diagnosed diabetes mellitus. *Journal of the American Medical Association* 270 (14): 1714-7.

Canadian Task Force on the Periodic Health Examination. 3 November 1979. The periodic health examination. *Canadian Medical Association Journal* 121: 1193-1254.

The Carter Center. July 1985. Closing the gap: The problem of diabetes mellitus in the United States. *Diabetes Care* 8 (4): 391-406.

Delahanty LM, and BN Halford. November 1993. The role of diet behaviors in achieving improved glycemic control in intensively treated patients in the Diabetes Control and Complications Trial. *Diabetes Care* 16 (11): 1453-8.

The Diabetes Control and Complications Trial Research Group. 30 September 1993. The effect of intensive treatment of diabetes on the development and progression of long-term complications in insulin-dependent diabetes mellitus. *New England Journal of Medicine* 329 (14): 977-86.

The Diabetes Control and Complications Trial Research Group. July 1993. Expanded role of the dietitian in the Diabetes Control and Complications Trial: Implications for clinical practice. *Journal of the American Dietetic Association* 93 (7): 758-67.

Garcia MJ, PM McNamara, T Gordon, et al. February 1974. Morbidity and mortality in diabetics in the Framingham population: Sixteen-year follow-up study. *Diabetes* 23 (2): 105-11.

Garnick DW, J Fowles, AG Lawthers, et al. 18 February 1994. Focus on quality: Profiling physicians' practice patterns. *In Press, Journal Ambulatory Care Management.*

Gerich JE. 2 November 1989. Oral hypoglycemic agents. *New England Journal of Medicine* 321 (18): 1231-45.

Golden MP, and DL Gray. 1992. Diabetes Mellitus. In *Textbook of Adolescent Medicine.* McAnarney ER, RE Kriepe, DP Orr, et al.,Philadelphia, PA: W. B. Saunders Company.

Goldstein DE, RR Little, H Wiedmeyer, et al. 1994. Is glycohemoglobin testing useful in diabetes mellitus? Lessons from the Diabetes Control and Complications Trial. *Clinical Chemistry* 40 (8): 1637-40.

Gordon D, CG Semple, and KR Paterson. 1991. Do different frequencies of self-monitoring of blood glucose influence control in type 1 diabetic patients. *Diabetic Medicine* 8: 679-82.

Gregerman RI. 1991. Diabetes mellitus. In *Principles of Ambulatory Medicine*, Third ed. Editors Barker LR, JR Burton, and PD Zieve, 913-51. Baltimore, MD: Williams and Wilkins.

Hamilton BP. October 1990. Diabetes mellitus and hypertension. *American Journal of Kidney Diseases* 16 (4-Suppl.1): 20-9.

Health and Public Policy Committee, and American College of Physicians. August 1983. Selected methods for the management of diabetes mellitus. *Annals of Internal Medicine* 99 (2): 272-4.

Kilo C, JP Miller, and JR Williamson. 1 February 1980. The Achilles heel of the University Group Diabetes Program. *Journal of the American Medical Association* 243 (5): 450-7.

Knatterud GL, CR Klimt, ME Levin, et al. 7 July 1978. Effects of hypoglycemic agents on vascular complications in patients with adult-onset diabetes. *Journal of the American Medical Association* 240 (1): 37-42.

Larsen ML, M Horder, and EF Mogensen. 11 October 1990. Effect of long-term monitoring of glycosylated hemoglobin levels in insulin-dependent diabetes mellitus. *New England Journal of Medicine* 323 (15): 1021-5.

Lederle RM. 1992. The effect of antihypertensive therapy on the course of renal failure. *Journal of Cardiovascular Pharmacology* 20 (Suppl. 6): S69-S72.

Muchmore DB, J Springer, and M Miller. 1994. Self-monitoring of blood glucose in overweight type 2 diabetic patients. *Acta Diabetologica* 31: 215-9.

Nathan DM. 1993. Diabetes mellitus. In *Scientific American Medicine.* Editor Rubenstein E, and D Federman, New York, NY: Scientific American Illustrated Library.

National Center for Health Statistics. 18 August 1994. *National Ambulatory Medical Care Survey: 1992 summary.* U.S. Department of Health and Human Services, Hyattsville, MD.

National Center for Health Statistics. 1994. *Vital statistics of the United States, 1990, vol. II: Mortality-part A.* U.S. Department of Health and Human Services, Hyattsville, MD.

Nerenz DR, DP Repasky, FW Whitehouse, et al. May 1992. Ongoing assessment of health status in patients with diabetes mellitus. *Medical Care Supplement* 30 (5, Supplement): MS112-MS123.

Palumbo PJ, LR Elveback, C Chu, et al. July 1976. Diabetes mellitus: Incidence, prevalence, survivorship, and causes of death in Rochester, Minnesota 1945-1970. *Diabetes* 25 (7): 566-73.

Patrick AW, GV Gill, IA MacFarlane, et al. 1994. Home glucose monitoring in type 2 diabetes: Is it a waste of time? *Diabetic Medicine* 11: 62-5.

Petitti DB, and K Grumbach. September 1993. Variation in physicians' recommendations about revisit interval for three common conditions. *Journal of Family Practice* 37 (3): 235-40.

Raz I, E Hauser, and M Bursztyn. 10 October 1994. Moderate exercise improves glucose metabolism in uncontrolled elderly patients with non-insulin-dependent diabetes mellitus. *Israel Journal of Medical Sciences* 30 (10): 766-70.

Reenders K, E De Nobel, H Van Den Hoogen, et al. 1992. Screening for diabetic retinopathy by general practitioners. *Scandinavian Journal of Primary Health Care* 10: 306-9.

Rubin RJ, WM Altman, and DN Mendelson. 1994. Health care expenditures for people with diabetes mellitus, 1992. *Journal of Clinical Endocrinology and Metabolism* 78 (4): 809A-F.

Singer DE, JH Samet, CM Coley, et al. 15 October 1988. Screening for diabetes mellitus. *Annals of Internal Medicine* 109: 639-49.

Singer DE, JH Samet, CM Coley, et al. 1991. Screening for diabetes mellitus. In *Common Screening Tests*. Editor Eddy DM, 154-78. Philadelphia, PA: American College of Physicians.

10. FAMILY PLANNING/CONTRACEPTION
Deidre Gifford, M.D.

The U.S. Preventive Services Task Force (USPSTF) review of "Counseling to Prevent Unintended Pregnancy" (1989), as well as the background papers in *Preventing Disease, Beyond the Rhetoric* (Feldman, 1990; Fielding and Williams, 1990, in Goldbloom and Lawrence, 1990) were used for the sections describing the importance of and recommendations for screening and counseling. For specific indicators regarding contraceptive methods, the relevant American College of Obstetricians and Gynecologists (ACOG) Committee Opinions and Technical Bulletins were consulted. In addition, *Contraceptive Technology* (Hatcher et al., 1994, pp. 233-284) and the textbook, *Infertility, Contraception and Reproductive Endocrinology* (Mishell, 1991, in Mishell et al., 1991) were used.

IMPORTANCE

Unintended and unwanted pregnancies are common in the United States. It has been estimated that 37 percent of births among women aged 15-44 are unintended, and just over one-quarter of those (10 percent of all births) are thought to be unwanted. As many as 18 percent of births to women aged 35-44 may be unwanted (USPSTF, 1989). Unwanted pregnancy is a risk factor for late entry into prenatal care, which has been associated with low birthweight and other poor pregnancy outcomes (USPSTF, 1989). Children born as a result of unwanted pregnancies are at increased risk for child abuse and neglect, and for behavioral and educational problems later in life. Unwanted pregnancies among adolescents are common, with as many as 10 percent of girls in the United States aged 15-19 becoming pregnant each year. Sixty-six percent of unmarried teenage girls are sexually active by the age of 19 (USPSTF, 1989).

EFFICACY OF INTERVENTION

Screening for Risk of Unintended Pregnancy

While there is no direct evidence available that taking a sexual history and offering contraception if desired lowers the rate of unintended pregnancy, counseling to prevent unintended pregnancy is widely recommended (USPSTF, 1989; Fielding and Williams, 1990, in Goldbloom and Lawrence, 1990). Except for abstinence, the most highly effective methods of contraception (hormonal methods, sterilization, and IUD) require a visit to a health professional. Providers who do not ask about sexual activity and contraceptive practices may miss the opportunity to offer an intervention (contraception) that prevents a serious adverse health outcome (unintended pregnancy). There is evidence that many providers do indeed miss that opportunity. One study of Canadian teens revealed that although 85 percent had seen their doctor in the preceding year, only one-third of sexually active girls had ever discussed contraception with their doctors (Feldman, 1990, in Goldbloom and Lawrence, 1990). According to a report by the World Health Organization, if all sexually active couples had routinely used effective contraception in 1980, there would have been almost 1 million fewer abortions, 340,000 fewer unintended births, 5,000 fewer infant deaths, and a reduction in the infant mortality rate of 10 percent (IOM, 1995). Furthermore, if the proportion of unintended pregnancies were reduced by 30 percent in the U.S., there would be 200,000 fewer unwanted births, and 800,000 fewer abortions each year (IOM, 1995).

Once it has been determined that an individual is at risk for unintended pregnancy (i.e., is sexually active without contraception or with ineffective contraception and does not desire pregnancy at that time), providers should discuss the risks and benefits of the various methods and offer the most acceptable contraceptive methods to her (USPSTF, 1989; Fielding and Williams, 1990, in Goldbloom and Lawrence, 1990). In a recent report on prevention of unintended pregnancy, the Institute of Medicine concluded that "...too few providers of health care...use all available opportunities to discuss contraception and the importance of intended pregnancy to the health and well-being of women and men, children and families" (IOM, 1995). The appropriate interval for screening for risk of unintended pregnancy has not been determined, but we propose that this be done annually.

Treatment

Effective methods exist for preventing unintended pregnancy. These include abstinence, sterilization, hormonal contraceptives (oral, injectable, and implants), intra-uterine devices and barrier methods. Other methods, such as periodic abstinence, coitus interruptus and spermicides are less effective. Oral contraceptives (OCs) are the most commonly used non-permanent form of contraception in the United States. Approximately 10 million women in the U.S. currently use this method (USPSTF, 1989). OCs generally contain both an estrogen and progestin component ("combination" OCs), although a progestin-only pill is also available. Combination OCs are highly effective in preventing pregnancy, with failure rates of 0.1 to 3.0 percent.

While oral contraceptives have many non-contraceptive benefits (e.g., reduction in menstrual flow, decreased dysmenorrhea, decreased anemia, lower risk of ovarian and endometrial cancer), they are also associated with health risks which may exceed their contraceptive benefit in some groups of women (ACOG Technical Bulletin, 1994). Specifically, women who smoke and take oral contraceptives are at increased risk of cardiovascular disease when compared to non-smoking OC users. The Royal College of General Practitioners' oral contraceptive study (Croft and Hannaford, 1989) recruited 1,400 OC users and 1,400 non-users in 1968 and followed this cohort to study the health effects of OC use. A nested case-control study using these data showed that neither current nor past OC use was a risk factor for myocardial infarction (MI) when other risk factors were controlled for. However, OC users who smoked were at increased risk of MI compared to non-smoking OC users. Those who smoked fewer than 15 cigarettes per day had a relative risk of MI of 3.5 (95 percent CI 1.3-9.5), and those who smoked more than 15 cigarettes per day had a relative risk of MI of 20.8 (95 percent CI 5.2-83.1). (These relative risks are not adjusted for age, hypertension or other risk factors for MI.) Although data on OC formulation were not reported, many of the pill users in this study were likely to have been using a 50 mcg OC at the time of recruitment. Data regarding the risk of smoking and low-dose OC use, stratified by age, are not available. Because earlier studies (primarily involving higher dose OCs) suggested that the increased risk of cardiovascular disease associated with OC use was concentrated in women over the age of 35, the consensus is that women over the age of 35 who smoke should not be prescribed oral contraceptives (ACOG Committee Opinion, 1985; ACOG Technical Bulletin, 1994; Mishell, 1991, in Mishell et al., 1991). Progestin-only contraceptives, IUDs, barrier methods or sterilization may be offered to women in this category (ACOG Technical Bulletin, 1994).

RECOMMENDED QUALITY INDICATORS FOR FAMILY PLANNING/CONTRACEPTION

The following criteria apply to all post-menarchal women.

Screening

	Indicator	Quality of evidence	Literature	Benefits	Comments
1.	A history to determine risk for unintended pregnancy should be taken yearly on all women. In order to establish risk, the following elements of the history need to be documented: a. Menstrual status (e.g., pre- or post-menopausal, history of hysterectomy, etc.), last menstrual period, or pregnancy test; b. Sexual history (presence or absence of current sexual intercourse); c. Current contraceptive practices; and d. Desire for pregnancy	III	USPSTF, 1989	Prevent unwanted pregnancies and births. Prevent abortions.	The USPSTF does not make a recommendation for screening interval. As many as 37% of births among women aged 15-44 are unintended and over one quarter are unwanted. The goal of these recommendations is to identify women at risk for unintended pregnancies and counsel appropriately those who are interested in contraception.

Treatment

	Indicator	Quality of evidence	Literature	Benefits	Comments
2.	Women at risk for unintended pregnancy should receive counseling about effective contraceptive methods.	III	USPSTF, 1989	Prevent unwanted pregnancies and births. Prevent abortions.	Women at risk for unintended pregnancy are those who are sexually active without effective contraception and who do not desire pregnancy. Effective contraception is defined as: 1) Hormonal contraception (OC, injectable prostaglandins or implants) 2) IUD 3) Barrier + spermicide 4) Sterilization 5) Complete abstinence
3.	The smoking status of women prescribed combination OCs should be documented in the medical record.	II	ACOG Technical Bulletin, 1994	Prevent myocardial infarction and other thromboembolic complications.*	Women who smoke and use combination oral contraceptives (containing both estrogen and progestin component) are at risk for myocardial infarction (relative risk is 20 times greater than in women who do not smoke). Therefore, if prescribing oral contraceptives, the smoking status should be documented.

143

4. Women who smoke and are prescribed oral contraceptives should be counseled and encouraged to quit smoking.	II-2	Croft and Hannaford, 1989; Kottke et al., 1988	Prevent myocardial infarction and other thromboembolic complications.*	Because smoking increases risk of MI among women using oral contraception, and also has other long term toxicities (lung cancer, chronic lung disease, etc.), women should be counseled to quit. Counseling by physicians has been shown to be effective.
5. Women over age 35 who smoke should not be prescribed combination oral contraceptives.	II-2	ACOG Technical Bulletin, 1994	Prevent myocardial infarction and other thromboembolic complications.*	The risk from oral contraceptives in smokers is probably highest for women over age 35.

*Thromboembolic complications include myocardial infarction, cerebrovascular accident, thrombophlebitis, and pulmonary emboli.

Quality of Evidence Codes:

I:	RCT
II-1:	Nonrandomized controlled trials
II-2:	Cohort or case analysis
II-3:	Multiple time series
III:	Opinions or descriptive studies

REFERENCES - FAMILY PLANNING/CONTRACEPTION

American College of Obstetricians and Gynecologists. December 1985. Contraception for women in their later reproductive years. *ACOG Committee Opinion* 41: 1-2.

American College of Obstetricians and Gynecologists. October 1994. Hormonal contraception. *ACOG Technical Bulletin* 198: 1-12.

Croft P, and PC Hannaford. 21 January 1989. Risk factors for acute myocardial infarction in women: Evidence from the Royal College of General Practitioners' oral contraception study. *British Medical Journal* 298: 165-8.

Feldman W. 1990. Unwanted teenage pregnancy: A Canadian perspective. In *Preventing Disease: Beyond the Rhetoric*. Editors Goldbloom RB, and RS Lawrence, 92-3. New York, NY: Springer-Verlag.

Fielding JE, and CA Williams. 1990. Unwanted teenage pregnancy: A US perspective. In *Preventing Disease: Beyond the Rhetoric*. Editors Goldbloom RB, and RS Lawrence, 94-100. New York, NY: Springe-Verlag.

Hatcher RA, J Trussell, F Stewart, et al. 1994. The pill: Combined oral contraceptives. In *Contraceptive Technology*, 16th revised ed. 223-84. New York, NY: Irvington Publishers, Inc.

Institute of Medicine, Committee on Unintended Pregnancy. 1995. *The Best Intentions: Unintended Pregnancy and the Well-Being of Children and Families*. Washington, DC: National Academy Press.

Kottke TE, RN Battista, GH DeFriese, et al. 20 May 1988. Attributes of successful smoking cessation interventions in medical practice: A meta-analysis of 39 controlled trials. *Journal of the American Medical Association* 259 (19): 2883-9.

Mishell DR. 1991. Oral steroid contraceptives. In *Infertility, Contraception and Reproductive Endocrinology*, Third ed. Editors Mishell DR, V Davajan, and RA Lobo, 839-71. Boston, MA: Blackwell Scientific Publications.

U.S. Preventive Services Task Force. 1989. *Guide to Clinical Preventive Services: An Assessment of the Effectiveness of 169 Interventions*. Baltimore, MD: Williams and Wilkins.

11. HEADACHE

Pablo Lapuerta, M.D., and Steven Asch, M.D., M.P.H.

Approach

We identified articles on the evaluation and management of headache by conducting a MEDLINE search of English language articles between 1990 and 1995 (keywords headache, diagnosis, treatment) and by reviewing two textbooks on primary care (Pruitt, 1995, in Goroll et al., 1995; Bleeker and Meyd, 1991, in Barker et al., 1991). Of the fourteen relevant articles that were retrieved, nine were review articles and five were observational studies. Several of these articles addressed the selection of diagnostic tests and principles of pharmacological management, with a focus on tension headache and migraine. We did not find controlled trials that analyzed elements of an appropriate history or physical examination, and for these topics expert opinion was the primary source of information.

IMPORTANCE

Headache accounts for 18 million outpatient visits per year. Approximately 73 percent of adults in the United States report having experienced a headache within the past year. Headaches lead to 638 million days of lost work per year, costing employers between $5.6 and $7.2 billion annually (Kumar and Cooney, 1995).

EFFICACY AND/OR EFFECTIVENESS OF INTERVENTIONS

Diagnosis

The International Headache Society (IHS) has developed a thorough and comprehensive etiologic classification system for headaches (Dalessio, 1994). Common categories include: tension, migraine, cluster, noncephalic infection (e.g., influenza), head trauma, intracranial vascular disorders (e.g., hemorrhage), intracranial nonvascular disorders (e.g., meningitis, neoplasm), substance withdrawal, and neuralgias. Much of the initial diagnostic work-up for headaches focuses on distinguishing benign etiologies like tension headaches from the more serious causes like meningitis, hemorrhage, or neoplasm. Once that distinction is made, clinicians should distinguish among the more common benign etiologies in order to prescribe the most efficacious treatment (Pruitt, 1995, in Goroll et al., 1995).

All sources recommended a detailed history as the first step in making these distinctions. Essential elements include: temporal profile (chronology, onset, frequency), associated symptoms (nausea, aura, lacrimation, fever), location (unilateral, bilateral, frontal, temporal), severity, and family history (Dalessio, 1994; Bleeker and Meyd, 1991, in Barker et al., 1991). There is less confusion about the essential elements of the neurologic examination, though most sources recommend at least an evaluation of the cranial nerves, a fundoscopic examination to rule out papilledema, and examination of reflexes (Dalessio, 1994; Larson et al., 1980; Frishberg, 1994).

One of the most difficult diagnostic decisions in the evaluation of new onset headache is the indication for computerized tomography (CT) and magnetic resonance imaging (MRI) of the head to find structural lesions like arteriovascular malformations, subdural hematomas, and tumors. Several observational studies suggest that a head CT scan is a low-yield evaluation tool in patients with normal neurological examinations (Larson et al., 1980; Masters et al., 1987; Becker et al., 1988; Nelson et al., 1992; Becker et al., 1993; Frishberg, 1994), though even in such patients severe headaches may indicate subarachnoid hemorrhage and constant headaches may indicate intracranial tumors. As a consequence, guidelines from a 1981 National Institutes of Health Consensus Panel on the use of CT recommended imaging only when the patient has an abnormal neurological examination or a severe or constant headache (NIH Consensus Statement, 1981). Others have expressed reservations that using severity alone as criteria for head imaging may lead to extensive overuse (Pruitt, 1995, in Goroll et al., 1995; Becker et al., 1988). The American Academy of Neurology (AAN) (1993) previously reviewed 17 case series to define the yield of pathology when CT or MRI scanning is used to evaluate headache patients. In 897 migraine patients, they found only 4 abnormalities, none of which were clinically unsuspected. Of the 1825 patients with headaches and normal neurologic examinations, 2.4 percent had intracranial pathology. Based on these data, the AAN recommended against scanning migraine patients, but concluded there was insufficient evidence to recommend for or against scanning other headache patients with normal neurologic examinations.

Head trauma is another strong indication for imaging. In a study of 3658 head trauma patients, the Skull X-Ray Referral Criteria Panel identified focal neurologic signs, decreasing level of consciousness and penetrating skull injury as indications for CT scanning (Masters et al., 1987). In a separate study of 374 blunt trauma patients, there were 7 abnormal head CT results in patients without abnormal neurological findings, but the best initial treatment for these cases was observation alone (Nelson et al., 1992).

While there is still some debate as to the proper indications for CT or MRI in headache patients, there is little controversy surrounding the use of skull radiographs in such patients. Clinical trials have shown skull radiographs to be poor predictors of adverse outcomes in patients with head trauma or others presenting for evaluation of headache (Masters et al., 1987).

Treatment

Our quality indicators address the two most common etiologies for headaches in women under 50: migraine and tension headaches.

The treatment of migraine headache depends on the frequency and severity of symptoms. Placebo-controlled trials support the use of aspirin, acetaminophen, and nonsteroidal anti-inflammatory medications in mild cases (Kumar and Cooney, 1995). For more severe pain, clinicians often rely on ergot preparations, antiemetics, opioids, and sumatriptan. Though clinical trials have found intravenous dihydroergotamine to be effective in reducing both pain and emergency room use, three clinical trials failed to find any effect of oral ergotamines on migraine pain (Kumar and Cooney, 1995). Metoclopramide and chlorpromazine also have clinical trial support in the treatment of acute migraine headaches (Kumar and Cooney, 1995). The newest agent in the migraine pharmacopoeia is sumatriptan, a 5-hydroxytryptamine 1D

agonist, available only in injectable form in the United States.
Sumatriptan reduced the pain and associated symptoms of migraine
headaches in 70 to 90 percent of subjects in several clinical trials
(Kumar and Cooney, 1995). However, sumatriptan should not be used
concurrently with ergotamine due to an interactive vasoconstrictive
effect (Raskin, 1994; Kumar and Cooney, 1995). Both sumatriptan and
ergotamine preparations should be avoided in patients with uncontrolled
hypertension, angina, or atypical chest pain for that same reason.

A consensus exists that, if a patient has more than two migraine
headaches per month, then prophylactic treatment is indicated, and this
concept has been endorsed by the International Headache Society. The
use of beta blockers, valproic acid, calcium channel blockers,
tricyclic antidepressants, naproxen, aspirin, cyprohepatadine and
valproate are supported by controlled clinical trials. No clinical
trials have compared any of these agents with another in preventing
migraines (Raskin, 1993; Sheftell, 1993; Raskin, 1994; Rapoport, 1994;
Kumar and Cooney, 1995).

Treatment options for tension headaches include aspirin,
acetaminophen, and nonsteroidal anti-inflammatory agents. At least one
clinical trial found prophylaxis with tricyclic antidepressants to be
beneficial. Tension headache and migraine have been considered to be
part of a continuum of the same process and as a result clear
distinctions between appropriate treatments for the two diagnoses are
not always present. While clinical trials support the effectiveness of
oral opioid agonists and barbiturates in these two conditions, most
sources recommend against initial therapy with these agents due to the
risk of dependence (Markley, 1994). Butorphonal nasal spray has been
encouraged as an outpatient opioid agent because it is less addictive
and has been shown to reduce emergency room visits for severe migraine
headache (Markley, 1994; Kumar, 1994).

Follow-up Care

The need for physician visits depends on the frequency and severity
of headache and cannot be precisely defined. Indeed, in the United
States most people who experience headaches do not seek evaluation or

treatment from physicians (Kumar and Cooney, 1995). Accepted guidelines for specialist referral are not present in the literature, and most cases of migraine and tension headache can be handled adequately by a primary care physician.

RECOMMENDED QUALITY INDICATORS FOR HEADACHE

These indicators apply to women aged 18-50.

Diagnosis

	Indicator	Quality of evidence	Literature	Benefits	Comments
1.	Patients with new onset headache should be asked about: a. Location of the pain (e.g., frontal, bilateral); b. Associated symptoms (e.g., aura); c. Temporal profile (e.g., new onset, constant); d. Severity; and e. Family history	III	Dalessio, 1994; Larson et al., 1980; Frishberg, 1994	Decrease symptoms of sinusitis (e.g., post nasal drip, fever) and prevent potential complications of mastoiditis, periosteal and epidural abscess. Decrease neurologic symptoms from migraines. Reduce tension headache symptoms and side effects of unwarranted therapy. Preserve neurologic function.	Location can distinguish sinus, tension, and cluster. Associated symptoms can distinguish migraine and cluster headaches. Temporal profile can distinguish cluster, tension, and tumors. Severity can distinguish hemorrhage. Family history can distinguish migraine. Accurate diagnosis of sinusitis can prompt antibiotic or decongestant treatment. Accurate diagnosis of migraine and cluster can prompt treatment (see below). Accurate diagnosis of tension headaches can prompt treatment (see below). Accurate diagnosis of tumors can prompt lifesaving radiation or surgery.
2.	Patients with new onset headache should have a neurological examination evaluating the: a. Cranial nerves, b. Fundi, and c. Deep tendon reflexes.	III	Dalessio, 1994; Larson et al., 1980; Frishberg, 1994	Preserve neurologic function.	Abnormal neurologic examination is an indication for CT or MRI scanning. Increased detection of tumors, cerebrovascular accidents and intracranial hemorrhage can lead to lifesaving radiation or surgery.
3.	CT or MRI scanning is indicated in patients with new onset headache and any of the following circumstances: Abnormal neurological examination, constant headache, or severe headache.	III	NIH Consensus Statement, 1981	Preserve neurologic function.	Recommendations of NIH Consensus Panel on Computed Tomographic Scanning of the Brain.
4.	Skull X-rays should not be part of an evaluation for headache.	II	Masters et al., 1987	Averts side effects (e.g., radiation) of skull X-ray. Averts delays in CT or MRI scanning where indicated.	Four observational trials found a combined incidence of pathology of 0.7% in patients who would not otherwise receive a CT or MRI scan.

Treatment

	Indicator	Quality of evidence	Literature	Benefits	Comments
5.	Patients with acute mild migraine or tension headache should receive aspirin, tylenol, or other nonsteroidal anti-inflammatory agents before being prescribed any other medication.	I	Kumar and Cooney, 1995	Reduced migraine symptoms* with fewest side effects from other potential agents.*	More effective than placebo in reducing headaches, nausea and photophobia, but no effect on vomiting.

152

#	Recommendation	Quality of Evidence	Reference	Benefit	Comments
6.	Patients with acute moderate or severe migraine headache should receive one of the following before being prescribed any other agent: intramuscular ketorolac, subcutaneous sumatriptan, intravenous dihydroergotamine, intravenous chlorpromazine, or Intravenous metaclopramide.	I	Kumar and Cooney, 1995; Raskin, 1993; Raskin, 1994; Sheftell, 1993; Rapoport, 1994	Reduced migraine symptoms.*	All listed agents have clinical trial support, but none have been compared against one another. Clinical trials did not find an effect for oral ergot preparations alone, though they have not been evaluated in their usual combination with caffeine or barbiturates.
7.	Recurrent moderate or severe tension headaches should be treated with a trial of tricyclic antidepressant agents.	I	Kumar and Cooney, 1995	Reduced rate of tension headache recurrence. Improve quality of life and functioning.	Clinical trials show reduction in pain scores.
8.	If a patient has more than 2 migraine headaches each month, then prophylactic treatment is indicated with one of the following agents: beta blockers, calcium channel blockers, tricyclic antidepressants, naproxen, aspirin, fluoxitene, valproate, or cyproheptadine.	I	Kumar and Cooney, 1995; Sheftell, 1993; Markley, 1994	Reduced rate of recurrent migraine symptoms.*	All listed agents have clinical trial support, but none have been compared against one another.
9.	Sumatriptan and ergotamine should not be concurrently administered.	III	Kumar and Cooney, 1995	Averts adverse effects of vasoconstriction: exacerbation of chest pain in ischemic disease, hypertension, painful extremties.	Synergistic effect may cause prolonged vasoconstriction.
10.	Opioid agonists and barbiturates should not be first-line therapy for migraine or tension headaches.	III	Markley, 1994; Kumar, 1994	Averts adverse effects of opiate theapy.*	Other less habit-forming alternative treatment should be tried first. If patient has already tried other medications at home, administration of opioid agonists is not considered first-line.
11.	Sumatriptan and ergotamine should not be given in patients with a history of: uncontrolled hypertension, atypical chest pain, or ischemic heart disease or angina.	II	Kumar and Cooney, 1995; Raskin, 1994	Averts adverse effects of vasoconstriction (see above).	Both drugs cause vasoconstriction.

* Side effects of migraine therapeutic agents include:
Ergotamines: vasoconstriction, exacerbation of coronary artery disease, nausea, abdominal pain, and somnolence;
Opiates: dependence, somnolence, and withdrawal;
Phenothiazines: dystonic reactions, anticholinergic reactions, and insomnia.

Migraine symptoms include: headache, nausea, photophobia, vomiting, phonophobia, scotomota, and other focal neurologic symptoms.

Quality of Evidence Codes:

I:	RCT
II-1:	Nonrandomized controlled trials
II-2:	Cohort or case analysis
II-3:	Multiple time series
III:	Opinions or descriptive studies

REFERENCES - HEADACHE

American Academy of Neurology. 1993. Summary statement: The Utility of Neuroimaging in the Evaluation of Headache in Patients With Normal Neurological Examinations. American Academy of Neurology, Minneapolis, MN.

Becker LA, LA Green, D Beaufait, et al. 1993. Use of CT scans for the investigation of headache: A report from ASPN, Part 1. Journal of Family Practice 37 (2): 129-34.

Becker L, DC Iverson, FM Reed, et al. 1988. Patients with new headache in primary care: A report from ASPN. Journal of Family Practice 27 (1): 41-7.

Bleecker ML, and CJ Meyd. 1991. Headaches and facial pain. In Principles of Ambulatory Medicine, Third ed. Editors Barker LR, JR Burton, and PD Zieve, 1082-96. Baltimore, MD: Williams and Wilkins.

Dalessio DJ. May 1994. Diagnosing the severe headache. Neurology 44 (Suppl. 3): S6-S12.

Frishberg BM. July 1994. The utility of neuroimaging in the evaluation of headache in patients with normal neurologic examinations. Neurology 44: 1191-7.

Kumar KL. 1994. Recent advances in the acute management of migraine and cluster headaches. Journal of General Internal Medicine 9 (June): 339-48.

Kumar KL, and TG Cooney. 1995. Headaches. Medical Clinics of North America 79 (2): 261-86.

Larson EB, GS Omenn, and H Lewis. 25 January 1980. Diagnostic evaluation of headache: Impact of computerized tomography and cost-effectiveness. Journal of the American Medical Association 243 (4): 359-62.

Markley HG. May 1994. Chronic headache: Appropriate use of opiate analgesics. Neurology 44 (Suppl. 3): S18-S24.

Masters SJ, PM McClean, JS Arcarese, et al. 8 January 1987. Skull x-ray examinations after head trauma: Recommendations by a multidisciplinary panel and validation study. New England Journal of Medicine 316 (2): 84-91.

National Institutes of Health. 1981. Computed tomographic scanning of the brain. NIH consensus statement (online), November 4-6 4 (2): 1-7.

Nelson JB, MA Bresticker, and DL Nahrwold. November 1992. Computed tomography in the initial evaluation of patients with blunt trauma. The Journal of Trauma 33 (5): 722-7.

Pruitt AA. 1995. Approach to the patient with headache. In Primary Care Medicine: Office Evaluation and Management of the Adult Patient, Third ed. Editors Goroll AH, LA May, and AG Mulley Jr., 821-9. Philadelphia, PA: J.B. Lippincott Company.

Rapoport AM. May 1994. Recurrent migraine: Cost-effective care. Neurology 44 (Suppl. 3): S25-S28.

Raskin NH. 1993. Acute and prophylactic treatment of migraine: Practical approaches and pharmacologic rationale. Neurology 43 (Suppl. 3): S39-S42.

Raskin NH. 1994. Headache. In: Neurology-from basics to bedside [Special Issue]. Western Journal of Medicine 161 (3): 299-302.

Sheftell FD. August 1993. Pharmacologic therapy, nondrug therapy, and counseling are keys to effective migraine management. Archives of Family Medicine 2: 874-9.

12. HYPERTENSION

Steven Asch, M.D., M.P.H.

We depended mainly on five sources in constructing quality
indicators for hypertension. For screening for hypertension, we used
three organizations' published guidelines: the Canadian Task Force on
Periodic Examination (CTF), the United States Preventive Services Task
Force (USPSTF) and the American College of Physicians (ACP) (CTF, 1984;
USPSTF, 1989; Hayward et al., 1991; Littenberg et al., 1991, in Eddy,
1991; Littenberg, 1995). For indicators of treatment and follow-up care
we relied upon the Fifth Report of the Joint National Committee on
Detection, Evaluation, and Treatment of High Blood Pressure (JNC V) and
a recently published meta-analysis of 14 studies of the treatment of
hypertension (NHBPEP, 1993; Collins et al., 1990). The JNC V has been
endorsed by more than 30 medical specialty organizations. When these
core references cited studies to support individual indicators, we have
referenced the original source. When the core references were unclear
in their support for a particular indicator, we performed a narrow
MEDLINE search for articles addressing that topic.

IMPORTANCE

Hypertension is one of the most common medical conditions. About
30 percent of adults suffer from it, perhaps as many as 58 million
people in all (USPSTF, 1989). Most of the morbidity from hypertension
derives from the damage it does to target organs. Epidemiologic studies
have shown hypertension to be a strong risk factor for two of the
leading causes of death in the United States: cardiovascular disease
and cerebrovascular disease. Uncontrolled hypertension also damages the
retina and kidney (USPSTF, 1989). Hypertension often goes undetected
and inadequately treated. The second National Health and Nutrition
Survey (NHANES II) found that among hypertensive adults, 54 percent were
aware of their condition, 33 percent took medications for it, and only
11 percent were under control (NHBPEP, 1985). Hypertension is also a
costly disease; patients under treatment spend about $900-$1400 annually

for drugs, laboratory tests, and provider visits (Hilleman et al., 1994).

EFFICACY AND/OR EFFECTIVENESS OF INTERVENTIONS

Screening

No randomized trials or observational studies have directly evaluated screening unselected patients for hypertension. Nonetheless, based on the demonstrated efficacy of treatment (see below), several widely accepted guidelines have been promulgated. The USPSTF recommends that all adults undergo blood pressure screening every 2 years for those with diastolic and systolic blood pressures below 85 mm Hg and 140 mm Hg, respectively, and every year for those with diastolic blood pressures of 85-89 mm Hg. The ACP makes no recommendations about the frequency of blood pressure measurement, but urges screening of all patients presenting for care. The CTF recommends that blood pressure be measured at every medical visit. (USPSTF, 1989; Littenberg et al., 1991, in Eddy, 1991; Hayward et al., 1991; Littenberg, 1995; CTF, 1984).

Estimates of the cost-effectiveness of screening patients for hypertension vary widely. While the screening test itself poses little risk to the patient's health, incorrectly labeling a patient as hypertensive may. Searching for secondary causes of hypertension may entail some invasive procedures and pharmacologic therapy may have side effects. Cost-effectiveness studies have supported case finding (the measurement of blood pressure in patients presenting for care for other reasons) over mass screening, finding that each quality-adjusted life-year saved costs about $15,000 (Weinstein, 1976). More recent studies have estimated the cost-effectiveness of screening middle-aged women to be in the range of $23,000 per quality-adjusted life year (Littenberg et al., 1991, in Eddy, 1991; Littenberg, 1995).

Initial Evaluation

Measurement Technique

The measurement of systolic and diastolic blood pressure using a mercury sphygmomanometer cuff is one of the oldest objective measures in medicine. Because its use predated modern experimental design, it is difficult to assess its efficacy. Studies have shown some difficulties in cuff measurements of the blood pressure of obese and elderly patients when compared to more invasive and impractical intra-arterial measurements, but virtually all studies of the natural history and treatment of the disease have been based on cuff measurements.

Classification

The JNC V introduced a new diagnostic staging system based on the degree of elevation of cuff measurements, which is shown in Table 12.1.

Table 12.1
High Blood Pressure Diagnostic Staging System

Category	Systolic (mm Hg)	Diastolic (mm Hg)
Normal	<130	<85
High normal	130-139	85-89
Stage 1 (mild)	140-159	90-99
Stage 2 (moderate)	160-179	100-109
Stage 3 (severe)	180-209	110-119
Stage 4 (very severe)	>210	>120

Source: National High Blood Pressure Education Program, 1993.

Diagnosis

Natural history studies of mild hypertension and the placebo arms of interventional studies have shown extreme variability in the blood pressures of Stages 1 to 2 hypertensives (Management Committee of the Australian National Blood Pressure Study, 1980; Medical Research Council Working Party, 1985). For that reason, the JNC V recommends using the average of three measurements documented over the course of several weeks to confirm the diagnosis.

Initial History and Physical

The initial history and physical of the newly diagnosed hypertensive patient searches for secondary causes, target organ disease and additional cardiac risk factors. A focused literature search revealed no direct evaluation of the value of the history and physical in preventing complications or death, so we have relied upon expert opinion. We modified the recommendations in the JNC V consensus statement to produce our proposed quality indicators.

Initial Laboratory Examination

Like the initial history and physical, initial laboratory tests search for secondary causes, target organ damage, and other cardiac risk factors. In addition, these tests may serve as a baseline for monitoring the side effects of pharmacotherapy. A focused literature review again revealed no direct evaluation of routine testing, so we again modified the JNC V recommendations when constructing our indicators.

Secondary Hypertension Due to Drugs

Clinical trials have associated many drugs with the development of hypertension, including oral contraceptives, steroids, nasal decongestants, appetite suppressants, cyclosporine, erythropoietin, tricyclic antidepressants, and monamine oxidase inhibitors. The JNC V recommends the discontinuation of these drugs (at least temporarily) to determine if they are the cause of the patient's hypertension.

Treatment

Lifestyle Changes

Most experts recommend nonpharmacologic lifestyle changes (e.g., weight reduction, low sodium diet, physical activity, alcohol avoidance) as the first line of treatment in Stage 1-3 hypertension. The evidence for such recommendations is fairly solid. An observational trial of 301 obese patients revealed significant declines in blood pressure in those who successfully lost weight (Schotte and Stunkard, 1990). A randomized trial of 878 Stage 1-2 patients who were more than 10 percent above their ideal body weight showed that weight loss enhances the antihypertensive effect of medication (Langford et al., 1991). Avoiding dietary sodium reduces systolic blood pressure by an average of 4.9 mm Hg and diastolic blood pressure by 2.6 mm Hg according to a meta-analysis of 23 randomized trials with 1536 subjects (Cutler et al., 1991). Patients with low levels of physical fitness, as measured by treadmill, developed hypertension 1.5 times more often in a cohort of 4820 men and 1219 women observed for 4 years (Blair et al., 1984).

Epidemiologic studies have linked excessive alcohol consumption and hypertension. In addition, a randomized controlled trial of 41 heavy drinkers supports this association. Though this randomized trial was plagued by a high dropout rate, it demonstrated that physicians simply advising patients to reduce their alcohol consumption resulted in an average drop of more than 5 mm Hg in systolic blood pressure (Maheswaran et al., 1991).

Pharmacotherapy

If nonpharmacologic measures do not lower the blood pressure to normal levels or if the patient has Stage 4 disease, the JNC V recommends the addition of medication to the patient's regimen. A meta-analysis of 14 randomized trials has demonstrated a 42 percent reduction in strokes, a 14 percent reduction in coronary heart disease and a 12 percent reduction in all-cause mortality over 4-6 years of follow-up (Collins et al., 1990; Hebert et al., 1988). These studies have predominantly used middle-aged or elderly men as subjects, somewhat limiting their application to women (Anastos et al., 1991). The benefits of pharmacologic treatment are most pronounced among those with Stage 4 hypertension, increasing five-year survival from close to zero to 75 percent (Hansson, 1988).

Choice of Pharmacologic Agent

Although many classes of drugs (e.g., angiotensin-converting enzyme inhibitors, calcium channel blockers, direct vasodilators, centrally acting alpha antagonists) have been proven effective at lowering blood pressure, only beta blockers and diuretics have demonstrated in randomized controlled trials that they effectively lower mortality. Indeed, recent observational data have given rise to the suspicion that calcium channel blockers may increase overall mortality (Psaty et al., 1995). All 14 trials cited in the above meta-analysis used beta blockers or diuretics to lower the blood pressure of the intervention group. While awaiting data expected in 2001 from ALLHAT (Antihypertensive and Lipid-Lowering Treatment to Prevent Heart Attack), a randomized trial evaluating ACE inhibitors, calcium channel blockers, centrally acting agents and cardiovascular morbidity and mortality, the

JNC V recommended initial pharmacologic therapy with either a diuretic or a beta blocker.

Concomitant Disease

The presence of concomitant disease may alter this JNC V recommendation. Both beta blockers and thiazide diuretics are associated with mild increases in serum lipids, though this effect has not been shown to persist (Grimm et al., 1981). For that reason, some experts recommend avoiding these agents in patients with known hyperlipidemia. Similarly, diabetics under treatment should avoid beta blockers because of the masking of hypoglycemic symptoms. Several randomized trials have shown ACE inhibitors and calcium channel blockers to delay the progression of diabetic nephropathy (Lederle, 1992; Baba et al., 1986; Bjorck et al., 1986; Marre et al., 1988; Hommel et al., 1986). Asthmatic patients should avoid beta blockers due to their bronchoconstrictive effect (Barker et al., 1991). Many thiazide diuretics increase uric acid and should thus be avoided as initial therapy for patients with gout (Barker et al., 1991). Patients with known coronary artery disease but no dilated cardiomyopathy (likely to be a rare group in our study population), should receive beta blockers preferentially over diuretics as initial therapy. Several randomized controlled trials have demonstrated that beta blockers reduce mortality in such patients (First International Study of Infarct Survival Collaborative Group, 1988).

Follow-up

No studies directly address the optimal follow-up period for hypertensive patients. The JNC V recommends two visits each year. The goal of antihypertensive therapy is to lower the blood pressure to normal levels. If hypertension persists despite treatment, most experts recommend altering the patient's regimen. However, there is no consensus as to the optimal algorithm for modifying the regimen. Increasing the dose, changing to another class of agents, adding an agent from another class, reducing the frequency of administration to improve compliance, and renewed efforts at lifestyle modification are all acceptable strategies.

RECOMMENDED QUALITY INDICATORS FOR HYPERTENSION

These indicators apply to nonpregnant women age 18-50.

Diagnosis

	Indicator	Quality of evidence	Literature	Benefits	Comments
	Screening				
1.	Systolic and diastolic blood pressure should be measured on adult women otherwise presenting for care at least once each year.	III	USPSTF, 1989; Hayward et al., 1991; Littenberg et al., 1991, in Eddy, 1991; Littenberg, 1995; CTF, 1984	Decrease hypertensive complications.*	Blood pressure measurement has been recommended by three widely accepted guidelines. Increased detection of asymptomatic hypertensives prompts treatment.
	Initial Assessment				
2.	Patients with a new diagnosis of stage 1-3 hypertension should have at least three measurements on different days with a mean SBP>140 and/or a mean DBP>90.	III	Management Committee of the Australian National Blood Pressure Study, 1980; Medical Research Council Working Party, 1985	Prevent medication side effects such as orthostatic hypotension, fatigue, and impotence.	Observational studies have shown variability in the blood pressure of patients with mild to moderate hypertension. False labeling of patients as hypertensive can lead to unnecessary treatment and potential medication side effects.
3.	Initial history and physical of patients with hypertension should document assessment of at least two items from each of the following groups by the third visit: a. Family or personal history of premature CAD, CVA, diabetes, hyperlipidemia; b. Personal history of tobacco abuse, alcohol abuse, or taking of medications known to cause hypertension;** and c. Examination of the fundi, heart sounds, abdomen for bruits, peripheral arterial pulses, neurologic system.	III	NHBPEP, 1993	Reduce or eliminate medication side effects. Prevent other symptoms from the underlying disease (e.g., renal failure from renal artery stenosis). Decrease synergistic risk of cardiovascular complications.* Prevent hypertensive complications.*	No controlled trials directly examine the elements of quality in the history and physical for hypertensives. These minimum recommendations from JNC V search for secondary causes, other cardiac risk factors, and target organ damage. Identification of secondary causes can eliminate the need for therapy. Staging of target organ damage should prompt more aggressive control of hypertension for advanced disease.

163

4.	Stage 1 hypertensive women taking drugs known to cause hypertension** should have the drug discontinued (at least temporarily) before pharmacotherapy is initiated.	I	NHBPEP, 1993	Prevent or reduce medication side effects.	Clinical trials have associated many drugs with hypertension. The JNC V recommends discontinuation of the implicated drugs to determine if they are causing hypertension. Drugs known to cause hypertension include: oral contraceptives, steroids, nasal decongestants, appetite suppressants, cyclosporine, monamine oxidase inhibitors, tricyclic antidepressants, and erythropoietin.
5.	Initial laboratory tests should include at least 5 of the following: a. Urinalysis, b. Glucose, c. Potassium, d. Calcium, e. Creatinine, f. Uric acid, g. Cholesterol, h. Triglyceride, i. Electrocardiogram, and j. Echocardiogram.	III	NHBPEP, 1993	Reduce or eliminate medication side effects. Prevent other symptoms from the underlying disease (e.g., renal failure from renal artery stenosis). Decrease synergistic risk of cardiovascular complications.* Prevent hypertensive complications.*	No clinical trials directly examine the efficacy of initial laboratory testing for hypertensive patients. These minimum recommendations from JNC V search for secondary causes, other cardiac risk factors, and end organ damage.

164

	Indicator	Quality of evidence	Literature	Benefits	Comments
6.	First-line treatment for Stage 1-3 hypertension is lifestyle modification. The medical record should indicate counseling for at least one of the following interventions prior to pharmacotherapy: weight reduction, increased physical activity, low sodium diet, or alcohol intake reduction.	I-II	Schotte and Stunkard, 1990; Langford, 1991; Blair et al., 1984; Cutler et al., 1991; Maheswaran et al., 1991	Avoids side effects of medical therapy. Decreases hypertensive complications.	Cohort data from 301 obese patients showed weight loss reduces blood pressure and a randomized trial of 878 obese patients showed that weight loss enhances antihypertensive pharmacotherapy. A meta-analysis of 23 randomized trials demonstrated that lowering dietary sodium lowers blood pressure. Cohort observational data indicates that sedentary patients develop hypertension more frequently. A randomized trial demonstrated that advising alcoholics to reduce their drinking reduced their blood pressure.
7.	First-line pharmacotherapy for Stage 1-3 hypertension is monotherapy with thiazide diuretics or beta blockers. The medical record should show failure on one of these agents or a contraindication*** before initiation of therapy with other agents.	I	Collins, 1990; Hebert, 1988; JNC V, 1993	Decreased hypertensive complications.	A meta-analysis of 14 randomized trials using these agents showed a 42% reduction in stroke, a 14% reduction in coronary heart disease, and a 12% reduction in mortality.
8.	First-line pharmacotherapy for diabetics should include an ACE inhibitor or a calcium channel blocker.	I	Lederle, 1992; Baba, 1987; Bjorck, 1986; Marre, 1988; Hommel, 1986	Decreased hypertensive complications (particularly nephropathy).	Randomized trials have shown these agents to reduce progression of proteinuria and diabetic nephropathy.

Follow-up

	Indicator	Quality of evidence	Literature	Benefits	Comments
9.	Hypertensive patients should visit the physician at least twice each year.	III	NHBPEP, 1993	Reduce hypertensive complications and medication side effects.	JNC V recommendations.
10.	Hypertensive patients with persistent elevations of SBP>160 or DBP>90 should have one of the following interventions recorded in the medical record: a. Change in dose or regimen of antihypertensives; or b. Repeated education regarding lifestyle modifications,	III	NHBPEP, 1993	Decrease hypertensive complications.	JNC V recommendations.

* Hypertensive complications include: cardiovascular disease, cerebrovascular disease, retinopathy and nephropathy. Cardiovascular disease can result in chest pain, shortness of breath, claudication, fatigue, and death. Cerebrovascular disease can result in neurologic symptoms (e.g., aphasia, paralysis) and death. Retinopathy can result in visual field defects and blindness. Nephropathy can result in edema, arrhythmias, nausea, vomiting, fatigue, dialysis, and death.

**Drugs known to cause hypertension include: oral contraceptives, steroids, nasal decongestants, appetite suppressants, cyclosporine, monamine oxidase inhibitors, tricyclic antidepressants, and erythropoietin.

***Relative contraindications to thiazide diuretics include hyperlipidemia and gout; relative contraindications to beta blockers include hyperlipidemia, diabetes and asthma.

NOTE: Stages 1-4 hypertension are defined as listed below. See Table 12.1 for the complete high blood pressure diagnostic staging system.

Stage of Hypertension	Systolic, mm Hg	Diastolic, mm Hg
Stage 1 (mild)	140-159	90-99
Stage 2 (moderate)	160-179	100-109
Stage 3 (severe)	180-209	110-119
Stage 4 (very severe)	>210	>120

Quality of Evidence Codes:

I: RCT
II-1:   Nonrandomized controlled trials
II-2:   Cohort or case analysis
II-3:   Multiple time series
III: Opinions or descriptive studies

166

REFERENCES - HYPERTENSION

Anastos K, P Charney, RA Charon, et al. 15 August 1991. Hypertension in women: What is really known? *Annals of Internal Medicine* 115 (4): 287-93.

Baba T, T Ishizaki, Y Ido, et al. November 1986. Renal effects of nicardipine, a calcium entry blocker, in hypertensive type II diabetic patients with nephropathy. *Diabetes* 35: 1206-14.

Barker LR. 1991. Hypertension. In *Principles of Ambulatory Medicine*, Third ed. Editors Barker LR, JR Burton, and PD Zieve, 789. Baltimore, MD: Williams and Wilkins.

Bjorck S, G Nyberg, H Mulec, et al. 23 August 1986. Beneficial effects of angiotensin converting enzyme inhibition on renal function in patients with diabetic nephropathy. *British Medical Journal* 293: 471-4.

Blair SN, NN Goodyear, LW Gibbons, et al. 27 July 1984. Physical fitness and incidence of hypertension in healthy normotensive men and women. *Journal of the American Medical Association* 252 (4): 487-90.

Canadian Task Force on the Periodic Health Examination. 15 May 1984. The periodic health examination: 2. 1984 update. *Canadian Medical Association Journal* 130 (10): 1278-85.

Collins R, R Peto, S MacMahon, et al. 1990. Blood pressure, stroke, and coronary heart disease. Part 2, short-term reductions in blood pressure: Overview of randomised drug trials in their epidemiological context. *Lancet* 335: 827-38.

Cutler JA, D Follmann, P Elliott, et al. 1991. An overview of randomized trials of sodium reduction and blood pressure. *Hypertension* 17 (Suppl. 1): I27-I33.

First International Study of Infarct Survival Collaborative Group. 23 April 1988. Mechanisms for the early mortality reduction produced by beta-blockade started early in acute myocardial infarction: ISIS-1. *Lancet* 1 (8591): 921-3.

Grimm RH, AS Leon, DB Hunninghake, et al. January 1981. Effects of thiazide diuretics on plasma lipids and lipoproteins in mildly hypertensive patients. *Annals of Internal Medicine* 94 (1): 7-11.

Hansson L. 10 February 1988. Current and future strategies in the treatment of hypertension. *The American Journal of Cardiology* 61: 2C-7C.

Hayward RSA, EP Steinberg, DE Ford, et al. 1 May 1991. Preventive care guidelines: 1991. *Annals of Internal Medicine* 114 (9): 758-83.

Hebert PR, NH Fiebach, KA Eberlein, et al. 1988. The community-based randomized trials of pharmacologic treatment of mild-to-moderate hypertension. *American Journal of Epidemiology* 127 (3): 581-90.

Hilleman DE, SM Mohiuddin, BD Lucas Jr., et al. 1994. Cost-minimization analysis of initial antihypertensive therapy in patients with mild-to-moderate essential diastolic hypertension. *Clinical Therapeutics* 16 (1): 88-102.

Hommel E, H Parving, E Mathiesen, et al. 23 August 1986. Effect of captopril on kidney function in insulin-dependent diabetic patients with nephropathy. *British Medical Journal* 293: 467-70.

Langford HG, BR Davis, D Blaufox, et al. 1991. Effect of drug and diet treatment of mild hypertension on diastolic blood pressure. *Hypertension* 17 (2): 210-7.

Lederle RM. 1992. The effect of antihypertensive therapy on the course of renal failure. *Journal of Cardiovascular Pharmacology* 20 (Suppl. 6): S69-S72.

Littenberg B. 15 June 1995. A practice guideline revisited: Screening for hypertension. *Annals of Internal Medicine* 122 (12): 937-9.

Littenberg B, AM Garber, and HC Sox. 1991. Screening for hypertension. In *Common Screening Tests*. Editor Eddy DM, 22-47 &397. Philadelphia, PA: American College of Physicians.

Maheswaran R, M Beevers, and DG Beevers. 1992. Effectiveness of advice to reduce alcohol consumption in hypertensive patients. *Hypertension* 19 (1): 79-84.

Management Committee of the Australian National Blood Pressure Study. 14 June 1980. The Australian therapeutic trial in mild hypertension. *Lancet* 1: 1261-7.

Marre M, G Chatellier, H Leblanc, et al. 29 October 1988. Prevention of diabetic nephropathy with enalapril in normotensive diabetics with microalbuminuria. *British Medical Journal* 297 (6656): 1092-5.

Medical Research Council Working Party. 13 July 1985. MRC trial of treatment of mild hypertension: Principal results. *British Medical Journal* 291: 97-104.

National High Blood Pressure Education Program. 25 January 1993. The fifth report of the Joint National Committee on Detection, Evaluation, and Treatment of High Blood Pressure (JNC V). *Archives of Internal Medicine* 153: 154-83.

National High Blood Pressure Education Program. 1985. Hypertension prevalence and the status of awareness, treatment, and control in the United States: Final report of the Subcommittee on Definition and Prevalence of the 1984 Joint National Committee. *Hypertension* 7 (3): 457-68.

Psaty BM, SR Heckbert, TD Koepsell, et al. 1 February 1995. The risk of incident myocardial infarction associated with anti-hypertensive drug therapies. *Circulation* 91 (3): 925.

Schotte DE, and AJ Stunkard. August 1990. The effects of weight reduction on blood pressure in 301 obese patients. *Archives of Internal Medicine* 150: 1701-4.

U.S. Preventive Services Task Force. 1989. *Guide to Clinical Preventive Services: An Assessment of the Effectiveness of 169 Interventions.* Baltimore, MD: Williams and Wilkins.

Weinstein, MC, and WB Stason. 1976. *Hypertension: A Policy Perspective.* Cambridge, MA: Harvard University Press.

13. LOW BACK PAIN (ACUTE)
Elizabeth A. McGlynn, Ph.D.

The principal reference for this review was the Clinical Practice Guideline (Number 14) produced by AHCPR titled *Acute Low Back Problems in Adults* (Bigos et al., 1994). The 23-member multidisciplinary panel based their findings and recommendations on a systematic review and analysis of the literature, their own expertise, public testimony, peer review, and some pretesting in outpatient settings.

IMPORTANCE

While there are a number of methodological challenges in estimating the prevalence of low back pain (Loeser and Volinn, 1991), studies concur that it is the second leading cause of work absenteeism in the United States (Deyo and Bass, 1989). The lifetime prevalence of low back pain has been estimated to be 60 to 80 percent and the one year prevalence is 15 to 20 percent (Andersson, 1991). Among the working age population, about half report symptoms of back pain during a one year period (Vallfors, 1985; Sternbach, 1986). About 5 to 10 percent of patients experience chronic problems (Lahad et al., 1994), but these individuals account for nearly 60 percent of expenditures for this problem.

There is evidence that many patients with low back pain who cannot perform their usual activities may be receiving care that is either inappropriate or suboptimal (Bigos et al., 1994). The evidence includes substantial variations in the rates of hospitalization and surgery for low back problems (Deyo, 1991; Kellett et al., 1991; Volinn et al., 1992) and variations in the use of diagnostic tests (Deyo, 1991). For example, in a study conducted in Washington state, the rate of surgery for low back pain varied 15-fold among the 39 counties in the state (Volinn et al., 1992). The likely explanation for this variation is difference in physician practice style. A study of the effect of practice style in managing back pain on patient outcomes found that a low-intensity intervention style characterized by self-care, fewer prescription medications, and less bed rest produced long term pain and functional outcomes that were similar to more intensive styles and were less costly and associated with higher levels of patient satisfaction (Von Korff et al., 1994). There are also patients that appear to have more disability after treatment than before, particularly those who have undergone surgery, those treated with extended bed rest, and those treated with extended use of high dose opioids (Bigos et al., 1994).

The lack of consensus on appropriate treatments for low back pain suggests that there is likely to be considerable variation in practice across the country. The recent promulgation of a clinical practice guideline by the AHCPR offers an opportunity for developing tools for monitoring the use of both recommended and nonrecommended practices. This may provide a substantial incentive for decreasing the variation in care and reducing poor quality care.

In 1990, the direct medical costs of low back pain treatment were $24 billion (Spengler et al., 1986) and the cost to the nation when work loss days are included increases substantially. It has been estimated that the work loss time plus disability payments cost more than three times the expenditures on medical treatment (Spengler et al., 1986), suggesting that the total annual costs of back pain may exceed $100 billion.

The costs of different approaches to treating back pain vary considerably. One study that examined the costs and outcomes of three different management styles for back pain described differences in the one-year costs of treatment ranging from $428 on average for patients seen by "low intensity" physicians to $768 on average for patients seen by "high intensity" physicians (Von Korff et al., 1994). The differences were reduced somewhat (from $340 to $277) when case mix variables were taken into account. Because the lower intensity practice style produced similar outcomes, that style would certainly be judged to be more cost effective.

EFFICACY AND/OR EFFECTIVENESS OF INTERVENTIONS

Primary Prevention

There is no strong evidence to suggest that preventive strategies for low back pain are effective. The literature evaluating the effectiveness of four prevention strategies was recently reviewed (Lahad et al., 1994). The strategies included: back and aerobic exercises, education, mechanical supports, and risk factor modification. The authors did not examine worksite-specific preventive measures, although all of the prevention studies included in the review were conducted in work settings.

Exercise may offer some protection against the development of back pain; four randomized trials of exercise interventions have been conducted (Gundewall et al., 1993; Donchin et al., 1990; Kellet et al., 1991; Linton et al., 1989). The studies were relatively small, ranging from 66 total subjects to 142 subjects, were conducted in specific worksites, and none of the studies followed subjects for longer than 18 months. The trials were consistent in their findings that fewer work loss days occurred in the preventive intervention group as compared to the control group. Among epidemiological studies, seven found an association between fitness or flexibility and decreased low back pain, but four of these studies showed no protective effect of exercise (Lahad et al., 1994). The authors of the review conclude that, taken together, the studies suggest that exercise is mildly protective (Lahad et al., 1994).

General education does not contribute to preventing low back pain; five randomized trials of educational interventions have been conducted (Daltroy et al., 1993; Walsh and Schwartz, 1990; Donchin et al., 1990; McCauley, 1990; Linton et al., 1989). Like the exercise studies, these trials also enrolled small numbers of subjects and were conducted in the workplace. Only one of the randomized trials of education found a decrease in subsequent low back pain (Linton et al., 1989) and because this trial included exercise, it is difficult to determine the independent role of education. Among the other four trials, three had intermediate positive outcomes and all had long-term negative outcomes.

The authors conclude that there is minimal support in the literature for the use of educational strategies (Lahad et al., 1994).

The use of orthotic devices has not been shown to prevent low back pain; two trials examining the use of corsets for the prevention of low back pain were conducted (Reddell et al., 1992; Walsh and Schwartz, 1990). One trial had a very low compliance rate for the intervention groups (58 percent of those assigned to wear a back belt stopped wearing it before the end of the study); based on an intention-to-treat analysis, the intervention group had a trend toward increased frequency of back pain (Reddell et al., 1992). The other trial found that subjects assigned to an educational plus corset intervention had a greater increase in knowledge and decrease in work loss days compared to controls (2.5 day decrease vs. 0.4 day increase). The authors of the review article conclude that, given the contradictory findings in these two trials, there is insufficient evidence to allow for a recommendation to be made regarding the use of orthotic devices for low back pain prevention (Lahad et al., 1994).

Several risk factors have been associated with increased risk of developing low back pain, including: smoking, obesity, and psychological functioning. Studies have shown an association between smoking and back pain that suggests risk is increased 1.5 to 2.5 times compared to nonsmokers (Deyo and Bass, 1989). Similarly, an association between obesity and back pain has been observed, but no interventions to change this risk factor as it relates to back pain have been conducted (Deyo and Bass, 1989). The psychological factors include depression, anxiety, and job stress but no intervention studies of changing psychological factors to prevent back pain have been conducted. The authors of the review article conclude that, while there are other health-related reasons to suggest the importance of interventions to modify these three risk factors, there is no evidence that demonstrates that a reduction in back pain will be the result (Lahad et al., 1994).

Diagnosis

The AHCPR's clinical practice guideline on the assessment and treatment of acute low back problems in adults (Bigos et al., 1994) indicates that the medical history is important in assessing whether the patient is suffering from a serious underlying condition such as cancer or spinal infection. The guideline recommends that the history include questions about: age, history of cancer, unexplained weight loss, immunosuppression, duration of symptoms responsiveness to previous therapy, pain that is worse at rest, history of intravenous drug use, and urinary or other infection. Symptoms of leg pain or problems walking due to leg pain may suggest neurological problems (e.g., herniated disc, spinal stenosis). The elements of the suggested medical history along with estimates of the sensitivity and specificity of those elements of the history are provided in the guideline document; an algorithm is provided for the use of responses to the initial assessment. The guideline panel noted that a number of factors (e.g., work status, educational level, workers compensation issues, depression) may affect patients' responses to questions on the history regarding symptoms and may also influence treatment outcomes (e.g., time for return to work).

Elements of the physical examination (e.g., inspection, palpation, observation, specialized neuromuscular evaluation) are also reviewed and estimates of their sensitivity and specificity for making differential diagnoses are provided. The guideline concludes that for 95 percent of patients with acute low back problems, no special interventions or diagnostic tests are required within the first month of symptoms.

Treatment

There are a wide variety of treatments for low back pain that are currently in use. The clinical care methods reviewed by the panel were: patient education about symptoms, structured patient education ("back school"), medications to control symptoms, physical treatments to control symptoms, and activity modifications, bed rest, exercise, special diagnostic tests, and surgery. A summary of the panel's findings and recommendations regarding lack of these treatment approaches follows.

Symptom education. The panel recommends educating patients about: expectations for recovery and recurrence, safe and effective methods of symptom control, reasonable activity modifications, methods for limiting recurrence of symptoms, no need for special investigations, and the effectiveness and risks of diagnostic and treatment measures if symptoms persist. The panel indicated that such educational intervention may reduce utilization of medical care, decrease patient apprehension, and increase the speed of recovery.

Medications. The panel concluded that both acetaminophen and NSAIDs were adequate for achieving pain relief; acetaminophen may have fewer side effects. Muscle relaxants were found to be no better than NSAIDs in reliving low back symptoms and they have greater side effects, especially drowsiness. Opioids were found to be no more effective than NSAIDs or acetaminophen in providing pain relief; side effects include decreased reaction time, clouded judgment, drowsiness and risk of physical dependence. A number of other medications (e.g., oral steroids, colchicine, antidepressants) were not recommended for the treatment of low back pain.

Physical treatments. Spinal manipulation for patients without radiculopathy is effective in reducing pain and may speed recovery within the first month. The evidence after one month is inconclusive. Transcutaneous electrical nerve stimulation (TENS), lumbar corsets and support belts, shoe lifts and supports, spinal traction, biofeedback, trigger point injections, ligamentous and sclerosant injections, facet joint injections, epidural injections, and acupuncture were not recommended for the treatment of acute back pain. For patients with radiculopathy, epidural steroid injections were considered an option after failure of conservative treatment and as a means of avoiding surgery.

Activity modifications. The panel recommended that patients with acute low back problems temporarily limit heavy lifting, prolonged sitting, and bending or twisting the spine. The activity limitations should take into account the age and clinical status of the patient as well as the demands of the patient's job. These modifications should be considered time-limited and the clinician may want to lay out goals for a return to normal activity.

Bed rest. Prolonged bed rest (i.e., more than 4 days) was not recommended because it may increase rather than decrease debilitation. The panel recommended a gradual return to normal activities and bed rest of short duration only for patients with severe initial symptoms of primary leg pain. A recently published randomized controlled trial found that continuing ordinary activities within the limits permitted by pain led to more rapid recovery than either bed rest or back mobilizing exercises (Malmivaara et al., 1995).

Exercise. The panel recommended that the initial goal of exercise programs be to prevent debilitation due to inactivity and then to improve activity tolerance with the goal of returning patients to their highest level of functioning. Exercise programs designed to improve general endurance (aerobic fitness) and muscular strength of the back and abdomen were considered particularly beneficial.

Special Diagnostic Tests. For patients whose symptoms with the recommended treatments listed above persist longer than one month, additional diagnostic and treatment procedures may be considered. The tests are of two types: tests for evidence of physiologic dysfunction and tests for evidence of anatomic causes of dysfunction. Tests in the former category include electromyography, sensory evoked potentials, thermography, general laboratory screening tests, and bone scan. The appropriate indications for and timing of these tests are provided in the guideline document. Tests in the latter category include plain myelography, MRI, CT, CT-myelography, discography, and CT-discography. These tests must be combined with information from the medical history, physical examination, and/or physiologic tests because these imaging studies can be difficult to interpret and many symptomatic patients may not show defects.

Surgery. Lumbar discectomy may provide faster pain relief in patients with severe and disabling leg symptoms who have failed to improve after one to two months of adequate nonsurgical treatment. However, there is little difference in long-term (4-10 years) outcomes of surgery as compared with conservative care and the procedure is quite expensive. Among methods of discectomy, direct methods of nerve root decompression were recommended over indirect methods. The role of patient preferences was emphasized, but only if adequate information about efficacy, risks and expectations is presented.

Surgery for spinal stenosis was not recommended within the first three months of symptoms. Decisions about this surgery should take into account the patient's lifestyle, preferences, other medical problems, and the risks associated with surgery.

Spinal fusion was not recommended during the first three months of symptoms in the absence of fracture, dislocation, or complications of tumor or infection. Spinal fusion was recommended for consideration following decompression in patients with combined degenerative spondylolisthesis, stenosis, and radiculopathy. Patients under age 30 with significant spondylolisthesis and severe leg pain may also be considered candidates for spinal fusion.

RECOMMENDED QUALITY INDICATORS FOR ACUTE LOW BACK PAIN

The following indicators apply to women age 18-50.

Assessment

	Indicator	Quality of evidence	Literature	Benefits	Comments
1.	Patients presenting with acute low back pain should receive a focused medical history and physical examination. The history should include questions about at least one of the following "red flags":	III	Bigos et al., 1994; Deyo et al., 1992; Waddell et al., 1982	Prevent disability and potential premature mortality.	A thorough exam and history will increase the likelihood of identifying serious systemic disease that requires further testing and specialized treatment.
	a. Spine fracture red flags: trauma, prolonged use of steroids	III	Deyo et al., 1992; Waddell et al., 1982	Prevent patient debilitation. Reduce pain.	Plain film or CT or MRI of the spine recommended if spine fracture suspected. Approximately 4% of patients in primary care will prove to have a spine fracture.
	b. Cancer red flags: history of cancer, unexplained weight loss, immunosuppression	III	Deyo et al., 1992; Waddell et al., 1982; Deyo and Diehl, 1988	Prevent patient debilitation. Reduce pain.	CT or MRI recommended if cancer suspected. Approximately 0.7% of patients presenting for acute low back pain have primary or metastatic bone cancer, which may be appropriately treated with radiation therapy.
	c. Infection red flags: fever, IV drug use	III	Deyo et al., 1992; Waddell et al., 1982	Prevent patient debilitation. Reduce pain.	Urinalysis recommended if infection is suspected. Approximately 0.01% of patients in primary care will prove to have an infection (e.g., urinary tract infection, skin infection), which may lead to epidermal abcess.
	d. Cauda equina syndrome or rapidly progressing neurologic deficit red flags: acute onset of urinary retention or overflow incontinence, loss of anal sphincter tone or fecal incontinence, saddle anesthesia, and global progressive motor weakness in the lower limbs.	III	Deyo et al., 1992; Waddell et al., 1982	Prevent permanent neurologic deficit. Reduce pain.	CT or MRI recommended if CES or neurologic deficit is suspected. Approximate prevalence of CES among patients with low back pain is 0.0004. A diagnosis of CES requires immediate surgery (or radiation therapy).
2.	The examination should include neurologic screening and straight leg raising.	III	Deyo et al., 1992; Waddell et al., 1982	Prevent debilitation.	Neurologic screening includes ankle and knee reflexes, ankle and great toe dorsiflexion strength, and distribution of sensory complaints. These examination procedures are undertaken to identify lumbar disk herniations and facilitate appropriate course of treatment (e.g., NSAIDs, brief bed rest, surgery). Surgery is indicated in approximately 2-10% of patients. Multiple findings increase the likelihood that a herniated disk will be found at surgery.

	Indicator	Quality of evidence	Literature	Benefits	Comments
3.	If no red flags identified, diagnostic testing should not be undertaken in first 4 weeks of symptoms.	III	Bigos et al., 1994	Prevent patient from undergoing unnecessary tests or procedures.	Diagnostic testing: EMG, SEPs, ESR, CBC, UA, bone scan, pain myelography, MRI, CT, CT-myelography, discography, CT-discography.

Treatment

	Indicator	Quality of evidence	Literature	Benefits	Comments
4.	If the patient is placed on medication for acute low back pain not due to spine fracture, cancer, infection, or cauda equina syndrome, one of the following should be used as a first-line agent: acetaminophen or NSAIDs.	I	Bigos et al., 1994; Postacchini et al., 1988; Amlie et al., 1987; Basmajian, 1989; Berry et al., 1982	Reduce pain.	No other medications listed as "options" were found to be superior to acetaminophen or NSAIDs (e.g., muscle relaxants, opiod analgesics) given the balance between effectiveness of pain relief and probability of serious side effects, although high doses of acetaminophen can lead to liver damage and gastrointestinal problems may be a side effect of NSAIDs.
5.	Patients should not be taking any of the following medications for treatment of acute low back pain:				
	a. phenylbutazone	III	Bigos et al., 1994	Avoid aplastic anemia and agranulocytosis.	Increased risk for bone marrow suppression.
	b. dexamethasone	I	Haimovic and Beresford, 1986	Prevent side effects.*	Effectiveness of pain relief has not been demonstrated.
	c. other oral steroids	III	Bigos et al., 1994	Prevent side effects.*	Has not been proven to be effective for pain relief.
	d. colchicine	I	Meek et al., 1985; Schnebel and Simmons, 1988; Simmons et al., 1990	Prevent side effects including gastrointestinal irritation, chemical cellulitis from intravenous infiltration, skin problems, and bone marrow suppression.	Evidence on pain relief for persons with gout is conflicting.
	e. anti-depressants	I	Alcoff et al., 1982; Goodkin et al., 1990; Jenkins et al., 1976	Prevent side effects such as urinary retention, orthostatic hypotension, constipation, and mania.	No studies have been done in patients with acute low back pain and no significant differences found in studies of chronic low back pain.
6.	Patients should not be receiving the following physical treatments for acute low back pain:				

Treatment		References	Benefits	Evidence/Risks
a. transcutaneous electrical nerve stimulation	I	Melzack et al., 1983; Deyo et al., 1990; Gemignani et al., 1991; Graff-Radford et al., 1989; Hackett et al., 1988; Lehmann et al., 1983; Lehmann et al., 1986; Thorsteinsson et al., 1977; Thorsteinsson et al., 1978	Benefits are inconclusive but the risks are low. Decrease time to recovery.	Evidence is inconclusive on effectiveness. Use of an ineffective treatment may delay recovery if more effective treatments are foregone.
b. lumbar corsets & support belts	I	Coxhead et al., 1981; Reddell et al., 1992; Walsh and Schwartz, 1990; Million et al., 1981	Decrease time to recovery.	No evidence of efficacy in patients with acute low back pain. Use of an ineffective treatment may delay recovery if more effective treatments are foregone.
c. spinal traction	I	Coxhead et al., 1981; Mathews et al., 1987; Mathews et al., 1988; Larsson et al., 1980; Mathews and Hickling, 1975; Pal et al., 1986; Weber et al., 1984	Prevent debilitation.	Prolonged traction may lead to debilitation.
d. biofeedback	I	Asfour et al., 1990; Bush et al., 1985; Flor et al., 1983; Nouwen, 1983	Decrease time to recovery.	No studies in patients with acute low back pain and conflicting evidence in patients with chronic low back pain. Use of an ineffective treatment may delay recovery if more effective treatments are foregone.
7. Patients should not be on prolonged bed rest (> 4 days).	I	Evans et al., 1987; Postacchini et al., 1988; Deyo et al., 1986; Gilbert et al., 1985	Prevent debilitation.	May lead to debilitation. Evidence that prolonged bed rest may increase probability of debilitation.

*Side effects from long-term use include fluid and electrolyte disturbance, hyperglycemia, pituitary-adrenal function, demineralization of bone, and immunosuppression. High-dose complications include avascular necrosis of bone, myopathy, subcapsular cataract formation, and central nervous system disturbance.

Quality of Evidence Codes:

I:	RCT
II-1:	Nonrandomized controlled trials
II-2:	Cohort or case analysis
II-3:	Multiple time series
III:	Opinions or descriptive studies

REFERENCES - LOW BACK PAIN

Alcoff J, E Jones, P Rust, et al. 1982. Controlled trial of imipramine for chronic low back pain. *Journal of Family Practice* 14 (5): 841-6.

Amlie E, H Weber, and I Holme. 1987. Treatment of acute low-back pain with piroxicam: Results of a double-blind placebo-controlled trial. *Spine* 12 (5): 473-6.

Andersson GBJ. 1991. The epidemiology of spinal disorders. In *The Adult Spine: Principles and Practice*. Editor Frymoyer JW, 107-46. New York, NY: Raven Press, Ltd.

Asfour SS, TM Khalil, SM Waly, et al. 1990. Biofeedback in back muscle strengthening. *Spine* 15 (6): 510-513.

Basmajian JV. April 1989. Acute back pain and spasm: A controlled multicenter trial of combined analgesic and antispasm agents. *Spine* 14 (4): 438-9.

Berry H, B Bloom, EBD Hamilton, et al. 1982. Naproxen sodium, diflunisal, and placebo in the treatment of chronic back pain. *Annals of the Rheumatic Diseases* 41: 129-32.

Bigos S, O Bowyer, Braen G., et al. December 1994. *Acute Low Back Problems in Adults: Clinical Practice Guideline No. 14.* AHCPR Publication No. 95-0642. Rockville, MD: Agency for Health Care Policy and Research, Public Health Service, U.S. Department of Health and Human Services.

Bush C, B Ditto, and M Feuerstein. 1985. A controlled evaluation of paraspinal EMG biofeedback in the treatment of chronic low back pain. *Health Psychology* 4 (4): 307-21.

Coxhead CE, H Inskip, TW Meade, et al. 16 May 1981. Multicentre trial of physiotherapy in the management of sciatic symptoms. *Lancet* 8229: 1065-8.

Daltroy LH, MD Iversen, MG Larson, et al. March 1993. Teaching and social support: Effects on knowledge, attitudes, and behaviors to prevent low back injuries in industry. *Health Education Quarterly* 20 (1): 43-62.

Deyo RA. October 1991. Nonsurgical care of low back pain. *Neurosurgery Clinics of North America* 2 (4): 851-62.

Deyo RA, and JE Bass. 1989. Lifestyle and low-back pain: The influence of smoking and obesity. *Spine* 14 (5): 501-6.

Deyo RA, and AK Diehl. May 1988. Cancer as a cause of back pain: Frequency, clinical presentation, and diagnostic strategies. *Journal of General Internal Medicine* 3: 230-8.

Deyo RA, AK Diehl, and M Rosenthal. 23 October 1986. How many days of bed rest for acute low back pain? A randomized clinical trial. *New England Journal of Medicine* 315 (17): 1064-1070.

Deyo RA, JD Loeser, and SJ Bigos. 15 April 1990. Herniated lumbar intervertebral disk. *Annals of Internal Medicine* 112 (8): 598-603.

Deyo RA, J Rainville, and DL Kent. 12 August 1992. What can the history and physical examination tell us about low back pain? *Journal of the American Medical Association* 268 (6): 760-5.

Donchin M, O Woolf, L Kaplan, et al. 1990. Secondary prevention of low-back pain: A clinical trial. *Spine* 15 (12): 1317-20.

Evans C, JR Gilbert, W Taylor, et al. March 1987. A randomized controlled trial of flexion exercises, education, and bed rest for patients with acute low back pain. *Physiotherapy Canada* 39 (2): 96-101.

Flor H, G Haag, DC Turk, et al. 1983. Efficacy of EMG biofeedback, pseudotherapy, and conventional medical treatment for chronic rheumatic back pain. *Pain* 17: 21-31.

Gemignani G, I Olivieri, G Ruju, et al. June 1991. Transcutaneous electrical nerve stimulation in ankylosing spondylitis: A double-blind study. *Arthritis and Rheumatism* 34 (6): 788-9.

Gilbert JR, DW Taylor, A Heldebrand, et al. 21 September 1985. Clinical trial of common treatments for low back pain in family practice. *British Medical Journal* 291: 791-6.

Goodkin K, CM Gullion, and WS Agras. August 1990. A randomized, double-blind, placebo-controlled trial of trazodone hydrochloride in chronic low back pain syndrome. *Journal of Clinical Psychopharmacology* 10 (4): 269-78.

Graff-Radford SB, JL Reeves, RL Baker, et al. 1989. Effects of transcutaneous electrical nerve stimulation on myofascial pain and trigger point sensitivity. *Pain* 37: 1-5.

Gundewall B, M Liljeqvist, and T Hansson. 1993. Primary prevention of back symptoms and absence from work. *Spine* 18 (5): 587-94.

Hackett GI, D Seddon, and D Kaminski. February 1988. Electroacupuncture compared with paracetamol for acute low back pain. *The Practitioner* 232: 163-4.

Haimovic IC, and HR Beresford. December 1986. Dexamethasone is not superior to placebo for treating lumbosacral radicular pain. *Neurology* 36: 1593-4.

Jenkins DG, AF Ebbutt, and CD Evans. 1976. Tofranil in the treatment of low back pain. *Journal of International Medical Research* 4 (Suppl. 2): 28-40.

Kellett KM, DA Kellett, and LA Nordholm. April 1991. Effects of an exercise program on sick leave due to back pain. *Physical Therapy* 71 (4): 283-93.

Lahad A, AD Malter, AO Berg, et al. 26 October 1994. The effectiveness of four interventions for the prevention of low back pain. *Journal of the American Medical Association* 272 (16): 1286-91.

Larsson U, U Choler, A Lidstrom, et al. 1980. Auto-traction for treatment of lumbago-sciatica: A multicenter controlled investigation. *Acta Orthopaedica Scandinavica* 51: 791-8.

Lehmann TR, DW Russell, and KF Spratt. 1983. The impact of patients with nonorganic physical findings on a controlled trial of transcutaneous electrical nerve stimulation and electroacupuncture. *Spine* 8 (6): 625-34.

Lehmann TR, DW Russell, KF Spratt, et al. 1986. Efficacy of electroacupuncture and TENS in the rehabilitation of chronic low back pain patients. *Pain* 26: 277-90.

Linton SJ, LA Bradley, I Jensen, et al. 1989. The secondary prevention of low back pain: A controlled study with follow-up. *Pain* 36: 197-207.

Loeser JD, and E Volinn. October 1991. Epidemiology of low back pain. *Neurosurgery Clinics of North America* 2 (4): 713-8.

Malmivaara A, U Hakkinen, T Aro, et al. 9 February 1995. The treatment of acute low back pain--bed rest, exercises or ordinary activity? *New England Journal of Medicine* 332 (6): 351-5.

Mathews JA, SB Mills, VM Jenkins, et al. 1987. Back pain and sciatica: Controlled trials of manipulation, traction, sclerosant and epidural injections. *British Journal of Rheumatology* 26: 416-23.

Mathews JA, and J Hickling. 1975. Lumbar traction: A double-blind controlled study for sciatica. *Rheumatology and Rehabilitation* 14: 222-5.

Mathews W, M Morkel, and J Mathews. 1988. Manipulation and traction for lumbago and sciatica: Physiotherapeutic techniques used in two controlled trials. *Physiotherapy Practice* 4: 201-6.

McCauley M. May 1990. The effect of body mechanics instruction on work performance among young workers. *The American Journal of Occupational Therapy* 44 (5): 402-7.

Meek JB, VW Guidice, JW McFadden, et al. October 1985. Colchicine confirmed as highly effective in disk disorders: Final results of a double-blind study. *Journal of Neurological and Orthopaedic Medicine and Surgery* 6 (3): 211-8.

Melzack R, P Vetere, and L Finch. April 1983. Transcutaneous electrical nerve stimulation for low back pain: A comparison of TENS and massage for pain and range of motion. *Physical Therapy* 63 (4): 489-93.

Million R, K Haavik Nilsen, MIV Jayson, et al. 1981. Evaluation of low back pain and assessment of lumbar corsets with and without back supports. *Annals of the Rheumatic Diseases* 40: 449-54.

Nouwen A. 1983. EMG biofeedback used to reduce standing levels of paraspinal muscle tension in chronic low back pain. *Pain* 17: 353-60.

Pal B, P Mangion, MA Hossain, et al. 1986. A controlled trial of continuous lumbar traction in the treatment of back pain and sciatica. *British Journal of Rheumatology* 25 (2): 181-3.

Postacchini F, M Facchini, and P Palieri. 1988. Efficacy of various forms of conservative treatment in low back pain: A comparative study. *Neuro-Orthopedics* 6: 28-35.

Reddell CR, JJ Congleton, RD Huchingson, et al. 1992. An evaluation of a weightlifting belt and back injury prevention training class for airline baggage handlers. *Applied Ergonomics* 23 (5): 319-29.

Schnebel BE, and JW Simmons. 1988. The use of oral colchicine for low-back pain: A double-blind study. *Spine* 13 (3): 354-7.

Simmons JW, WP Harris, CW Koulisis, et al. July 1990. Intravenous colchicine for low-back pain: A double-blind study. *Spine* 15 (7): 716-7.

Spengler DM, SJ Bigos, NA Martin, et al. 1986. Back injuries in industry: A retrospective study. I. Overview and cost analysis. *Spine* 11 (3): 241-5.

Sternbach RA. 1986. Pain and 'hassles' in the United States: Findings of the Nuprin Pain Report. *Pain* 27: 69-80.

Thorsteinsson G, HH Stonnington, GK Stillwell, et al. 1978. The placebo effect of transcutaneous electrical stimulation. *Pain* 5: 31-41.

Thorsteinsson G, HH Stonnington, GK Stillwell, et al. January 1977. Transcutaneous electrical stimulation: A double-blind trial of its efficacy for pain. *Archives of Physical Medicine and Rehabilitation* 58: 8-12.

Vallfors, B. 1985. *Acute, Subacute and Chronic Low Back Pain: Clinical Symptoms, Absenteeism and Working Environment*. Goteborg, Sweden: Kompendietryckeriat-Kallered.

Volinn E, J Mayer, P Diehr, et al. 1992. Small area analysis of surgery for low-back pain. *Spine* 17 (5): 575-9.

Von Korff M, W Barlow, D Cherkin, et al. 1 August 1994. Effects of practice style in managing back pain. *Annals of Internal Medicine* 121 (3): 187-95.

Waddell G, CJ Main, EW Morris, et al. 22 May 1982. Normality and reliability in the clinical assessment of backache. *British Medical Journal* 284: 1519-23.

Walsh NE, and RK Schwartz. October 1990. The influence of prophylactic orthoses on abdominal strength and low back injury in the workplace. *American Journal of Physical Medicine and Rehabilitation* 69 (5): 245-50.

Weber H, AE Ljunggren, and L Walker. 1984. Traction therapy in patients with herniated lumbar intervertebral discs. *Journal of the Oslo City Hospitals* 34: 61-70.

14. PRENATAL CARE

Deidre Gifford, M.D., Paul Murata, M.D., and Elizabeth A. McGlynn, Ph.D.

This review is based primarily on a review of the processes and outcomes of prenatal care that was done for a previous RAND study (Murata et al., 1992). In addition, we sought to update the literature by conducting a targeted MEDLINE search on specific topics. We conducted a MEDLINE search covering the years 1980 to 1990 to identify articles related to process and outcomes of prenatal care. We supplemented these articles by examining some reference lists in the recent literature and major obstetrical textbooks; articles published before 1980 were included in this step if they represented important research findings. Articles not published in English were excluded. Since this report focuses on prenatal care, intrapartum and postpartum processes and outcomes are addressed only to the extent that they directly relate to prenatal care.

We also reviewed recommendations made by a number of organizations regarding the content of prenatal care. The American College of Obstetricians and Gynecologists (ACOG) periodically publishes Technical Reports on various topics and, in conjunction with the American Academy of Pediatrics (AAP), has published *Guidelines for Perinatal Care* (Frigoletto and Little, 1988). The United States Preventive Services Task Force (USPSTF) has published a review of preventive health services in the United States, some of which pertain to prenatal care (USPSTF, 1989). The United States Public Health Service (USPHS) also convened an expert panel that completed a review of the content of prenatal care (USPHS, 1989; Merkatz and Thompson, 1990). These recommendations differ from each other as to the importance placed on various prenatal care processes. Because these reviews were conducted at nearly the same time and therefore would have made their recommendations based on much of the same information, the differences between them probably reflect varying value judgments used in weighing the information (Eddy et al., 1988).

IMPORTANCE

In this section, we will review the evidence for including various processes in prenatal care. Most of these processes have been discussed in the United States Preventive Services Task Force and the United States Public Health Service Prenatal Care Panel reports (USPSTF, 1989; USPHS, 1989). This report differs in that the processes emphasized are those for which objective quality of care measures can be developed using information from a medical records chart audit. Several processes that are commonly performed during prenatal care because of the opportunity to screen the mother for certain health problems not related to the pregnancy (e.g., cervical cancer) will not be discussed.

We will first consider the timing and frequency of prenatal care visits and the processes that should be routinely performed during these visits. Separate sections will discuss the problem of substance abuse during pregnancy, screening and treatment of infections during pregnancy including sexually-transmitted diseases, screening for congenital abnormalities, and screening and management of common prenatal obstetrical complications. These conditions and their prevalence during pregnancy are summarized in Table 14.1.

Table 14.1

Prevalence of Conditions Affected by Prenatal Care

Condition	Prevalence	Major Risk Factors	Literature
Routine Prenatal Care			
Anemia	9-10%	Race, SES, parity, nutritional status	USPSTF, 1989; Horn, 1988; Merkatz et al., 1980
Substance Abuse			
Smoking	30-40%	Race, education level	Stewart and Dunkley, 1985; Kleinman and Kopstein, 1987; Kleinman et al., 1988; Williamson et al., 1989; Fingerhut et al., 1990; Osterloh and Lee, 1989
Alcohol	3% of women average more than 1 drink/day		Strecher et al., 1989; Olsen et al., 1991; Ernhart et al., 1988; Morrow-Tlucak et al., 1989; Waterson and Murray-Lyon, 1989; Rosett and Weiner, 1981
Drug Abuse	Cocaine 3.4-18.0% Marijuana 11.9-27.0% Opiates 0.3%		Zuckerman et al., 1989; Osterloh and Lee, 1989; Main and Gabbe, 1987
Infections and Sexually-Transmitted Diseases			
Rubella Nonimmune	10-20%		Williamson et al., 1989
Asymptomatic Bacteriuria	3-10%	Black race, multiparity	Stenqvist et al., 1989; Romero et al., 1989; Campbell-Brown et al., 1987
Group B Streptococcus	8-31%		Daugaard et al., 1988; Siegel et al., 1980
Hepatitis B Carrier	0.1-0.5%	IV drug use, homosexual males, hemodialysis patients, clients and staff in mental institutions, Asians, household contacts of carriers, and health care workers	Malecki et al., 1986; Summers et al., 1987; Kumar et al., 1987; Cruz et al., 1987; Alexander, 1988; Rothenberg, 1979; Friedman et al., 1988; Greenspoon et al., 1989; Christian and Duff, 1989; Arevalo and Arevalo, 1989; Immunization Practices Advisory Committee, 1985; Immunization Practices Advisory Committee, 1988
Syphilis	0.02%		CDC, 1988a

(Continued)

Condition	Prevalence	Major Risk Factors	Literature
Gonorrhea	1-4%		Alexander, 1988; Investigators of the Johns Hopkins Study of Cervicitis and Adverse Pregnancy Outcome, 1989
Chlamydia	5-15%	Adolescents, unmarried, history of STD	Harrison et al., 1983; Martin et al., 1982; Investigators of the Johns Hopkins Study of Cervicitis and Adverse Pregnancy Outcome, 1989; Schachter et al., 1986a; McMillan et al., 1985; Schachter et al., 1986b
Herpes Simplex	0.2%	Previous episode of genital herpes (1.4%)	Arvin et al., 1986; Prober et al., 1988; Gibbs et al., 1988
Human Immunodeficiency Virus	0.1-0.8%	IV drug use, transfusion recipient, sex partner of IV drug user or bisexual male, multiple sex partners, or emigrant from endemic area	Hoff et al., 1988; Lindsay et al., 1989; Barton et al., 1989
Inherited Disorders			
Down Syndrome	0.3% @ 35y 3% @ 45y	Age, family history of Down syndrome	USPSTF, 1989
Neural Tube Defects	0.1%	Previous or family history of NTD	U.K. Collaborative Study, 1977; Ward et al., 1981; Macri and Weiss, 1982; Burton et al., 1983; Hooker et al., 1984; Milunsky and Alpert, 1984; Robinson et al., 1989; Milunsky, 1989a, Milunsky, 1989b
Rh Negative	9-10%	White race	USPSTF, 1989
Sickle Cell Carrier	8%	Black race, family history	USPSTF, 1989; BCSH General Haematology Task Force, 1988
Common Pregnancy Complications			
Intrauterine Growth Retardation	3-10%	Multiple gestation, hypertension, diabetes, chronic disease	Goldenberg et al., 1989a, Goldenberg et al., 1989b
Post-term Pregnancy	4-12%		Goldenberg et al., 1989a; McClure-Brown, 1963; Vorherr, 1975
Pregnancy-Induced Hypertension	5-10%	Nulliparity, black race, chronic hypertension	Lindheimer and Katz, 1985
Gestational Diabetes Mellitus	2-3%	Age, previous macrosomic infant or GDM, obesity, family history	CDC, 1989; O'Sullivan et al., 1973; Merkatz et al., 1980

EFFICACY AND/OR EFFECTIVENESS OF INTERVENTIONS

Timing and Frequency of Visits

The most commonly used standard for prenatal care is an index described by Kessner which prescribes prenatal care for normal pregnancies in terms of timing and frequency of visits and includes the type of hospital delivery service, private or general (Kessner et al., 1973). After adjusting for differences in gestational length, prenatal care is classified into three levels: adequate, intermediate, or inadequate. Adequate care at 36 weeks is defined as nine visits with the first visit occurring in the first trimester. Many studies using minor modifications of this index have shown pregnancy outcomes are related to the three levels of care (Institute of Medicine, 1985; Showstack et al., 1984; Gorsky and Colby, 1989).

Although studies have consistently shown that some prenatal care is better than no prenatal care, the number of visits considered to be sufficient is still subject to debate. The USPHS panel supported reducing the recommended number of prenatal visits for normal-risk pregnancies (USPHS, 1989). In contrast to the Kessner Index, they recommended that more prenatal care visits occur early in the pregnancy—including a preconceptual visit—to perform better risk assessment and to target high-risk pregnancies for more frequent follow-up. Fewer visits were recommended for the second trimester and overall. By 36 weeks, for uncomplicated nulliparous pregnancies, they recommended only seven visits compared to nine using the Kessner Index. For multiparous women, the USPHS panel recommended six visits; the Kessner Index does not differ based on parity.

Past recommendations have emphasized that prenatal care should begin in the first trimester. In the USPHS Panel Report, however, a preconceptual visit was proposed (USPHS, 1989). This visit would provide the opportunity to treat specific preexisting conditions such as diabetes or hypertension (Hollingsworth et al., 1984) and provide anticipatory guidance such as genetic counseling. For example, better glucose control of diabetes in the periconceptual period may prevent

some congenital malformations (Miller et al., 1981; Steel et al., 1990).
Similarly, evidence suggests that folate supplementation in the first
six weeks of gestation may prevent neural tube defects (Milunsky et al.,
1989a and 1989b).

Evidence supporting the role of the preconceptual visit, however,
is still lacking. The extent to which preconceptual risk assessment and
counseling are cost-effective in addressing problems, such as
appropriate interpregnancy intervals, maternal weight, anemia, substance
abuse and environmental teratogens, remains to be determined. The USPHS
report, while recommending the preconceptual visit, acknowledged that
further research is needed to substantiate its benefits. It is probably
premature to use a preconceptual visit as an indicator of prenatal care
quality. An initial visit during the first trimester would be a more
reasonable standard for which there is some evidence supporting a
relationship to pregnancy outcomes (Sokol et al., 1980).

Gestational Age Determination

An accurate determination of the gestational age is a very
important process because it ensures that key prenatal care
interventions are properly timed and that pregnancy complications can be
appropriately identified and managed. Accurate dating of a pregnancy
maximizes the likelihood that an infant will be delivered as close to
term as possible, thus avoiding the multitude of complications related
to either premature or postterm births. For a number of problems such
as premature rupture of membranes, multiple gestations, intrauterine
growth retardation and pregnancy-induced hypertension, the risk of
potential complications must be weighed against the complications of
premature delivery in deciding upon the appropriate time to effect
delivery; this is best done when the gestational age of the infant is
known precisely.

In pregnancies with an accurate last menstrual period (LMP), the
day of delivery can be predicted within fourteen days in over 85 percent
of pregnancies. Other clinical parameters such as early uterine sizing,
fundal height, auscultated fetal heart tones, and quickening are useful
adjuncts to confirm the accuracy of the gestational age determination

based on the LMP (Andersen et al., 1981). The addition of ultrasound dating can further improve the accuracy of the delivery date prediction, but only modestly (Campbell et al., 1985). One study found that even with an accurate LMP, ultrasounds were more likely to result in a revision of the estimated date delivery in those pregnancies where precise dating is the most important--i.e., in preterm and postterm gestations (Kramer et al., 1988). Although the routine use of ultrasonography in early pregnancy to establish an accurate gestational age might identify a higher proportion of preterm and postterm pregnancies, this has not been recommended because of the added costs to prenatal care, the limited overall benefit, and the problems with incorrectly predicting normal gestations as preterm or postterm (USPHS, 1989; Goldenberg et al., 1989a; Consensus Conference, 1984).

In contrast, in pregnancies with uncertain LMP dates or with early physical examinations not consistent with the LMP, ultrasound examinations are essential in more accurately predicting the delivery date. Ultrasounds performed in the first trimester are accurate to within five days. From the second trimester through 26 weeks, the estimates are accurate to within ten days, but after 26 weeks the accuracy declines to within two to three weeks (Cunningham et al., 1989).

Nutrition and Anemia

The importance of nutrition for adequate fetal growth during pregnancy was first shown in studies from the Dutch famine during World War II. Extreme nutritional deprivation reduced infant birthweights by 300 to 400 grams. Excess premature births and perinatal mortality also occurred. Under conditions of moderate malnutrition seen in developing countries, nutritional supplementation appears to improve birthweights by 60 grams. However, under the less extreme conditions seen in most developed countries, improved infant birthweights and perinatal mortality from better maternal nutrition have been more difficult to show (Rush et al., 1980; Susser, 1981; Sweeney et al., 1985; Orstead et al., 1985; Ershoff et al., 1983).

Studies in the United States have shown an association between low maternal weight gain during pregnancy and adverse pregnancy outcomes including low birthweight and perinatal mortality among women beginning the pregnancy underweight (Brown et al., 1981; Naeye, 1979). The Special Supplemental Food Program for Women, Infants and Children (WIC) has been implemented to improve pregnancy outcomes in high-risk populations through better maternal nutrition. Women enrolled in WIC have lower rates of low birthweight and premature births compared to similar women not enrolled; its greatest benefit occurs among women at highest nutritional risk. It is unclear, however, whether the benefits from the WIC program are the result of better nutritional status, self-selection by participants, or better prenatal care, a secondary benefit of the program (Stockbauer, 1987; Kotelchuck et al., 1984; Kennedy and Kotelchuck, 1984; Rush et al., 1988; Collins et al., 1985; Rush, 1981). One prospective, randomized controlled trial in a high-risk population has shown that WIC supplementation increased birthweights by 91 grams, after adjusting for the adequacy of prenatal care (Metcoff et al., 1985). For women who are not at high nutritional risk, adequate nutrition is prudent but routine nutritional counseling has not been shown to be beneficial (Robitaille and Kramer, 1985). Factors such as maternal height, pre-pregnancy weight, and smoking history can be used to identify women who are at high nutritional risk and for whom nutritional counseling might be recommended. Monitoring maternal weight gain during pregnancy may be helpful, but may also produce unnecessary anxiety without improving pregnancy outcomes (Dawes and Grudzinskas, 1991; Committee on Nutritional Status During Pregnancy and Lactation, 1990; Worthington-Roberts and Klerman, 1990).

Vitamin and mineral supplementation during pregnancy has become a routine obstetrical practice. In the 1980 National Natality Survey, 97 percent of married pregnant women took a vitamin-mineral supplement, usually on the advice of their physician (Hemminki, 1988). A review in 1978 identified seventeen controlled trials of vitamin and/or mineral supplementation (Hemminki and Starfield, 1978). Few showed any utility in their routine use. One study showed vitamin and mineral supplements decreased rates of preeclampsia, low birthweight and deliveries before

39 weeks; another showed decreased preeclampsia only. A third study
showed that women had decreased rates of dental caries. The remaining
studies all failed to show any differences in birthweight, preterm
delivery, infant or maternal morbidity and mortality with routine
vitamin or mineral supplementation. Many of these studies had design
problems, the most apparent being insufficient power to conclude a lack
of effect. A more recent case-control study in Finland failed to show
an association between limb anomalies and vitamin intake during early
pregnancy (Aro et al., 1984). A recent well-designed study was able to
show that folate supplementation decreased the incidence of neural tube
defects. A large sample size and a careful dietary history were
important in showing this benefit (Milunsky et al., 1989b). Another
large study of neural tube defects, however, failed to show benefit from
vitamin supplementation (Mills et al., 1989).

Another very common obstetrical practice has been to screen for
anemia because women of child-bearing age are at greater risk. Anemia
(defined as hematocrit < 34 percent or hemoglobin < 10.4 g/dl) has been
associated with adverse outcomes such as preterm delivery and perinatal
mortality (Lieberman et al., 1988; Murphy et al., 1986). Higher
hemoglobin levels may be important in maximizing fetal growth potential
and in providing pregnant women with adequate reserve in the event of
excess blood loss during delivery. Anemia, however, may be only
indirectly related to poor outcomes. Women with anemia are likely to
have other risk factors such as inadequate prenatal care and low
socioeconomic status explaining their greater risk of preterm delivery
and perinatal mortality. One study that corrected for some of these
other factors showed that anemia during the third trimester is only
weakly associated, if at all, with preterm delivery (Klebanoff et al.,
1989). Iron supplementation during pregnancy, while improving
hemoglobin levels, has not been shown to improve perinatal outcomes
(Hemminki and Starfield, 1978; Reece et al., 1987).

Currently, there is insufficient evidence to conclude that routine
vitamin or mineral supplements during pregnancy are necessary (Hibbard,
1988; Horn, 1988). The one exception may be the use of folate in the
first six weeks of pregnancy (Milunsky et al., 1989). For the purposes

of assessing prenatal quality of care, measuring the use of supplements
is not likely to be helpful, given that most women already take vitamin
or mineral supplements (Hemminki, 1988). The USPSTF, USPHS Panel, the
Canadian Task Force and ACOG have all recommended screening for anemia
during pregnancy, despite little evidence showing clear benefits. Even
if early detection of anemia were beneficial, the benefits from
screening would be diminished since most women already routinely take
iron supplements.

Substance Abuse

Three main categories of substance abuse have an important impact
upon pregnancy outcomes: smoking, alcohol use, and illicit drug use.
In recent years, substance abuse in pregnancy has been recognized as an
important cause of perinatal morbidity and mortality. Physicians may
have difficulty identifying individuals with a substance abuse problem
because women may not accurately report their behavior. Many women will
have problems with multiple substances.

Smoking

The most commonly used substance in pregnancy is tobacco. About 30
to 40 percent of women in their child-bearing years smoke (Stewart and
Dunkley, 1985; Kleinman and Kopstein, 1987; Kleinman et al, 1988;
Williamson et al., 1989; Fingerhut et al., 1990). Pregnant smokers have
a 25 to 56 percent greater chance of perinatal mortality compared to
nonsmokers, after controlling for other maternal risk factors.
Perinatal mortality rates could be lowered by an estimated 7 to 10
percent if all women stopped smoking during pregnancy (Kleinman et al,
1988; McIntosh and Chir, 1984; Cnattingius et al., 1988).

Infants whose mothers smoke also have significantly lower
birthweights (150 to 300 grams less on average) (Wainright, 1983).
Birthweights appear to be correlated with the duration of smoking during
pregnancy. Compared to nonsmokers, pregnant women who smoked but quit
had a 1.3 relative risk of delivering a low birthweight infant; women
who smoked throughout pregnancy had a relative risk of 3.1 (Petitti and
Coleman, 1990). The risk of low birthweight is partly due to increased
rates of preterm birth, particularly births prior to 33 weeks (Shiono et

al., 1986). Congenital anomalies have not been consistently associated with smoking (Khoury et al., 1987; Malloy et al., 1989).

Self-report of cigarette smoking in the general population appears to be generally valid (Strecher et al, 1989). Identifying pregnant smokers is a much easier task than identifying pregnant alcohol and drug users. Many women will stop smoking once they learn that they are pregnant (Ershoff et al., 1983; Fingerhut et al., 1990). For others, smoking cessation interventions have been shown to be effective in a variety of patient populations once the smoking problem has been identified. Pregnant smokers in a WIC clinic were entered into a randomized, controlled trial of a multiple component intervention, which included twenty-minute individual counseling sessions and printed materials. By the ninth month of pregnancy, 11.1 percent of women receiving the intervention had quit smoking, compared to 2.6 percent in the control group (Mayer et al., 1990). In an HMO setting, pregnant smokers were randomized to receive a series of mailings containing printed smoking cessation materials; 22.2 percent of the treatment group quit smoking compared to 8.6 percent of controls (Ershoff et al., 1989). The most impressive results were shown in a group of women who smoked ten or more cigarettes per day who were seen by private or university hospital obstetricians. These women were randomly assigned to receive an intensive personalized intervention with individual counseling sessions and multiple mail and phone follow-up contacts. Forty-three percent of women in the treatment group quit smoking by the eighth month of their pregnancy compared to 20 percent of controls. Infants born to women in the treatment group weighed an average of 92 grams more than control infants. Improvements in average gestational age at birth and very low birthweight rates, however, were not seen (Sexton and Hebel, 1984; Hebel et al., 1985).

Effective smoking cessation interventions are available and can improve pregnancy outcomes, but most of the available methods rely largely on time-consuming counseling (Ershoff et al., 1983). Physicians generally recommend that pregnant women cease smoking, but most physicians are not trained or do not have the time to directly provide smoking cessation services using the best available approaches (Hickner et al., 1990). Other types of interventions such as nicotine gum and clonidine are contraindicated during pregnancy. Smoking cessation has been widely recommended for all persons regardless of whether they are pregnant. The USPSTF and the USPHS panel have specifically recommended routine prenatal assessment of cigarette smoking with appropriate intervention.

Alcohol Use

Jones and Smith (1973) first recognized that heavy alcohol consumption during pregnancy could cause problems in fetal development. They described the fetal alcohol syndrome, the main features of which are growth retardation, mild to moderate mental retardation, and congenital anomalies, usually craniofacial (Jones and Smith, 1973). FAS is the leading known cause of congenital mental retardation, ahead of Down syndrome and spina bifida, affecting 1 to 3 infants per 1,000 live births (Abel and Sokol, 1986).

Alcohol intake during pregnancy can cause perinatal morbidity in addition to the complete fetal alcohol syndrome (FAS). Several congenital anomalies of the extremities and cardiovascular system have been associated with alcohol intake (Ouellette et al., 1977). One study found that one drink per day was associated with an average decrease in birthweight of 91 grams (Little, 1977). A prospective study showed a clear linear relationship between maternal alcohol intake and the proportion of infants born who were small-for-gestational-age. Among infants whose mothers were non-drinkers, 5.8 percent had birthweights below the 10th percentile. This percentage increased linearly to 17.7 percent for infants whose mothers had six or more drinks per day; their adjusted odds ratio of delivering a small-for-gestational-age infant compared to non-drinkers was 2.3 (Mills et al., 1984). In another prospective study, alcohol consumption was related to increased still birth rates and lower birth weights (Kaminski, 1978). There is also evidence to suggest that alcohol consumption interacts adversely with smoking in further reducing birthweights (Olsen et al., 1991). It does not appear that occasional alcohol intake (fewer than two drinks weekly) affects infant birthweights (Mills et al., 1984; Halmesmaki et al., 1987; Ernhart et al., 1989), but the precise level at which problems begin to occur is not known. Results have varied as to whether alcohol consumption increases the risk of preterm birth (Shiono et al., 1986; Halmesmaki et al., 1987). Women who drink or use drugs have also been shown to be at greater risk for being victims of violence (Amaro et al., 1990).

Decreasing alcohol consumption during pregnancy depends on identifying women with alcohol problems. Self-report of alcohol intake in nonpregnant and pregnant patients often underestimates actual consumption (Strecher et al., 1989; Ernhart et al., 1988; Morrow-Tlucak et al., 1989). Because many women know that alcohol consumption during pregnancy is not good, there may be greater bias in self-report among pregnant women because of social desirability. Standard alcoholism screening surveys used in the general population also may not be sensitive enough for use in pregnant patients because accurate measurement of lower levels of consumption may be required. Better measures of alcohol intake applicable to prenatal patients are needed (Waterson and Murray-Lyon, 1989; Rosett and Weiner, 1981).

Many women spontaneously decrease their alcohol consumption once they learn that they are pregnant out of concern for the infant's health (Kruse et al., 1986; Waterson and Murray-Lyon, 1989; Allen and Ries, 1985). For those who continue to drink, the usual interventions used for nonpregnant problem drinkers often cannot be used during pregnancy. Medications used to treat withdrawal symptoms, such as benzodiazepines and anticonvulsants, have potential risks for the fetus. Disulfiram for abstinence maintenance therapy has also been identified as a potential teratogen. Most treatment programs during pregnancy have relied upon individualized counseling and close follow-up. Although these methods may help to reduce alcohol consumption (Rosett et al., 1983; Halmesmaki, 1988), better strategies tested in studies with randomized designs are needed. Among women decreasing their intake, improved pregnancy outcomes are seen (Rosett and Weiner, 1981; Rosett et al., 1983; Halmesmaki, 1988).

Alcohol consumption during pregnancy has a significant impact on infant morbidity, specifically mental retardation. There are problems in identifying pregnant women with drinking problems and better alcohol cessation techniques are needed. As the USPHS Panel, USPSTF, and ACOG have all concluded, there is sufficient evidence to recommend that pregnant women should be counseled to decrease and preferably avoid alcohol during pregnancy.

Drugs

Use of illicit drugs during pregnancy has been associated with a wide range of adverse pregnancy outcomes including low birthweight, preterm delivery and perinatal mortality (O'Connor, 1987; Joyce, 1990). Opiates have been associated with premature delivery, intrauterine growth retardation, premature rupture of membranes, and other complications (Kaye et al., 1989; Doberczak et al., 1987). Methamphetamine and marijuana use have been associated with similar complications (Oro and Dixon, 1987; Little et al., 1988; Zuckerman et al., 1989).

In recent years, problems related to cocaine use have increased. A review of toxicological screening in a public teaching hospital showed cocaine to be the most common drug detected (Osterloh and Lee, 1989). Cocaine use in pregnancy is associated with an average 93 gram decrease in birthweight (Zuckerman et al., 1989). Use throughout pregnancy is associated with a four-fold increased risk of delivering a low birthweight infant. Petitti et al. estimated that 10 percent of the low birthweight deliveries in their county were due to cocaine use (Petitti and Coleman, 1990). Cocaine use has also been associated with preterm labor, premature rupture of membranes, intrauterine growth retardation (Chasnoff et al., 1989; Cherukuri et al., 1988; Chouteau et al., 1988; Keith et al., 1989; Chasnoff et al., 1987), maternal and infant cerebral hemorrhage (Mercado et al., 1989), neurobehavioral abnormalities in newborn infants (Chasnoff et al., 1989), and congenital syphilis (Worthington-Roberts and Klerman, 1990; Nanda et al., 1990).

A major problem in treating drug use during pregnancy is that many drug users are not seen for prenatal care (Cherukuri et al., 1988). Even when seen, self-report greatly underestimates actual drug use. Despite consenting to drug testing, 26 percent of women who tested positive for marijuana denied using it. Forty-five percent of women testing positive for cocaine denied its use (Zuckerman et al., 1989).

Few prospective studies have been conducted to demonstrate whether
drug treatment programs during pregnancy can decrease drug use and
improve pregnancy outcomes. Methadone can be used to treat mothers
addicted to heroin, decreasing obstetrical problems related to acute
narcotic withdrawal and the drug-seeking life style (O'Connor, 1987).
No similar maintenance substitute is available for cocaine or other
drugs. Providing comprehensive prenatal care and psychosocial services
are thought to be important in encouraging decreased drug use (Chavkin,
1990). Uncontrolled studies have reported mixed results. One study
enrolled 109 cocaine users before their twelfth week of pregnancy.
Although these women averaged fourteen visits throughout their
pregnancies, 21 percent successfully discontinued their cocaine use,
while 48 percent used cocaine throughout the pregnancy and the remainder
used cocaine sporadically (Chasnoff et al., 1989). Another intervention
study of 58 pregnant opiate addicts reported achieving normal
distributions of newborn weight, length and head circumference, and no
perinatal deaths. Their low birthweight rate was 17.7 percent and very
low birthweight rate was 1.6 percent (Rosner et al., 1982).
Interpreting these two rates, however, is difficult without an adequate
control group; the rates are high relative to the general population,
but may be comparable to women of similar socioeconomic status who are
not drug users.

Circumstantial evidence for benefit with drug treatment comes from
other studies which show a relationship between duration of drug use
during pregnancy and outcomes. Women who continued to use drugs
throughout their pregnancy had the greatest risk of poor outcomes, those
who discontinued use for part of the pregnancy were at intermediate
risk, and those who completely stopped using drugs from the first
trimester were at lowest risk (Petitti and Coleman, 1990; Zuckerman et
al., 1989).

For the purposes of developing process measures of prenatal care,
the literature on drug use during pregnancy is lacking in several areas.
Drug use is clearly a major preventable cause of adverse pregnancy
outcomes. As the USPHS panel and the USPSTF have recommended, routine
inquiries into drug use as part of the prenatal assessment is important,

but it is probably unreliable. Better means of identifying pregnant drug users are greatly needed (Chasnoff, 1989). In some settings, implementing routine or random urine screening for drug use has increased the numbers of pregnant women identified who are using drugs (Chasnoff, 1989; Chasnoff et al., 1990). Given the profound impact of drug use on the fetus, broader use of prenatal drug screening may need to be considered (Graham et al., 1989). Once drug use has been identified as a problem, these women need to receive adequate prenatal care and appropriate social services. It is not clear what constitutes an effective prenatal drug treatment program. Access to existing programs is limited (Chavkin, 1990). Programs for nonpregnant patients which have longer term goals may need significant modifications to meet the more immediate needs of the pregnant patient. Although it is likely that pregnancy outcomes will improve once successful prenatal drug use cessation programs have been developed, this has not yet been demonstrated conclusively.

Infections and Sexually Transmitted Diseases
Asymptomatic Bacteriuria

Asymptomatic bacteriuria occurs in 3 to 10 percent of pregnancies (Stenqvist et al., 1989). Of these pregnancies, 20 to 40 percent will later develop symptomatic urinary tract infections which are associated with an increased risk of pyelonephritis and preterm labor (Kincaid-Smith and Bullen, 1965; Patterson and Andriole, 1987). A meta-analysis of seventeen cohort studies found that women treated for asymptomatic bacteriuria had a lower relative risk of LBW (0.65) and lower relative risk of preterm delivery (0.50) compared to untreated women (Romero et al., 1989).

Screening for bacteriuria can be done with urinalyses and screening dipstick tests, but in comparison to the urine culture, they are less sensitive and specific. The nitrite dipstick test has a sensitivity ranging from 35 to 85 percent and a specificity of 92 to 100 percent. The leukocyte esterase test has better sensitivity ranging from 72 to 97 percent, but with poorer specificity, 64 to 82 percent (Pels et al., 1989). In one screening program, 5.1 percent of 4,470 pregnant women

had positive dipslide tests; only 2.6 percent of the total were
confirmed positive on urine culture (Campbell-Brown et al., 1987).

Women identified as having asymptomatic bacteriuria can benefit
from treatment. Most of the randomized controlled trials of treatment
for asymptomatic bacteriuria have shown decreases in low birthweight
rates. A meta-analysis of eight trials found that treated patients had
a 0.56 relative risk of LBW birth compared to untreated patients (Romero
et al., 1989).

There is good consensus that pregnant women should be screened for
asymptomatic bacteriuria. The USPSTF, the USPHS panel, and the Canadian
Task Force recommend using urine cultures, whereas ACOG accepts
urinalyses as the initial screening method.

Rubella

Congenital rubella infection can cause considerable morbidity
including fetal wastage, cataracts, deafness, microcephaly, congenital
heart defects, mental retardation and thrombocytopenia. About 80
percent of infants whose mothers are infected in early pregnancy develop
manifestations. Second trimester infections are less likely to cause
abnormalities (Hardy et al., 1969). Ten to twenty percent of women of
child-bearing age lack evidence of immunity to rubella (Centers for
Disease Control, 1989). Congenital rubella in the children of these
women can be prevented by screening and vaccinating the women before
they become pregnant (Griffiths and Baboonian, 1982). The serologic
tests to screen for rubella immunity are 95 to 99 percent sensitive and
specific (USPSTF, 1989). Effective live-attenuated vaccines are
available which have been shown to cause successful seroconversion in 98
percent of women when given in the postpartum period (Black et al.,
1983). Inadvertent administration of the vaccine to pregnant women has
not been shown to cause congenital rubella syndrome (Centers for Disease
Control, 1989). Postpartum vaccination generally avoids this risk.

Optimally, susceptible women should be immunized more than three
months before becoming pregnant. Postpartum vaccination misses the
opportunity to prevent congenital rubella in the current pregnancy, but
one-third to one-half of congenital rubella cases occur in pregnancies
subsequent to the first (CDC, 1987; CDC, 1986b). Rubella screening of

pregnant women with postpartum vaccination has been supported by the
USPHS panel, the USPSTF, the AAP and ACOG (ACOG, 1992).

Group B Streptococcus

Group B streptococcus (GBS) is associated with severe perinatal
morbidity and mortality. Women infected with GBS have increased rates
of preterm delivery and fetal deaths (Regan et al., 1981; Boyer and
Gotoff, 1988). One to three per 1,000 live births will be affected by
early-onset GBS infections; these carry a case fatality rate of 25 to 80
percent (Daugaard et al., 1988).

Prenatal screening and prophylaxis have proven to be impractical.
GBS can be found in the urogenital tract of 20 percent of pregnant
women. Antibiotic therapy has little effect on GBS carriage. Many of
the women reacquire the infection later in pregnancy, even with
treatment of their sex partner. An alternative strategy of treating
women near term reduces maternal carriage but does not reduce newborn
colonization. Waiting until near term also has the disadvantage of
missing the pregnancies with the greatest neonatal morbidity and
mortality due to GBS, those delivering before 38 weeks (Boyer and
Gotoff, 1988).

Several strategies for preventing GBS infections in newborns may
become available. Developing a vaccine against GBS for pregnant women
could help prevent GBS disease (Baker et al., 1988). Rapid methods of
diagnosing maternal GBS infections during the intrapartum period may
permit the early use of antibiotics to reduce neonatal colonization and
early-onset group B streptococcal disease (Boyer and Gotoff, 1986).
However, in studies of antenatal screening for GBS, early treatment of
neonates at risk has not been shown to prevent early-onset streptococcal
disease nor reduce excess mortality (Pyati et al., 1983; Siegel et al.,
1980). In certain high-risk pregnancies--e.g., preterm labor or
premature rupture of membranes--intrapartum screening and treatment of
GBS infections may be beneficial. Currently, no organization recommends
routine antepartum screening for GBS.

Hepatitis B

Pregnant women carrying the hepatitis B virus (HBV) are at risk for
transmitting the virus to their baby at birth. Forty to forty-five

percent of infants born to chronic hepatitis B carriers become infected; this risk increases to 65 to 90 percent if the mother also carries the hepatitis B virus e antigen (HBeAg) (Stevens et al., 1975; Xu et al., 1985). Although these perinatal infections infrequently cause acute hepatitis in the neonate, they often result in the development of a chronic HBV carrier state. Among perinatally-infected infants, 85 to 90 percent develop chronic HBV infections (Xu et al., 1985; Stevens et al., 1985). The long-term consequences of these infections include chronic active hepatitis, cirrhosis, and primary hepatocellular carcinoma (PHC). In a prospective study, chronic HBV carriers had a 390-fold greater risk of developing primary hepatocellular carcinoma (Beasley, 1982). Ultimately, 40 to 50 percent of chronic carriers have been estimated to die from either PHC or liver cirrhosis (Beasley and Hwang, 1984).

Hepatitis B vaccines with hepatitis B immune globulin given to neonates can prevent 85 to 95 percent of perinatal HBV infections and provide long-term protection (Xu et al., 1985; Stevens et al., 1985; Beasley et al., 1983; Schalm et al., 1989). Even among infants at the highest risk of becoming infected, those whose mothers carried the e antigen, the risk of infection can be decreased from 65 to 90 percent to between 7 and 30 percent (Poovorawan et al., 1989). Initial efforts to identify at-risk infants for vaccination focused on selective screening for HBV carriers among high-risk pregnant women (Table 15.1) (CDC, 1985). Several reports, however, have shown that selective screening may miss 50 to 67 percent of pregnant HBV carriers (Malecki et al., 1986; Summers et al., 1987; Kumar et al., 1987; Cruz et al., 1987; Jonas et al., 1987; McQuillan et al., 1987; Friedman et al., 1988; Greenspoon et al., 1989). Their prenatal care provider may not be adequately determining their risk status or carriers may be reluctant to report their high-risk behaviors. Some HBV carriers also do not belong to any of the high-risk groups.

Consequently, routine screening of all prenatal patients has been recommended in an effort to more effectively prevent perinatal HBV transmission. There has been some criticism of this approach because the studies showing the high proportion of missed carriers with selective screening were conducted in inner-city public hospitals with

low socioeconomic status populations, likely to have higher carrier
rates than the general population. Two more recent studies conducted in
lower-risk populations suggest that selective screening may be
sufficient. One study screened all enlisted military personnel and
their dependents seen for prenatal care. No cases of chronic HBV would
have been missed using the CDC risk factors (Table 15.1); all of the HBV
carriers were of Asian descent (Christian and Duff, 1989). A smaller
study of 430 prenatal patients seen in a family practice clinic
identified 38 women as being chronic carriers. All but two of these
would have been detected using a single high-risk factor, Asian descent
(Table 15.1) (Arevalo and Arevalo, 1989).

Long-term morbidity and mortality due to perinatal transmission of
HBV infections can be effectively prevented through the use of HBV
vaccines in the peripartum period. Mothers at high risk for being HBV
carriers should be screened to determine whether their child needs
neonatal vaccination. Additional studies in low-risk populations are
needed to resolve conclusively whether all prenatal patients should be
screened routinely. However, the USPHS Panel, the USPSTF, ACOG, AAP,
CDC, and the Canadian Task Force recommend that all pregnant women be
screened routinely for HBV.

Syphilis

In recent years, there has been a resurgence in the incidence of
syphilis in the general population. As a result, there has also been a
rise in the rate of congenital syphilis. In the second half of 1987,
the congenital syphilis rate increased 21 percent to 10.5 cases per
100,000 live births. Sixty-seven percent of these cases occurred in the
three states (Florida, California, and New York) with the highest
syphilis rates for the general population (CDC, 1988a). Untreated
congenital syphilis causes perinatal deaths in about 40 percent of
affected pregnancies (Schulz et al., 1987), although it is not known how
many fetal deaths are currently caused by syphilis infections. Infants
born with congenital syphilis can have a variety of manifestations
including osteochondritis, gummas, hepatosplenomegaly, and neurosyphilis
(CDC, 1988b).

Screening for syphilis in mothers is very effective. Non-treponemal screening tests vary in sensitivity depending on the stage at presentation. In secondary syphilis, sensitivity approaches 100 percent; lower sensitivities are seen in other stages. When combined with treponemal syphilis tests, specificity of these tests approaches 100 percent. Diagnosis and proper treatment of syphilis in early pregnancy can effectively prevent many of the manifestations of congenital syphilis (CDC, 1988a).

The USPHS Panel, the USPSTF, the Canadian Task Force, CDC, and ACOG all recommend routine screening for syphilis at the first prenatal visit (CDC, 1988a). For high-risk women, a second test at the beginning of the third trimester is also recommended.

Gonorrhea

Routine screening for gonorrhea has been commonly performed in pregnancy. Its main benefit is preventing ophthalmia neonatorum with its associated risk of blindness. Untreated gonorrhea during pregnancy can also develop into an acute pelvic infection with its associated morbidity. Septic abortions, chorioamnionitis, and premature rupture of membranes with premature delivery are associated with gonorrhea infections during pregnancy (Schulz et al., 1987; Hook and Holmes, 1985; Alexander, 1988).

Successful screening and treatment of gonorrhea have made its complications during pregnancy relatively rare events (Rothenberg, 1979). The efficacy of prenatal screening has not been studied. Ethical considerations make it difficult to study issues such as whether neonatal conjunctivitis prophylaxis is sufficient or if maternal screening and treatment is also important. Routine screening for gonorrhea in pregnancy continues to receive wide support from most organizations including the USPHS Panel, the USPSTF, the CDC, ACOG, and the Canadian Task Force.

Chlamydia

Chlamydia trachomatis infections are estimated to occur in 8 to 12 percent of pregnancies. Women who are adolescent, unmarried or low socioeconomic status are at greater risk (Harrison et al., 1983; Martin et al., 1982). *Chlamydia trachomatis* infections may cause a number of adverse outcomes in pregnancy. In one prospective study, stillbirths or neonatal death occurred in 33 percent of pregnancies complicated by *C. trachomatis* infections compared to 3 percent of uninfected women (relative risk = 9.9); premature delivery occurred in 28 percent of infected women compared to 6 percent of uninfected women (relative risk = 4.4) (Martin et al., 1982). Another prospective study found an increased risk of IUGR (OR = 2.4) and preterm delivery (OR = 1.6) with chlamydial infections (Investigators of the Johns Hopkins Study of Cervicitis and Adverse Pregnancy Outcome, 1989). Harrison et al. found an increased risk of prematurity and perinatal death, but only among IgM-seropositive women, indicating those with more recent infection (Harrison et al., 1983). Premature rupture of membranes, preterm labor, postpartum endometritis and fever have been linked in other studies to *C. trachomatis* infections (Sweet et al., 1987).

Chlamydia can be transmitted from the mother to the infant in the peripartum period. Infants born to mothers carrying *C. trachomatis* have an 18 percent chance of developing chlamydial conjunctivitis and a 16 percent chance of developing chlamydial pneumonia (Schachter et al., 1986a). Pregnant women can be screened for chlamydia and treated with erythromycin to prevent antepartum complications and perinatal acquisition of chlamydia by the newborn infant (McMillan et al., 1985; Schachter et al., 1986b; Cohen et al., 1990). However, chlamydial infections not detected by screening usually can be treated with antibiotics in the neonatal period without adverse outcomes (Schachter et al., 1986a).

Chlamydia screening in pregnancy is recommended for high-risk groups including adolescents, unmarried women, and those reporting multiple sex partners or a history of other sexually-transmitted disease (CDC, 1985). Groups supporting this recommendation include the USPHS Panel, the USPSTF, the CDC, ACOG, and the Canadian Task Force.

Human Immunodeficiency Virus (HIV)

A woman carrying the HIV virus has an estimated 30 percent chance of transmitting it to her fetus (AAP Task Force on Pediatric AIDS, 1988). Congenital HIV infections have very poor prognoses and are increasing in frequency (Scott et al., 1989). Until recently, the value of screening for HIV infection in pregnant women derived mostly from providing women with information to inform choices about the continuation of pregnancy. However, recent data have provided an additional reason for identifying women at risk of transferring HIV infection to their fetuses.

One study demonstrated that HIV-infected women who were treated with the anti-retroviral drug zidovudine during pregnancy had a significantly lower risk of transmitting the infection to their newborns (Connor et al., 1994). In this randomized, double-blind, placebo-controlled trial of HIV-infected pregnant women with CD4+ counts about 200, women treated with zidovudine transmitted the infection to 8.3 percent of their infants, whereas women treated with placebo transmitted the infection to 25.5 percent of their infants. This 67.5 percent reduction in perinatal transmission is statistically significant (P<0.01). Further, minimal short term toxic effects were observed in either mothers or infants treated with zidovudine.

These data on the effectiveness of zidovudine in preventing perinatal HIV transmission provide a compelling rationale for identifying HIV-infected pregnant women. The USPHS (1989) has recommended offering HIV testing to all pregnant women. All pregnant women should receive counseling about their individual risk of HIV infection, and should be offered testing so that antiretroviral therapy can be instituted in women found to be positive.

Congenital Fetal Disorders

Down Syndrome

Antenatal screening for Down syndrome in women over 35 years of age has long been an accepted prenatal care process. The risk of a Down syndrome infant increases exponentially when the mother is 35 years or older; the rate is 1 in 375 births at age 35 and 1 in 30 births at age 45. Karyotyping of the fetus, from amniocentesis and more recently chorionic villus sampling, is a sensitive and specific means of prenatal detection. The main disadvantage to antenatal detection is the risk of inducing abortions in normal pregnancies. This occurs following about 0.5 percent of amniocenteses. Amniocentesis may also rarely cause

orthopedic deformities and respiratory distress syndrome in the fetus
(Campbell, 1987). Alternatively, chorionic villus sampling can be
performed earlier in the pregnancy with equal or slightly higher
abortion rates (American Medical Association, 1987). For women aged 35
years, this means one normal fetus is aborted for every one or two Down
syndrome infant(s) detected.

Offering amniocentesis to women over 35 years old has been
recommended by the USPSTF, the USPHS panel, ACOG, and AAP. Newer, less
invasive, methods of screening for Down syndrome are being investigated
such as maternal serum AFP screening and ultrasound, but none have yet
been proven to be accurate enough to replace amniocentesis.

Neural Tube Defects

Neural tube defects (NTDs) are among the most common congenital
anomalies, occurring in approximately 1 in every 1000 pregnancies in the
United States. Some women are at higher risk of having an infant with a
NTD, but 90 percent of NTDs occur in low-risk groups. About half of the
NTDs are anencephalie and do not survive. The remainder are mostly
spina bifidas and myelomeningoceles which can cause significant
neurologic impairment including paraplegia and bowel and bladder
incontinence (USPSTF, 1989; Campbell, 1987).

Measuring maternal serum alpha-fetoprotein (AFP) can be used to
detect NTDs in early pregnancy. Screening using serum AFP
determinations is performed by first measuring the maternal level
usually between 16 and 18 weeks gestation. Based on this initial
screen, 2.5 to 7.0 percent of serum AFP samples, depending on the
criteria used, will be abnormally high. Abnormal screening AFP levels
are then evaluated by either repeating the AFP determination to confirm
or performing an ultrasound to identify a NTD or to exclude incorrect
gestational age and multiple gestations as a cause for the abnormality
(Nadel et al., 1990). For elevated AFPs not explained by the
ultrasound, amniocentesis may be performed to measure amniotic fluid AFP
and acetylcholinesterase levels. About 1.5 percent of all pregnancies
receiving an AFP screen are subsequently offered amniocentesis. For
women who complete this evaluation, the sensitivity of AFP screening for
anencephaly has been 83 to 100 percent and 50 to 100 percent for open

spina bifida (see Table 15.2). The specificity of AFP screening is nearly 100 percent. Almost no normal pregnancies have been terminated based on abnormal results from an amniocentesis or ultrasound evaluation--although the risk of inducing an abortion in performing amniocentesis is estimated to be 0.5 percent (Campbell, 1987). The feasibility of AFP screening has been demonstrated in numerous large-scale trials initially in the United Kingdom and later in the United States (Table 14.2). Reports have been published on over 100,000 pregnancies screened (UK Collaborative Study, 1977; Ward et al., 1981; Macri and Weiss, 1982; Burton et al., 1983; Hooker et al., 1984; Milunsky and Alpert, 1984; Milunsky et al., 1989a).

Table 14.2

Summary of Serum Alpha-Fetoprotein Screening for Neural Tube Defects in Pregnancy

Author	Study Setting	Number of Patients	NTD Rate (per 1,000)	Elevated AFPs No. (%) [Criteria]	Offered Amniocentesis No. (%)	Proportion of Anencephaly Detected	Proportion of Open Spina Bifida Detected*
U.K. Collaborative Study, 1977	19 U.K. centers	19,148	1.6	N.R. (3.3%) [2.5x median]	N.R.	88%	79%
Ward, 1981	1 U.K. center	5,668	1.9	129 (2.3%) [Varied]	19 (0.3%)	100%	50%
Macri, 1982	Long Island, NY screening program	17,703	1.2	692 (3.9%) [2x median]	365 (2.1%)	83.3%	100%
Burton, 1983	No. Carolina screening prgm.	12,084	1.5	452 (3.7%) [2.5x median]	148 (1.2%)	80%	85%
Hooker, 1984	1 U.K. center	6,344	1.3	88 (1.4%) [2.5x median]	45 (0.7%)	None occurred	100%
Milunsky, 1984	New England private practices	21,442	1.2	249 (1.2%) [2.5x median]	56 (0.3%)	86%	63%
Robinson, 1989	California AFP program	35,787	0.9	560 (1.6%) [2.5x median]	413 (1.2%)	N.R.	N.R.
Milunsky, 1989	New England private practices	13,486	1.6	530 (3.9%) [2.0x median]	N.R.	100%	91%

* Excludes closed neural tube defects
N.R. = not reported

Maternal serum AFP screening has other advantages besides detecting NTDs. About 40 percent of patients with elevated AFPs are determined by ultrasound to have incorrect dates or twin gestations. Whether having this information improves pregnancy management and outcome has not been determined. Patients with elevated AFP levels with subsequent normal amniotic AFP levels have also been identified as having a greater risk of perinatal loss (Robinson, 1989). Finally, pregnancies with abnormally low AFP levels are at greater risk for chromosome abnormalities, including Down syndrome (Milunsky et al., 1989; DiMaio et al., 1987). Amniocentesis for genetic analysis has been recommended to evaluate low serum AFP levels, although the value of this approach is still considered investigational (American Medical Association, 1988).

ACOG, USPHS panel, the USPSTF and an international consensus meeting (Boppart et al., 1985) have all supported well-coordinated AFP programs which provide mothers with appropriate counseling services if any abnormalities are detected. Antenatal detection of NTDs enables pregnant women to make more informed choices about their pregnancy and to receive appropriate counseling. Concerns about the value of AFP screening have been raised because half of the anomalies detected are anencephaly, for which early detection does not alter the ultimate outcome (fetal or early neonatal death), although considerable emotional trauma from the unexpected delivery of a severely deformed fetus may be avoided. Also, AFP screening can result in the termination of normal pregnancies, the greatest risk being related to the performance of amniocentesis. For cases of spina bifida detected, the parents are faced with what can be a difficult ethical decision regarding pregnancy termination since these pregnancies can result in a mentally intact, but chronically disabled, infant. AFP screening programs must take into consideration individual perspectives about how to value life and the burden of suffering imposed on an afflicted infant.

Sickle Cell Disease

Sickle cell disease and its variants are genetic abnormalities transmitted in an autosomal recessive pattern; both parents must carry an abnormal gene for the disease to be fully manifest. The disease causes severe hemolytic anemia, painful vasoocclusive crises,

cholelithiasis, renal dysfunction, cerebral thromboses, and decreased
life expectancy. It afflicts about 0.15 percent of blacks. About 8
percent of blacks are asymptomatic heterozygous carriers. This places
one in 150 black couples at risk for giving birth to a child with sickle
cell disease.

Parents can be screened to determine whether they carry the trait.
If both members of a couple carry the trait, antenatal testing of the
fetus for sickle cell disease can be performed either using
amniocentesis (Boehm et al., 1983; Driscoll et al., 1987; Embury et al.,
1987) or chorionic villus sampling (Goossens et al., 1983). The
sensitivity and specificity of these tests appear to be very good
although no large scale studies have yet been reported (USPSTF, 1989).

As with other genetic abnormalities, antenatal diagnosis of sickle
cell disease allows the family to make informed decisions about whether
to carry the pregnancy to term (Anionwu et al., 1988). Patients should
be counseled about their options including termination of the pregnancy.
The USPSTF supports routine screening of pregnant women at risk. ACOG
and the British Society for Haematology (BCSH General Haematology Task
Force, 1988) recommend that pregnant women with abnormal red cell
indices be screened for sickle cell and other hemoglobinopathies.

Rh Isoimmunization

The incidence of Rh isoimmunization, which causes such fetal
complications as hemolytic anemia, hyperbilirubinemia, hydrops fetalis
and fetal death, has declined dramatically since the introduction of
Rh(D) immune globulin (Rhogam) prophylaxis. About 9 to 10 percent of
women are Rh-negative. Of these women, 8 to 15 percent would become
isoimmunized in the postpartum period without prophylaxis. Rhogam has
been used so successfully that only 14.3 of every 100,000 pregnancies
are now affected (USPSTF, 1989).

With postpartum prophylaxis reducing the number of women
isoimmunized in the postpartum period, isoimmunization occurring in the
antepartum period has increased in relative importance (Tovey and
Taverner, 1981). From 0.7 to 1.8 percent of Rh-negative women are
isoimmunized if they do not receive Rhogam antenatally. Studies of

antepartum administration of the Rh immune globulin have found it to be effective in preventing antepartum isoimmunization (Hensleigh, 1983).

Screening for Rh-negative women and Rh immune globulin prophylaxis, both antenatally and postpartum, are unanimously recommended by the USPSTF, the USPHS panel, ACOG, AAP, and the Canadian College of Obstetricians and Gynecologists. Performing an indirect Coombs test to detect other less common types of isoimmunizations has also been recommended.

Common Pregnancy Complications
Intrauterine Growth Retardation

Intrauterine growth retardation (IUGR) complicates about 5 percent of pregnancies. These infants are at greater risk for obstetrical complications including fetal distress during labor, meconium aspiration, hypoglycemia and hypothermia, and perinatal mortality. Growth-retarded infants accounted for 18 percent of total perinatal mortality and 31 percent of fetal loss (Tejani and Mann, 1977).

The simplest means of screening for IUGR is serial measurements of symphysis-fundal height (SFH). SFH measurements are safe and inexpensive, but are subject to several problems. One problem is its relatively poor reliability. Repeated SFH measurements for a given patient can vary between observers by as much as 4 cm (S.D. = 1 cm) (USPSTF, 1989; Rogers and Needham, 1985). Another difficult problem is deciding upon the specific SFH-gestational age discrepancy to define abnormal since this greatly influences the sensitivity and specificity of this method. A three- or four-centimeter discrepancy between the SFH and that expected for a given gestational age is the criterion generally recommended with reported sensitivities ranging from 65 to 85 percent and specificities from 80 to 93 percent (USPSTF, 1989; Cunningham et al., 1989; Goldenberg et al., 1990). A lower criterion could be used to increase the sensitivity of the test but this would also decrease the test's specificity and positive predictive value. Finally, the utility of the test will vary with the prevalence of IUGR in the population. Assuming a sensitivity of 75 percent and specificity of 90 percent, the positive predictive value in a population with a prevalence of 5 percent would be about 28 percent. Using the same sensitivities and specificities in a higher-risk population with a prevalence of 10 percent, the positive predictive value increases to 45 percent.

The relatively low sensitivity of SFH measurements (as many as 35 percent of IUGR will not be detected) has led to the consideration of an alternative means of screening for IUGR, obstetrical ultrasound. Its sensitivity compares favorably to physical examination, with sensitivities of 80 to 96 percent and specificities of 80 to 90 percent (USPSTF, 1989; Seeds, 1984). Again, the low prevalence of IUGR in the general population limits its positive predictive value. Even assuming a sensitivity of 95 percent and specificity of 90 percent, the positive predictive value is improved to only 33 percent. In pregnancies with complicating maternal or fetal conditions that increase the risk of IUGR, the improved positive predictive value may warrant ultrasound screening. Of note, a single ultrasound examination is often not sufficient to diagnose IUGR. Many pregnancies will require two or more ultrasound examinations to evaluate problems adding considerably to the cost of prenatal care. For example, women in Norway where routine ultrasonography is widely accepted have an average of 2.45 examinations per pregnancy (Nesheim et al., 1987). Studies of the safety and long-term effects of obstetrical ultrasounds so far have not shown any harmful consequences, but many authors warn of possible unobserved effects (Kremkau, 1984).

Arguments for the routine use of ultrasound to screen for IUGR are supported by its benefit in detecting other obstetrical problems such as: incorrect gestational age based on LMP, congenital anomalies, multiple gestations, placenta previa, and abnormal fetal presentation. By screening for these problems and IUGR, earlier interventions could be implemented to improve pregnancy outcomes. A number of controlled clinical trials have tested the overall benefit of routine obstetrical ultrasounds (Campbell et al., 1985; Goldenberg et al., 1989a; Bennett et al., 1982; Cochlin, 1984; Neilson et al., 1984; Eik-Nes et al., 1984; Bakketeig et al., 1984; Waldenstrom et al., 1988; Reading and Cox, 1982; Field et al., 1985; Ewigman et al., 1990). Some benefits were noted such as fewer inductions of postterm pregnancies, earlier detection of multiple gestations and placenta previas. Only limited benefits in terms of perinatal outcomes, however, were noted. Eik-Nes found nonsignificantly higher birthweights for twin gestations and lower perinatal mortality rates among women receiving routine ultrasounds (Eik-Nes et al., 1984). Bakketeig found a nonsignificant improvement in birthweights for twin gestations (Bakketeig et al., 1984). Waldenstrom et al. (1988) found slightly fewer infants with low birthweight. These studies are limited by their sample sizes in their ability to show statistically significant differences with routine ultrasound. Pooled analysis was still inconclusive showing nonsignificant improvements in both perinatal death rate and Apgar scores (Thacker, 1985).

Other methods of detecting IUGR are being tested. Doppler ultrasound of umbilical artery flow has been used to evaluate uteroplacental perfusion. Fetuses with abnormal Doppler studies are at greater risk of poor pregnancy outcomes. Its present role, however, is in confirming abnormal growth patterns suggesting IUGR, and not as a screening test (Reuwer et al., 1987).

In the United States, serial physical examinations continue to be the primary method of screening for IUGR. Although obstetrical ultrasounds are used for medical indications, their use for routine screening has not been advocated by any major organizations in the United States. The USPSTF recommends ultrasound examinations be performed routinely for women at increased risk of delivering a growth-retarded infant. They should also be considered for pregnancies with uncertain menstrual dates. A National Institutes of Health consensus development conference (Consensus Conference, 1984) and ACOG have made similar recommendations for the use of ultrasound. The Canadian Task Force also does not recommend routine serial ultrasounds in normal pregnancies. Even in Norway where 94 percent of women receive ultrasound examinations, a consensus group could not recommend implementing ultrasound screening citing concerns about overutilization, uncertain quality, and unknown risks (Nesheim et al., 1987). The only organization currently recommending routine ultrasound examinations is the Royal College of Obstetricians and Gynaecologists in Britain.

Management of IUGR relies mostly upon treating the underlying cause, such as cigarette smoking. A precise cause for the IUGR, however, is often not known. Patients are advised to limit their strenuous activities and optimize their nutritional intake. Fetuses with IUGR are at greater risk for fetal distress; signs of fetal distress on serial fetal monitoring would be an indication to effect delivery. Depending upon the severity of the IUGR and fetal maturity, early delivery should be considered (Seeds, 1984).

Postterm Pregnancy

From 4 to 12 percent of pregnancies continue beyond 42 weeks after the last menstrual period (McClure Browne, 1963; Vorherr, 1975). The process by which labor is initiated remains unknown, but many of these postterm pregnancies are likely due to inaccurate recall of the last menstrual period or to delayed ovulation (Saito et al., 1972). True postterm pregnancies, however, are at increased risk of perinatal morbidity and mortality. Rates of perinatal mortality increase at 41 weeks, double by 42 weeks and quadruple by 44 weeks. Postterm infants are at greater risk for cesarean delivery due to fetal distress and failed progress in labor related to higher birthweights (McClure Browne, 1963; Arias, 1987).

Studies have shown that appropriate management of postterm pregnancies can prevent much of the perinatal mortality (Yeh and Read, 1982; Eden et al., 1982; Shime et al., 1984; Dyson et al., 1987; Johnson et al., 1986; Bochner et al., 1987; Khouzami et al., 1983;). These studies vary somewhat in their obstetrical management and few comparisons of approaches have been made to identify the optimal strategy. Much of the management of postterm pregnancy depends on the accuracy of the fetal gestational age.

For patients with good dates, labor can be routinely induced at 42 weeks, particularly if the cervix is favorable (Witter and Weitz, 1987). If not induced, fetal monitoring should be performed regularly beginning no later than 42 weeks (Benedetti and Easterling, 1988). Some authors recommend beginning fetal monitoring at 41 weeks because some fetal deaths occur between 41 and 42 weeks (Bochner et al., 1988). A variety of different antepartum fetal monitoring methods are used including nonstress test, contraction stress test, biophysical profiles, serum estriols, and ultrasound. When the cervix is not favorable, the decision to deliver is based on repeated fetal monitoring and estimated fetal weight; fetal distress or oligohydramnios are indications for induction of labor, or possibly primary cesarean section (see Chapter 6). Pregnancies with good dates should rarely continue beyond 43 weeks (Dyson, 1988; ACOG, 1989).

For patients with poor dates, management is more difficult. Inducing labor in a pregnancy with inaccurate determination of gestational age could result in the delivery of a premature infant. A more conservative approach is used to manage these pregnancies. Antepartum fetal monitoring is used to assess the status of the fetus while awaiting spontaneous labor. Once the pregnancy reaches a stage at which fetal maturity can be assured based on clinical information or fetal distress is noted, induction may occur (Dyson, 1988).

Pregnancy-Induced Hypertension

Pregnancy-induced hypertension (PIH) is one of the more common medical complications during pregnancy. It occurs in about 5 to 10 percent of pregnancies with manifestations ranging from isolated mild elevations in blood pressure to eclamptic seizures, disseminated intravascular coagulopathy, and maternal or fetal death. Most cases occur among primiparous women or those with preexisting hypertension.

Several studies have suggested primary prevention of PIH may be possible, but further studies are needed (Klonoff-Cohen et al., 1989; Benigni et al., 1989; Schiff et al., 1989). Prenatal care currently plays an important role in the secondary and tertiary prevention of complications due to PIH. Failure to diagnose and treat preeclampsia appropriately is an important factor in maternal mortality from PIH and eclampsia (Evans et al., 1983).

Screening for PIH is based primarily on noting an increase in blood pressure, preferably before the second trimester of pregnancy. The most commonly used criteria are systolic blood pressure above 140 mm Hg and diastolic above 90 mm Hg, or increases in blood pressure during pregnancy of more than 30 mm Hg systolic or 15 mm Hg diastolic. Elevated blood pressure alone, however, does not reliably predict which women will develop complications. Many women with even moderately elevated blood pressures will have no other manifestations of PIH; women who develop eclamptic seizures, however, will sometimes have only mild elevations of blood pressure. The presence of proteinuria or peripheral edema with elevated blood pressures helps to confirm the diagnosis of preeclampsia. Neither proteinuria nor peripheral edema alone or combined have sufficient sensitivity and specificity (Chesley, 1985). Other methods have been suggested to refine the screening for PIH such as mean arterial blood pressure, uric acid levels, and platelet counts. Preeclampsia still remains a clinical diagnosis based primarily on blood pressure criteria, but taking into consideration other clinical information such as proteinuria and edema (Sibai, 1988; Redman and Jefferies, 1988; Fay et al., 1985).

Early detection and appropriate treatment of preeclampsia almost certainly helps to avert many of its complications (ACOG, 1986). However, the weight of scientific evidence and expert consensus ethically precludes such a trial from being conducted. Management of PIH depends on its severity and when during pregnancy it is diagnosed. When the pregnancy is near term, efforts are usually made to deliver the fetus. When the pregnancy is remote from term, however, management of PIH may vary. Disease severity can be assessed by physical examination, and laboratory tests including complete blood counts, coagulation tests, liver function tests and renal function tests (Thiagarajah et al., 1984). For milder cases, bedrest can usually be prescribed, but it is not clear at what point hospitalization becomes necessary (Sibai, 1988). In more severe cases, immediate delivery should be considered when fetal maturity can be demonstrated, conservative management fails, signs of fetal distress or growth retardation develop, or gestational age exceeds 32 to 34 weeks (Thiagarajah et al., 1984; Lindheimer and Katz, 1985; Cunningham and Pritchard, 1984; Sibai et al., 1985). Magnesium sulfate or other anti-seizure measures should be implemented to prevent eclampsia (Cunningham and Pritchard, 1984; Sibai et al., 1984; Slater et al., 1987). Antihypertensive medications can be used to treat severe hypertension (diastolic blood pressure over 110 mm Hg) (Cunningham and Pritchard, 1984). Antihypertensive medications do not appear to

influence outcomes in milder preeclampsia (Sibai et al., 1987).
Disseminated intravascular coagulation should be appropriately diagnosed
and treated (Thiagarajah et al., 1984).

Screening for preeclampsia with periodic blood pressure
measurements during pregnancy has been supported by the USPSTF, USPHS,
ACOG and the Canadian Task Force. Although most groups recommend that
blood pressure be taken at every visit, the optimal frequency of
measurement recommended varies among the different groups because they
differ in their recommended number and frequency of prenatal visits.
The USPSTF leaves the recommended frequency to clinical discretion
noting that the optimal frequency has not been determined.

Gestational Diabetes Mellitus

Gestational diabetes is a relatively common problem, developing in
2 to 3 percent of pregnancies, usually in the second or third trimester
(O'Sullivan et al., 1973; Merkatz et al., 1980; CDC, 1986). By
comparison, only 0.3 percent of pregnant women have a previous diagnosis
of diabetes. Gestational diabetes is associated with increased risk of
perinatal mortality, fetal macrosomia and associated delivery
complications, and neonatal morbidities including hypoglycemia,
hypocalcemia, polycythemia and hyperbilirubinemia (O'Sullivan et al.,
1966; American Diabetes Association, 1986).

In order to identify women with gestational diabetes, risk factors
such as age, obesity, family history, and previous delivery of a
macrosomic or congenitally malformed infant can be used to select women
for screening. Most women with gestational diabetes, however, will not
have any risk factors (O'Sullivan et al., 1973). For selective or
routine screening for gestational diabetes, a 50 gram glucose challenge
test is generally given at 24 to 28 weeks gestation. Plasma glucose
levels drawn one hour after ingestion are abnormal if greater than 140
mg/dl. Abnormal screening tests are confirmed with a three-hour glucose
tolerance test. This method is about 80 to 85 percent sensitive and
specific. Other diabetes screening methods such as urine dipsticks for
glucose and glycosylated hemoglobins are not sensitive enough for
screening (USPSTF, 1989; CDC, 1988b; ACOG, 1994).

Treatment of gestational diabetes usually includes diabetes education, diet, and exercise (CDC, 1986; ACOG, 1994). Although routine use of insulin helps prevent macrosomia and related complications of delivery (Coustan and Lewis, 1978; Coustan and Imarah, 1984), there may not be any advantage over treating with diet initially and reserving insulin therapy for women whose fasting or postprandial glucoses are not well-controlled (e.g., fasting plasma glucose > 65 ml/dl or two-hour postprandial glucose > 120 mg/dl) (ACOG, 1994; Persson et al., 1985). Oral hypoglycemic medications are generally not used during pregnancy. Because of the complications associated with gestational diabetes, fetal monitoring is generally initiated at term and delivery is usually effected close to term (CDC, 1988b; ACOG, 1994; Langer, 1990).

The improvement in outcomes from screening and treating gestational diabetes are relatively limited. Two experimental controlled trials and a number of observational studies have shown that treatment of gestational diabetes can significantly reduce the incidence of fetal macrosomia. In the experimental trials, however, decreased macrosomia was not associated with improvements in perinatal mortality and birth trauma rates (O'Sullivan et al., 1966; Coustan and Lewis, 1978; Singer et al., 1988). Thus, the benefits from screening for gestational diabetes are limited to avoiding some short-term morbidity related to the delivery of a macrosomic infant and do not appear to include improved long-term morbidity nor perinatal mortality.

The USPHS panel, the USPSTF, the American Diabetes Association, the CDC, and the Second International Workshop-Conference on Gestational Diabetes Mellitus support routine screening for diabetes in pregnancy. ACOG, however, does not recommend routine screening; rather, screening is recommended only for women over age 30 or for those who have specific risk factors which include glucosuria, hypertension, family history of diabetes, previous delivery of a macrosomic, malformed, or stillborn infant, or obesity (ACOG, 1994).

RECOMMENDED QUALITY INDICATORS FOR PRENATAL CARE

Screening

Indicator	Quality of evidence	Literature	Benefits	Comments
Routine Prenatal Care				
1. The first prenatal visit should occur in the first trimester.	II-1	USPHS, 1989	Prevent morbidity/mortality associated with complications in pregnancy.	An early first prenatal visit has been associated with decreased low birth weight. First trimester blood pressure assessment allows more accurate diagnosis of pre-eclampsia later in pregnancy. High-risk factors for which intervention is available can be identified (e.g., smoking, substance abuse, chronic hypertension, diabetes).
2. The physician should make an accurate determination of gestational age using: a. An ultrasound in the 1st or 2nd trimester, or b. Reliable LMP and size within 2 wks indicated by dates in the 1st trimester, or c. No 1st trimester exam, but reliable LMP & 2 of the following: 1) size w/in 2 wks. of dates in 2d trimester; 2) quickening by 20 wks.; 3) fetal heart tones by fetoscope before 20 weeks, or d. If unreliable LMP, then an ultrasound is required.	III	USPHS, 1989; Cunningham et al., 1989; Campbell et al., 1985; Andersen et al., 1981; Kramer et al., 1988; Goldenberg et al., 1989a; NIH Consensus Conference, 1984	Prevent or identify complications of pregnancy such as post-datism and intrauterine growth retardation. Prevent prematurity. Prevent unnecessary induction of labor.	Diagnosis of inappropriate fetal growth and post-dates require accurate knowledge of gestational age. The timing of induction of labor for post-dates is dependent on accurate gestational age information. Scheduled cesarean deliveries prior to term can be avoided if accurate dating is available.
3. Pregnant women should be screened for anemia at the first prenatal visit.	III	USPSTF, 1989; USPHS, 1989; Hemminki and Starfield, 1978; Lieberman et al., 1988; Murphy et al., 1986; Klebanoff et al., 1989; Reece et al., 1987; Hibbard, 1988; Horn, 1988; Shapiro and Lyons, 1989	Prevent low and very low birthweight births.	Early identification of anemia allows for treatment during pregnancy. Severe anemia has been associated with low birthweight. The risk of untreated mild anemia is not well defined, but screening and iron supplementation have become routine.

225

#	Recommendation	Rating	References	Objective	Comments
4.	Pregnant women should be rescreened for anemia after 24 weeks.	III	Lieberman et al., 1988; Murphy et al., 1986	Prevent low and very low birthweight births.	Allows identification of anemias which may have developed during pregnancy and require treatment.
Substance Abuse					
5.	A smoking history should be obtained at the first prenatal visit.	I+	Mayer et al., 1990; Ershoff et al., 1989; Sexton and Hebel, 1984; Hebel et al., 1985;	Reduce incidence of low birthweight.	Identifying women who smoke can lead to counseling about cessation which in turn can contribute to preventing low birthweight.
6.	An alcohol history should be obtained at the first prenatal visit.	II-2	USPSTF, 1989; USPHS, 1989; Rosett and Weiner, 1981; Kruse et al., 1986; Waterson and Murray-Lyon, 1989; Allen and Ries, 1985; Rosett et al., 1983; Halmesmaki, 1988;	Decrease the incidence and severity of fetal alcohol syndrome.	Poor reliability of self-report. Identifying problem drinkers can facilitate treatment which can prevent fetal alcohol syndrome.
7.	A drug history should be obtained during the first prenatal visit.	III	USPSTF, 1989; Petitti and Coleman, 1990; O'Connor, 1987; Zuckerman et al., 1989; Chasnoff et al., 1989; Chavkin, 1990; Rosner et al., 1982	Prevent intrauterine growth retardation, congenital anomalies, neonatal withdrawal, and abruptio placentae.	Poor reliability of self-report. Identification of substance abusing women can lead to counseling and treatment. Literature on effectiveness of treatment inconclusive.
Infections and STDs					
Asymptomatic Bacteriuria					
8.	Pregnant women should receive a urine culture at the first prenatal visit.	I+	Romero et al., 1989; Pels et al., 1989; Campbell-Brown et al., 1987; Wadland and Plante, 1989;	Prevent pyelonephritis and its complications (e.g., preterm delivery, hospitalization).	ACOG recommends culture for high-risk only; UA for all others. Sensitivity and specificity of urine culture superior to UA or screening dipstick for detecting asymptomatic bacteriuria.

Rubella

#	Recommendation	Level	References	Benefit	Comments
9.	Pregnant women should receive a serologic test for rubella immunity before delivery.	II-2+	USPSTF, 1989; Griffiths and Baboonian, 1982; Black et al., 1983; CDC, 1987; CDC, 1986; ACOG, 1992	Prevent congenital rubella syndrome in subsequent pregnancies.	Allows for vaccination after pregnancy. May alert women to avoid exposure in current pregnancy.

Hepatitis B Carriers

#	Recommendation	Level	References	Benefit	Comments
10.	Pregnant women should be screened for HBsAg before delivery.	II-2	Xu et al., 1985; Stevens et al., 1985; Beasley et al., 1983; Schalm et al., 1989; Poovorawan and Sanpavat, 1989; CDC, 1985; Arevalo and Washington, 1988	Decrease incidence of hepatitis infection in newborns.	Many HBsAg carriers can be detected using risk factor screening, but in practice this has not been effective. Routine screening allows for early vaccination of newborns, as well as Ig prophylaxis, which can effectively prevent vertical transmission.

Syphilis

#	Recommendation	Level	References	Benefit	Comments
11.	A non-treponemal screening test (e.g., VDRC) should be performed on pregnant women at the first prenatal visit.	II-3+	CDC, 1988b; Stray-Pedersen, 1983; Williams, 1985	Prevent congenital syphyllis	Screening only high risk women has not proven effective.

Gonorrhea

#	Recommendation	Level	References	Benefit	Comments
12.	A cervical gonorrhea culture should be performed on pregnant women at the first prenatal visit.	III+	USPSTF, 1989; Alexander, 1988; Rothenberg, 1979	Prevent ophthalmia neonatorum and associated risk of blindness. Prevent septic abortions, chorioamnionitis, premature rupture of membranes and premature delivery.	Ethical considerations preclude controlled studies of GC screening.

Chlamydia

#	Recommendation	Level	References	Benefit	Comments
13.	Pregnant Women at high risk (adolescents, unmarried, those with multiple sex partners, low SES, other STD diagnosed) should receive a cervical chlamydia culture or antigen detection at the first prenatal visit.	III	CDC, 1985	Reduce neonatal chlamydial infection.	Chlamydial infections in newborns include pneumona and conjunctivitis.

Human Immunodeficiency Virus

#	Recommendation	Level	References	Benefit	Comments
14.	Pregnant women should be counseled about their individual risk for HIV infection at the first prenatal visit.		Minkoff and Landesman, 1988	Reduce perinatal transmission of HIV.	In order to inform their decision to accept or reject HIV testing, women need to know if they fall into a high-risk category.

15.	Pregnant women should be offered HIV testing at the first prenatal visit.	I/III	Connor, 1994; USPHS, 1989	Reduce perinatal transmission of HIV.	Based on data that show that zidovudine therapy can effectively reduce perinatal transmission. Also allows for PCP prohpylaxis or early treatment of those pregnant women infected with HIV.

Inherited Disorders

Down Syndrome

| 16. | Pregnant women age 35 and over, or who have had a previous Down syndrome infant, should receive amniocentesis or chorionic villus sampling (CVS), or should explicitly decline such a test after genetic counseling. | II-2+ | USPSTF, 1989; Sadovnick and Baird, 1982 | Facilitate patient-informed choice. | Allows women who would consider terminating their pregnancy early access to information about chromosomal abnormalities. The age cutoff is designed to balance the risk of a spontaneous abortion with a chosen abortion and the chance of an affected child. |

Neural Tube Defects (NTDs)

| 17. | Pregnant women under age 35 should be offered serum AFP; this should be performed between 15 and 20 weeks. | II-2+ | USPSTF, 1989; USPHS, 1989; Campbell, 1987; Nadel et al., 1990; American Medical Association, 1988; Boppart et al., 1985; Sadovnick and Baird, 1983; Sadovnick and Baird, 1982; Layde et al., 1979 | Allows parents who would consider termination of pregnancy to do so. Prepares parents and health care team for birth of affected infant. | See Table 14.1. Early detection of fetuses with open neural tube defects. Serum AFP can also detect Down Syndrome, twins, and incorrect dating. |

| 18. | Pregnant women who have had a previous NTD infant should receive amniocentesis or should explicitly decline such a test after genetic counseling. | II-2+ | Boppart et al., 1985 | Identify fetuses with NTD early. Allow parents who would consider termination to do so. Prepares parents and health care team for birth of affected infant. | These women are at increased risk of having fetuses affected with neural tube defects. |

#	Recommendation	Grade	References	Purpose	Comment
Sickle Cell Disease					
19.	Pregnant women who are African American or have a family history of sickle cell disease should be screened at the first prenatal visit.	II-2+	Boehm et al., 1983; Driscoll et al., 1987; Embury et al., 1987; Goossens et al., 1983; Anionwu et al., 1988; BCSH General Haematology Task Force, 1988	Identify fetuses at risk for sickle cell disease and allow for diagnosis and termination of pregnancy, if desired.	If a woman is a sickle cell carrier, testing of the partner and appropriate counseling can take place.
20.	For pregnant women with the sickle cell trait, the baby's father should be screened.	II-2+	See above.	Identify fetuses at risk for sickle cell disease and allow for diagnosis and termination of pregnancy, if desired.	Allows for the quantification of the risk of sickle cell disease in the fetus.
Rh Isoimmunization					
21.	Pregnant women should receive an Rh factor and antibody screen at the first prenatal visit.	II-2+	Tovey and Taverner, 1981; Hensleigh, 1983; Torrance and Zipursky, 1984; Adams et al., 1984;	Prevent isoimmunization. Prevent complications (e.g., hydrops fetalis, fetal death) in women previously isoimmunized.	Unsensitized women can be administered anti-D immunoglobulin at the appropriate interval. Sensitized women can be monitored with antibody titers and amniocentesis.
Common Pregnancy Complications					
Intrauterine Growth Retardation					
22.	Measurements of the symphysis-fundal height should be made at each visit from 20-32 weeks.	III+	Wennergren and Karlsson, 1982; Rogers and Needham, 1985	Prevent intrauterine fetal death.	Although not a highly-specific test, this measurement can identify a subset of infants at risk for intrauterine growth retardation, who can be followed and diagnosed with ultrasound. Without intervention, a growth-retarded fetus is at risk for intrauterine death.
Post-term Pregnancy					
23.	Weekly fetal monitoring should begin at 41.5 weeks and continue until labor (spontaneous or induced) begins.	II-1+	Arias, 1987; Dyson et al., 1987; Bochner et al., 1988; Dyson, 1988	Reduce risk of intrauterine fetal death.	Risk of intrauterine fetal death at greater than 41 weeks is increased and can be lowered to the risk at 40 weeks with testing and an induction protocol.
Pregnancy-Induced Hypertension (PIH)					
24.	Blood pressure measurements should be taken at each visit.	II-2+	Sibai, 1988; ACOG, 1986	Prevent complications of pre-eclampsia (e.g., seizure, abruptio placentae, fetal and maternal death).	Early identification of PIH may result in better outcomes.

Indicator	Quality of evidence	Literature	Benefits	Comments
Gestational Diabetes Mellitus				
25. A one-hour, 50g glucose challenge test should be performed on pregnant women with risk factors at 24-28 weeks.	I+	CDC, 1986; ADA, 1986; ACOG, 1994; Persson et al., 1985	Decrease fetal macrosomia.	ACOG recommends screening high risk only. Screening and treatment of gestational diabetes decreases morbidity from macrosomia but no mortality benefit. ACOG risk factors include: age > 30; glucosuria; hypertension; family history of diabetes; previous delivery of a macrosomic, malformed, or stillborn infant; or obesity.

Diagnosis

Indicator	Quality of evidence	Literature	Benefits	Comments
Infections and STDs				
Hepatitis B Carriers				
26. For pregnant women carrying HBsAg, carrier status should be documented in delivery record.	I+	Xu et al., 1985; Stevens et al., 1985	Decrease incidence of hepatitis B infection in newborns.	Newborn can be vaccinated at birth and given Hb immunoglobulin if maternal carrier status is known.
Syphilis				
27. Pregnant women whose non-treponemal tests are weakly reactive or reactive should receive a treponemal test to confirm presence of syphilis.	II-3+	CDC, 1988	Reduce risk of side effects from unnecessary syphilis medications.	Pregnancy and other conditions can result in a false positive test. This confirmatory test avoids unnecessary treatment.
Inherited Disorders				
Neural Tube Defects (NTDs)				
28. Pregnant women with an abnormal serum AFP should receive an ultrasound to evaluate gestational age and possible multiple gestation.	II-2+	Nadel et al., 1990	Avoid erroneous diagnosis of neural tube defect.	Prevents unnecessary intervention (i.e., termination or increased surveillance) based on improper test interpretation.
Sickle Cell Disease				
29. Pregnant women with the sickle cell trait should receive either amniocentesis or chorionic villus sampling, unless the baby's father is known to be negative for the sickle trait.	II-2+	Driscoll et al., 1987; Embury et al., 1987; Goosens et al., 1983	Identify affected fetuses. Allow termination of pregnancy if desired.	Sensitivity and specificity of these tests for detecting fetuses with sickle cell disease is good.
Common Pregnancy Complications				
Intrauterine Growth Retardation				
30. Pregnant women whose symphysis-fundal height is 4cm less than indicated by their gestational age between 20-32 weeks should have an ultrasound.	III+	USPSTF, 1989; Seeds, 1984	Decrease the risk of intrauterine fetal death.	Ultrasound will improve specificity of symphysis-fundal height measurement. A fetus with growth retardation can be delivered early if intrauterine compromise is evident.

Pregnancy-induced Hypertension (PIH)

#	Recommendation				Comments
31.	For elevated BPs (systolic > 140mm Hg, or diastolic > 90mm Hg, OR systolic rise >30mm Hg or diastolic rise > 15mm Hg), proteinuria and peripheral edema should be assessed.	II-2+	Sibai, 1988; Redman and Jeffries, 1988; Fay et al., 1985	Prevent complications of pre-eclampsia (e.g., seizure, placental abruption, or fetal or maternal death).,	Pregnancy complicated by hypertension and proteinuria has an increased risk of maternal and fetal complication (e.g., seizure, placental abruption, death), whereas hypertension alone does not confer as great a risk.
32.	For pregnant women with elevated BP and either proteinuria (1+ or more) or edema (> trace), PIH diagnosis should be made.	II-2+	Sibai, 1988; Redman and Jeffries, 1988; Fay et al., 1985	Prevent complications of pre-eclampsia (e.g., seizure, placental abruption, or fetal or maternal death).,	Diagnosis allows for increased surveillance and delivery at earliest time determined to be appropriate. Delivery is the only "cure".

Gestational Diabetes Mellitus

#	Recommendation				Comments
33.	Pregnant women with abnormal glucose challenge tests (≥140 mg/dL or 7.8 mmol/L) should have a 3-hour plasma glucose tolerance test performed.	I+	ACOG, 1994	Decrease macrosomia.	An abnormal glucose challenge test has a low specificity for women at risk of complications. A 3-hr. plasma glucose tolerance test increases specificity and appropriate treatment of gestational diabetes.

231

	Indicator	Quality of evidence	Literature	Benefits	Comments
	Substance Abuse				
34.	Pregnant women identified as smokers should receive counseling to stop smoking from their physician.	I+	Kleinman et al., 1988; McIntosh and Chir, 1984	Decrease low birthweight births.	Counseling will help increase the percentage of women who quit and consequently decrease the associated risks (e.g., low birth weight).
35.	Pregnant women identified as smokers should be referred to a smoking cessation clinic, group, or counselor.	I+	Kleinman et al., 1988; McIntosh and Chir, 1984	Decrease low birthweight births.	Intervention will help increase the percentage of wome n who quit and consequently decrease the associated risks (e.g., low birth weight).
36.	Pregnant women who indicate they use any amount of alcohol should be counseled to eliminate alcohol consumption during pregnancy.	II	Little, 1977; Halmesmaki, 1988	Prevent fetal alcohol syndrome.	No threshold level has been identified and therefore the risk of fetal alcohol syndrome may exist at any level of consumption.
37.	Pregnant women who indicate they use cocaine or heroin should be counseled by their physician to cease use during pregnancy.	II	Zuckerman et al., 1989	Decrease abruptions and preterm labor (cocaine). Decrease the chance of fetal death (heroin).	Counseling may increase rate of cessation of drug use.
38.	Pregnant women who indicate they use drugs should be referred to a drug treatment clinic, group, or counselor.	II	Keith et al., 1989; Pettiti and Coleman, 1990	Decrease abruptions and preterm labor (cocaine). Decrease the chance of fetal death (heroin).	Specialized facilities are better equiped to counsel patients.
	Infections and Sexually Transmitted Diseases				
	Asymptomatic Bacteriuria				
39.	Pregnant women with positive cultures (>100,000 bacteria/cc) should receive an appropriate antibiotic.	I+	Romero et al., 1989	Prevent pyelonephritis and its complications (e.g., preterm delivery, hospitalization).	Untreated bacteriuria has been associated with these adverse outcomes.
	Rubella				
40.	Pregnant women not immune to rubella should receive postpartum immunization.	I	Black et al., 1983	Prevent congenital rubella syndrome.	Opportunistic method for protecting against problems in future pregnancies.
	Syphilis				
41.	Pregnant women with confirmed positive serology should be treated with penicillin appropriate for the stage of disease; tetracycline and doxycycline are contraindicated.	II-3+	CDC, 1988	Prevent congenital syphyllis.	Tetracycline and doxycycline are teratogens.
	Gonorrhea				
42.	Pregnant women with positive cultures should be treated as recommended by the PHS Guidelines on STD (250 mg IM once of ceftriaxone and erythromycin base 500 mg orally 4x/day for 7 days).	III+	CDC, 1988	Prevent opthalmia neonatorum, septic abortions, chorioamnionitis, premature rupture of membranes and premature delivery.	Untreated gonorrhea has been associated with each of these complications.

#	Recommendation	Grade	Reference		
	Human Immunodeficiency Virus				
43.	Pregnant women known to be HIV positive with CD4+ counts of 200 or greater should be treated with zidovudine during pregnancy and intrapartum.	I	Connor, 1994	Reduce perinatal transmission of HIV.	Based on data that show that zidovudine therapy can effectively reduce perinatal transmission.
	Inherited Disorders				
	Down Syndrome				
44.	Pregnant women whose amniocentesis shows infant with abnormal karyotype should receive additional genetic counseling.	II-2+	USPSTF, 1989; USPHS, 1989	Allows women to chose the most appropriate option given current information about their test results and risks.	Genetic counseling is considered a necessary way of helping patients understand their options.
	Neural Tube Defects (NTDs)				
45.	Pregnant women with abnormal serum AFP and normal ultrasound should be offered an amniocentesis and genetic counseling.	II-2+	USPSTF, 1989; USPHS, 1989; AMA, 1988	Enhance patient-informed choice.	Genetic counseling should be present throughout this diagnostic process.
46.	Pregnant women whose amniotic fluid AFP shows infant with probable NTD should be offered additional genetic counseling.	II-2+	Boppart et al., 1985	Enhance patient-informed choice.	Genetic counseling can facilitate informed choice.
	Sickle Cell Disease				
47.	Pregnant women whose amniocentesis shows an infant with sickle cell disease should be offered genetic counseling.	II-2+	Anionwu et al., 1988	Enhance patient-informed choice.	Genetic counseling can facilitate informed choice.
	Rh Isoimmunization				
48.	Pregnant women who are Rh negative should receive Rhogam between 26 and 30 weeks antenatally and postpartum.	II-2+	Hensleigh, 1983	Prevents isoimmunization.	Avoiding isoimmunization will prevent possible hydrops fetalis in future pregnancies.
	Common Pregnancy Complications				
	Post-Term Pregnancy				
49.	Labor should be induced when fetus shows signs of distress or oligohydramnios.	II-1+	Dyson, 1988	Prevent fetal death.	A post-term fetus with signs of distress or oligohydramnois is at high risk for intrauterine fetal death.
50.	Pregnancies with reliable dates should not extend beyond 44 weeks.	II-1+	Shime et al., 1984; Dyson et al., 1987; Witter and Weitz, 1987; Dyson, 1988	Prevent fetal death.	Risk of fetal death increased in pregnancies greater than 44 weeks.
	Pregnancy-Induced Hypertension (PIH)				
51.	If PIH diagnosed and patient is not admitted, bedrest should be recommended & a return visit should occur w/in 1 week.	II-2+	Sibai, 1988	Prevent complications of PIH (e.g., seizure, placental abruption, or fetal or maternal death).	May allow delay of delivery until maturity.
52.	If PIH diagnosed and pregnancy is at term (> 37 weeks), either labor should be induced or delivery by cesarean section should take place.	II-2+	Thiagarajah et al., 1984; Cunningham and Pritchard, 1984	Reduce risk of seizure, placental abruption, and death.	Increased risk of induction and cesarean delivery when compared to spontaneous vaginal delivery. Risk probably offset by reducing PIH complications.

233

53.	If severe PIH is diagnosed by any of the following: (systolic >160 mm Hg, diastolic >110 mm Hg, 3-4+ proteinuria, pulmonary edema, oliguria, RUQ pain or seizures), patient should be admitted to induce labor or deliver by cesarean section.	II-2+	ACOG, 1986; Lindheimer and Katz, 1985	Decreases risk of PIH complications (see above).	Should consider transfering cases to a tertiary care center.

Gestational Diabetes Mellitus

54.	Pregnant women with abnormal 3-hour glucose tolerance tests should receive dietary counseling from a dietician.	I+	CDC, 1986; ACOG, 1994	Reduce blood glucose levels and eliminate the need for insulin therapy.	Gestational diabetes can often be managed with diet alone.
55.	Pregnant women on dietary therapy with 2 or more consecutive abnormal fasting (>105 mg/dL) or postprandial (>120 mg/dL one-hour post) plasma glucose tests should be placed on insulin therapy.	I+	ADA, 1986; ACOG, 1994	Reduce risk of macrosomia and neonatal complications (e.g., hypogylcemia, hypocalcemia).	If hyperglycemia persists on dietary therapy, insulin is indicated.
56.	An oral agent should not be used in diabetic pregnant women.	I+	ADA, 1986; ACOG, 1994	Prevent birth defects.	Oral hypoglycemics are teratogenic.

Follow-up

	Indicator	Quality of evidence	Literature	Benefits	Comments
	Infections and Sexually Transmitted Diseases				
	Asymptomatic Bacteriuria				
57.	Pregnant women treated for positive cultures should receive a post-treatment follow-up culture within one month of completing treatment.	I+	Patterson and Andriole, 1987	Prevent pyelonephritis and its complications (e.g., preterm birth, hospitalization).	Testing for failure of initial treatment.
	Syphilis				
58.	Pregnant women diagnosed with syphilis in pregnancy should be followed up with monthly serology and retreated if necessary.	II-3+	CDC, 1988	Prevent congenital syphilis.	Assures adequate treatment.
	Gonorrhea				
59.	Pregnant women with positive cultures should receive a post-treatment follow-up culture 4-7 days after treatment is completed.	III+	Hook and Holmes, 1985	Prevent spread of disease to infant and other sexual partners.	Testing for failure of initial treatment.
	Chlamydia				
60.	Pregnant women with positive cultures should receive a post-treatment follow-up culture 4-7 days after treatment is completed.	III	CDC, 1993	Prevent spread of disease to infant and other sexual partners.	Allows identification of treatment failures and further follow-up.
	Common Pregnancy Complications				
	Gestational Diabetes Mellitus				
61.	Pregnant women with abnormal 3-hour plasma glucose tolerance tests who are on dietary therapy should have biweekly fasting or postprandial glucose tests.	I+	ACOG, 1994	Prevent fetal macrosomia.	Identify those women at increased risk for macrosomia and treat with insulin. Biweekly glucose testing will indicate whether or not dietary treatment requires modification.

Quality of Evidence Codes:

I: RCT
II-1:   Nonrandomized controlled trials
II-2:   Cohort or case analysis
II-3:   Multiple time series
III: Opinions or descriptive studies

+:   Individual process studied only as part of an overall intervention

235

REFERENCES - PRENATAL CARE

Abel EL, and RJ Sokol. 22 November 1986. Fetal alcohol syndrome is now leading cause of mental retardation. *Lancet* 2: 1222.

Adams MM, JS Marks, and JP Koplan. 1984. Cost implications of routine antenatal administration of Rh immune globulin. American Journal of Obstetrics and Gynecology 149 (6): 633-8.

Alexander ER. 1988. Gonorrhea in the newborn. *Annals of the New York Academy of Sciences* 549: 180-6.

Allen CD, and CP Ries. May 1985. Smoking, alcohol, and dietary practices during pregnancy: Comparison before and after prenatal education. *Journal of the American Dietetic Association* 85: 605-6.

Amaro H, LE Fried, H Cabral, et al. May 1990. Violence during pregnancy and substance use. *American Journal of Public Health* 80 (5): 575-9.

American Academy of Pediatrics, and Task Force on Pediatric AIDS. December 1988. Perinatal human immunodeficiency virus infection. *Pediatrics* 82 (6): 941-44.

American College of Obstetricians and Gynecologists. 1994. Diabetes and Pregnancy. *ACOG Technical Bulletin* 200: 1-8.

American College of Obstetricians and Gynecologists. July 1989. Diagnosis and management of postterm pregnancy. *ACOG Technical Bulletin* 130: 1-4.

American College of Obstetricians and Gynecologists. February 1986. Management of preeclampsia. *ACOG Technical Bulletin* 91: 1-5.

American College of Obstetricians and Gynecologists. 1992. Rubella and Pregnancy. *ACOG Technical Bulletin* 171: 1-6.

American Diabetes Association. 1986. Gestational diabetes mellitus. *Annals of Internal Medicine* 105: 461.

American Medical Association. 25 December 1987. Questions and answers: Diagnostic and therapeutic technology assessment (DATTA). *Journal of the American Medical Association* 258 (24): 3560-3.

American Medical Association. 23 September 1988. Questions and answers: Diagnostic and therapeutic technology assessment (DATTA). *Journal of the American Medical Association* 260 (12): 1779-82.

Andersen HF, TRB Johnson, JD Floar, et al. 1 August 1981. Gestational age assessment. II. Prediction from combined clinical observations. *American Journal of Obstetrics and Gynecology* 140: 770-4.

Anionwu EN, N Patel, G Kanji, et al. 1988. Counselling for prenatal diagnosis of sickle cell disease and beta thalassaemia major: A four year experience. *Journal of Medical Genetics* 25: 769-772.

Arevalo JA, and M Arevalo. 1989. Prevalence of hepatitis B in an indigent, multi-ethnic community clinic prenatal population. *Journal of Family Practice* 29 (6): 615-9.

Arevalo JA, and AE Washington. 15 January 1988. Cost-effectiveness of prenatal screening and immunization for hepatitis B virus. *Journal of the American Medical Association* 259 (3): 365-9.

Arias F. July 1987. Predictability of complications associated with prolongation of pregnancy. *Obstetrics and Gynecology* 70 (1): 101-6.

Aro T, J Haapakoski, OP Heinonen, et al. 1984. Lack of association between vitamin intake during early pregnancy and reduction limb defects. *American Journal of Obstetrics and Gynecology* 150 (4): 433.

Baker CJ, MA Rench, MS Edwards, et al. 3 November 1988. Immunization of pregnant women with a polysaccharide vaccine of group B streptococcus. *New England Journal of Medicine* 319 (18): 1180-5.

Bakketeig LS, SH Eik-Nes, G Jacobsen, et al. 28 July 1984. Randomised controlled trial of ultrasonographic screening in pregnancy. *Lancet* 2: 207-11.

Barton JJ, TM O'Connor, MJ Cannon, et al. 1989. Prevalence of human immunodeficiency virus in a general prenatal population. *American Journal of Obstetrics and Gynecology* 160 (6): 1316-24.

BCSH General Haematology Task Force. 1988. Guidelines for haemoglobinopathy screening. *Clinical and Laboratory Haematology* 10: 87-94.

Beasley RP, and L Hwang. 1984. Epidemiology of Hepatocellular Carcinoma. In *Viral Hepatitis and Liver Disease*. Editor Vyas GN, 209-24. Orlando, Fl: Grune & Stratton.

Beasley RP, L Hwang, GC Lee, et al. 12 November 1983. Prevention of perinatally transmitted hepatitis B virus infections with hepatitis B immune globulin and hepatitis B vaccine. *Lancet* 2: 1099-1102.

Benedetti TJ, and T Easterling. March 1988. Antepartum testing in postterm pregnancy. *Journal of Reproductive Medicine* 33 (3): 252-8.

Benigni A, G Gregorini, T Frusca, et al. 10 August 1989. Effect of low-dose aspirin on fetal and maternal generation of thromboxane by platelets in women at risk for pregnancy-induced hypertension. *New England Journal of Medicine* 321 (6): 357-62.

Bennett MJ, G Little, J Sir Dewhurst, et al. May 1982. Predictive value of ultrasound measurement in early pregnancy: A randomized controlled trial. *British Journal of Obstetrics and Gynecology* 89: 338-41.

Black NA, A Parsons, JB Kurtz, et al. 29 October 1983. Post-partum rubella immunisation: A controlled trial of two vaccines. *Lancet* 2: 990-2.

Bochner CJ, AL Medearis, J Davis, et al. August 1987. Antepartum predictors of fetal distress in postterm pregnancy. *American Journal of Obstetrics and Gynecology* 157 (2): 353-8.

Bochner CJ, J Williams III, L Castro, et al. September 1988. The efficacy of starting postterm antenatal testing at 41 weeks as compared with 42 weeks of gestational age. *American Journal of Obstetrics and Gynecology* 159 (3): 550-4.

Boehm CD, SE Antonarakis, JA Phillips, et al. 5 May 1983. Prenatal diagnosis using DNA polymorphisms: Report on 95 pregnancies at risk for sickle-cell disease or beta-thalassemia. *New England Journal of Medicine* 308 (18): 1054-8.

Boppart I, D Brook, L Dallaire, et al. 1985. Maternal serum alpha-fetoprotein screening for neural tube defects: results of a consensus meeting. *Prenatal Diagnostics* 77: 77-83.

Boyer KM, and SP Gotoff. December 1988. Antimicrobial prophylaxis of neonatal group B streptococcal sepsis. *Clinics in Perinatology* 15 (4): 831-50.

Boyer KM, and SP Gotoff. 26 June 1986. Prevention of early-onset group B streptococcal disease with selective intrapartum chemoprophylaxis. *New England Journal of Medicine* 314 (26): 1665-9.

Braveman P, G Oliva, MG Miller, et al. 24 August 1989. Adverse outcomes and lack of health insurance among newborns in an eight-county area of California, 1982 to 1986. *New England Journal of Medicine* 321 (8): 508-13.

Brown JE, HN Jacobson, LH Askue, et al. January 1981. Influence of pregnancy weight gain on the size of infants born to underweight women. *Obstetrics and Gynecology* 57 (1): 13-7.

Browne JCM. 1 March 1963. Postmaturity. *American Journal of Obstetrics and Gynecology* 85 (5): 573-82.

Burton BK, SG Sowers, and LH Nelson. 15 June 1983. Maternal serum alpha-fetoprotein screening in North Carolina: Experience with more than twelve thousand pregnancies. *American Journal of Obstetrics and Gynecology* 146 (4): 439-44.

Campbell-Brown M, IR McFadyen, DV Seal, et al. 20 June 1987. Is screening for bacteriuria in pregnancy worth while? *British Medical Journal* 294: 1579-82.

Campbell S, SL Warsof, D Little, et al. May 1985. Routine ultrasound screening for the prediction of gestational age. *Obstetrics and Gynecology* 65 (5): 613-20.

Campbell TL. 1987. Maternal serum alpha-fetoprotein screening: Benefits, risks, and costs. *Journal of Family Practice* 25 (5): 461-7.

Centers for Disease Control. 24 September 1993. 1993 sexually transmitted diseases treatment guidelines. *Morbidity and Mortality Weekly Report* 42 (RR-14): 1-102.

Centers for Disease Control. 23 August 1985. Chlamydia trachomatis infections. *Morbidity and Mortality Weekly Report* 34 (3S): 53S-74S.

Centers for Disease Control. 15 January 1988. Guidelines for the prevention and control of congenital syphilis. *Morbidity and Mortality Weekly Report* 37 (S-1): 1-13.

Centers for Disease Control. 1986. Perspectives in disease prevention and health promotion: Public health guidelines for enhancing diabetes control through maternal and child-health programs. *MMWR* 35 (13): 201-212.

Centers for Disease Control. 10 June 1988. Prevention of perinatal transmission of hepatitis B virus: Prenatal screening of all pregnant women for hepatitis B surface antigen. *Morbitiy and Mortality Weekly Report* 37 (22): 341-51.

Centers for Disease Control. 7 June 1985. Recommendations for protection against viral hepatitis. *Morbidity and Mortality Weekly Report* 34 (22): 313-35.

Centers for Disease Control. 19 December 1986. Rubella and congenital rubella syndrome--New York City. *Morbidity and Mortality Weekly Report* 35 (50): 770-9.

Centers for Disease Control. 16 October 1987. Rubella and congenital rubella--United States, 1984-1986. *Morbidity and Mortality Weekly Report* 36 (40): 664-76.

Centers for Disease Control. 5 May 1989. Rubella vaccination during pregnancy--United States, 1971-1988. *Morbidity and Mortality Weekly Report* 38 (17): 289-93.

Centers for Disease Control. 19 August 1988. Syphilis and congenital syphilis--United States, 1985-1988. *Morbidity and Mortality Weekly Report* 37 (32): 486-9.

Chasnoff IJ, KA Burns, and WJ Burns. 1987. Cocaine use in pregnancy: Perinatal morbidity and mortality. *Neurotoxicology and Teratology* 9: 291-3.

Chasnoff IJ, DR Griffith, S MacGregor, et al. 1989. Temporal patterns of cocaine use in pregnancy. *Journal of the American Medical Association* 261 (12): 1741-4.

Chasnoff IJ, HJ Landress, and ME Barrett. 26 April 1990. The prevalence of illicit-drug or alcohol use during pregnancy and discrepancies in mandatory reporting in Pinellas County, Florida. *New England Journal of Medicine* 322 (17): 1202-6.

Chavkin W. April 1990. Drug addiction and pregnancy: Policy crossroads. *American Journal of Public Health* 80 (4): 483-7.

Cherukuri R, H Minkoff, J Feldman, et al. August 1988. A cohort study of alkaloidal cocaine ("crack") in pregnancy. *Obstetrics and Gynecology* 72 (2): 147-51.

Chesley LC. March 1985. Diagnosis of preeclampsia. *Obstetrics and Gynecology* 65 (3): 423-5.

Chouteau M, BP Namerow, and P Leppert. September 1988. The effect of cocaine abuse on birth weight and gestational age. *Obstetrics and Gynecology* 72 (3, Part 1): 351-4.

Christian SS, and P Duff. August 1989. Is universal screening for hepatitis B infection warranted in all prenatal populations? *Obstetrics and Gynecology* 74 (2): 259-61.

Cnattingius S, B Haglund, and O Meirik. 23 July 1988. Cigarette smoking as risk factor for late fetal and early neonatal death. *British Medical Journal* 297: 258-61.

Cochlin DL. September 1984. Effects of two ultrasound scanning regimens on the management of pregnancy. *British Journal of Obstetrics and Gynecology* 91: 885-90.

Cohen I, J Veille, and BM Calkins. 20 June 1990. Improved pregnancy outcome following successful treatment of chlamydial infection. *Journal of the American Medical Association* 263 (23): 3160-3.

Collins TR, ST DeMellier, JD Leeper, et al. May 1985. Supplemental food program: Effects on health and pregnancy outcome. *Southern Medical Journal* 78 (5): 551-5.

Connor EM, RS Sperling, R Gelber, et al. 3 November 1994. Reduction of maternal-infant transmission of human immunodeficiency virus type 1 with zidovudine treatment. *New England Journal of Medicine* 331 (18): 1173-80.

Coustan DR, and J Imarah. 1 December 1984. Prophylactic insulin treatment of gestational diabetes reduces the incidence of macrosomia, operative delivery, and birth trauma. *American Journal of Obstetrics and Gynecology* 150 (7): 836-42.

Coustan DR, and SB Lewis. March 1978. Insulin therapy for gestational diabetes. *Obstetrics and Gynecology* 51 (3): 306-10.

Cruz AC, BH Frentzen, and M Behnke. May 1987. Hepatitis B: A case for prenatal screening of all patients. *American Journal of Obstetrics and Gynecology* 156 (5): 1180-3.

Cunningham, FG, PC MacDonald, and NF Gant. 1989. *Williams Obstetrics*. Norwalk, CT: Appleton and Lange.

Cunningham FG, and JA Pritchard. March 1984. How should hypertension during pregnancy be managed. *Medical Clinics of North America* 68 (2): 505-26.

Daugaard HO, AC Thomsen, U Henriques, et al. 1988. Group B streptococci in the lower urogenital tract and late abortions. *American Journal of Obstetrics and Gynecology* 158: 28-31.

Dawes MG, and JG Grudzinskas. February 1991. Repeated measurement of maternal weight during pregnancy. Is this a useful practice? *British Journal of Obstetrics and Gynaecology* 98: 189-94.

DiMaio MS, A Baumgarten, RM Greenstein, et al. 6 August 1987. Screening for fetal down's syndrome in pregnancy by measuring maternal serum alpha-fetoprotein levels. *New England Journal of Medicine* 317 (6): 342-78.

Doberczak TM, JC Thornton, J Bernstein, et al. November 1987. Impact of maternal drug dependency on birth weight and head circumference of offspring. *American Journal of Diseases in Children* 141: 1163-7.

Driscoll MC, N Lerner, K Anyane-Yeboa, et al. 1987. Prenatal diagnosis of sickle hemoglobinopathies: The experience of the Columbia University Comprehensive Center for Sickel Cell Disease. *American Journal of Human Genetics* 40: 548-58.

Dyson DC. 1988. Fetal surveillance vs. labor induction at 42 weeks in postterm gestation. *Journal of Reproductive Medicine* 33 (3): 262-70.

Dyson DC. April 1987. Management of prolonged pregnancy: Induction of labor versus antepartum fetal testing. *American Journal of Obstetrics and Gynecology* 156 (4): 928-34.

Eddy DM, V Hasselblad, W McGivney, et al. 11 March 1988. The value of mammography screening in women under age 50 years. *Journal of the American Medical Association* 259 (10): 1512-9.

Eden RD, RZ Gergely, BS Schifrin, et al. 15 November 1982. Comparison of antepartum testing schemes for the management of the postdate pregnancy. *American Journal of Obstetrics and Gynecology* 144 (6): 683-92.

Eik-Nes SH, O Okland, JC Aure, et al. 16 June 1984. Ultrasound screening in pregnancy: A randomised controlled trial. *Lancet* 1: 1347.

Embury SH, SJ Scharf, RK Saiki, et al. 12 March 1987. Rapid prenatal diagnosis of sickle cell anemia by a new method of DNA analysis. *New England Journal of Medicine* 316 (11): 656-61.

Ernhart CB, M Morrow-Tlucak, RJ Sokol, et al. July 1988. Underreporting of alcohol use in pregnancy. *Alcoholism: Clinical and Experimental Research* 12 (4): 506-11.

Ernhart CB, RJ Sokol, JW Ager, et al. 1989. Alcohol-related birth defects: Assessing the risk. *Annals of the New York Academy of Sciences* 562: 159-72.

Ershoff DH, NK Aaronson, BG Danaher, et al. November 1983. Behavioral, health, and cost outcomes of an HMO-based prenatal health education program. *Public Health Reports* 98 (6): 536-47.

Ershoff DH, PD Mullen, and VP Quinn. February 1989. A randomized trial of a serialized self-help smoking cessation program for pregnant women in an HMO. *American Journal of Public Health* 79 (2): 182-7.

Evans S, FD Frigoletto Jr., and JF Jewett. 29 December 1983. Report from the Committee on Maternal Welfare-Mortality of eclampsia: A case report and the experience of the Massachusetts Maternal Mortality Study, 1954-1982. *New England Journal of Medicine* 309 (26): 1644-7.

Ewigman B, M LeFevre, and J Hesser. August 1990. A randomized trial of routine prenatal ultrasound. *Obstetrics and Gynecology* 76 (2): 189-194.

Fay RA, DR Bromham, JA Brooks, et al. 15 August 1985. Platelets and uric acid in the prediction of preeclampsia. *American Journal of Obstetrics and Gynecology* 152 (8): 1038-9.

Field T, D Sandberg, TA Quetel, et al. October 1985. Effects of ultrasound feedback on pregnancy anxiety, fetal activity, and neonatal outcome. *Obstetrics and Gynecology* 66 (4): 525-8.

Fingerhut LA, JC Kleinman, and JS Kendrick. May 1990. Smoking before, during, and after pregnancy. *American Journal of Public Health* 80 (5): 541-4.

Friedman SM, L DeSilva, HE Fox, et al. March 1988. Hepatitis B screening in a New York City obstetrics service. *American Journal of Public Health* 78 (3): 308-10.

1988. *Guidelines for Perinatal Care*, Second ed. Editors Frigoletto FD, and GA Little,Elk Grove Village, IL: American Academy of Pediatrics and American College of Obstetricians and Gynecologists.

Fuhrmann W. 1985. Maternal serum alpha-fetoprotein screening for neural tube defects: Results of a consensus meeting. *Prenatal Diagnosis* 5: 77-83.

Gibbs RS, MS Amstey, RL Sweet, et al. May 1988. Management of genital herpes infection in pregnancy. *Obstetrics and Gynecology* 71 (5): 779-80.

Goldenberg RL. 1990. Intrauterine growth retardation. In *New Perspectives on Prenatal Care*. Editors Merkatz IR, and JE Thompson, 461-79. New York, NY: Elsevier Science Publishing Co., Inc.

Goldenberg RL, GR Cutter, HJ Hoffman, et al. 1989. Intrauterine growth retardation: Standards for diagnosis. *American Journal of Obstetrics and Gynecology* 161 (2): 271-7.

Goldenberg RL, RO Davis, GR Cutter, et al. 1 1989. Prematurity, postdates, and growth retardation: The influence of use of ultrasonography on reported gestational age. *American Journal of Obstetrics and Gynecology* 160 (2): 462-70.

Goossens M, Y Dumez, L Kaplan, et al. 6 October 1983. Prenatal diagnosis of sickle-cell anemia in the first trimester of pregnancy. *New England Journal of Medicine* 309 (14): 831-3.

Gorsky RD, and JP Colby Jr. December 1989. The cost effectiveness of prenatal care in reducing low birth weight in New Hampshire. *Health Services Research* 24 (5): 583-98.

Graham K, G Koren, J Klein, et al. 15 December 1989. Determination of gestational cocaine exposure by hair analysis. *Journal of the American Medical Association* 262 (23): 3328-30.

Greenspoon JS, J Martin, RL Greenspoon, et al. September 1989. Necessity for routine obstetric screening for hepatitis B surface antigen. *Journal of Reproductive Medicine* 34 (9): 655-8.

Griffiths PD, and C Baboonian. 1982. Is post partum rubella vaccination worthwhile? *Journal of Clinical Pathology* 35: 1340-4.

Halmesmaki E, KO Raivio, and O Ylikorkala. April 1987. Patterns of alcohol consumption during pregnancy. *Obstetrics and Gynecology* 69 (4): 594-7.

Halmesmaki E. March 1988. Alcohol counseling of 85 pregnant problem drinkers: Effect on drinking and fetal outcome. *British Journal of Obstetrics and Gynecology* 95: 243-7.

Hardy JB, GH McCracken, MR Gilkeson, et al. 31 March 1969. Adverse fetal outcome following maternal rubella after the first trimester of pregnancy. *Journal of the American Medical Association* 207 (13): 2414-20.

Harrison HR, ER Alexander, L Weinstein, et al. 7 October 1983. Cervical chlamydia trachomatis and mycoplasmal infections in pregnancy: Epidemiology and outcomes. *Journal of the American Medical Association* 250 (13): 1721-7.

Hebel JR, P Nowicki, and M Sexton. 1985. The effect of antismoking intervention during pregnancy: An assessment of interactions with maternal characteristics. *American Journal of Epidemiology* 122 (1): 135-48.

Hemminki E. February 1988. Content of prenatal care in the United States: A historic perspective. *Medical Care* 26 (2): 199-210.

Hemminki E, and B Starfield. 1978. Routine administration of iron and vitamins during pregnancy: Review of controlled clinical trials. *British Journal of Obstetrics and Gynaecology* 85: 404-10.

Hensleigh PA. 1 August 1983. Preventing rhesus isoimmunization: Antepartum Rh immune globulin prophylaxis versus a sensitive test for risk identification. *American Journal of Obstetrics and Gynecology* 146 (7): 749-55.

Hibbard BM. 19 November 1988. Iron and folate supplements during pregnancy: Supplementation is valuable only in selected patients. *British Medical Journal* 297: 1324-5.

Hickner J, A Cousineau, and S Messimer. 1990. Smoking cessation during pregnancy: Strategies used by Michigan family physicians. *Journal of the American Board of Family Practice* 3 (1): 39-42.

Hoff R, VP Berardi, BJ Weiblen, et al. 3 March 1988. Seroprevalence of human immunodeficiency virus among childbearing women: Estimation by testing samples of blood from newborns. *New England Journal of Medicine* 318 (9): 526-30.

Hollingsworth DR, OW Jones, and R Resnik. 15 August 1984. Expanded care in obstetrics for the 1980s: Preconception and early postconception counseling. *American Journal of Obstetrics and Gynecology* 149 (8): 811-4.

Hook III EW, and KK Holmes. 1985. Gonococcal infections. *Annals of Internal Medicine* 102 (2): 229-43.

Hooker JG, M Lucas, BA Richards, et al. 1984. Is maternal alpha-fetoprotein screening still of value in a low risk area for neural tube defects? *Prenatal Diagnosis* 4: 29-33.

Horn E. 19 November 1988. Iron and folate supplements during pregnancy: Supplementing everyone treats those at risk and is cost effective. *British Medical Journal* 297: 1325-7.

Institute of Medicine. 1985. *Preventing Low Birthweight*. Washington, DC: National Academy Press.

Investigators of the Johns Hopkins Study of Cervicitis and Adverse Pregnancy Outcome. 1989. Association of chlamydia trachomatis and mycoplasma hominis with intrauterine growth retardation and preterm delivery. *American Journal of Epidemiology* 129 (6): 1247-57.

Johnson JM, CR Harman, IR Lange, et al. February 1986. Biophysical profile scoring in the management of the postterm pregnancy: An analysis of 307 patients. *American Journal of Obstetrics and Gynecology* 154 (2): 269-73.

Jonas MM, ER Schiff, MJ O'Sullivan, et al. 1987. Failure of Centers for Disease Control criteria to identify hepatitis B infection in a large municipal obstetrical population. *Annals of Internal Medicine* 107 (3): 335-7.

Jones KL, and DW Smith. 3 November 1973. Recognition of the fetal alcohol syndrome in early infancy. *Lancet* 2: 999-1001.

Joyce T. June 1990. The dramatic increase in the rate of low birthweight in New York City: An aggregate time-series analysis. *American Journal of Public Health* 80 (6): 682-4.

Kaminski M, C Rumeau, and D Schwartz. April 1978. Alcohol consumption in pregnant women and the outcome of pregnancy. *Alcoholism: Clinical and Experimental Research* 2 (2): 155-63.

Kaye K, L Elkind, D Goldberg, et al. May 1989. Birth outcomes for infants of drug abusing mothers. *New York State Journal of Medicine* 89: 256-61.

Keith LG, S MacGregor, S Friedell, et al. May 1989. Substance abuse in pregnant women: Recent experience at the Perinatal Center for Chemical Dependence of Northwestern Memorial Hospital. *Obstetrics and Gynecology* 73 (No. 5, Part 1): 715-20.

Kennedy ET, and M Kotelchuck. 1984. The effect of WIC supplemental feeding on birth weight: A case-control analysis. *American Journal of Clinical Nutrition* 40: 579-85.

Kessner, DM, J Singer, CE Kalk, et al. 1973. *Infant Death: An Analysis by Maternal Risk and Health Care*. Washington, DC: National Academy of Sciences.

Khoury MJ, A Weinstein, S Panny, et al. 1987. Maternal cigarette smoking and oral clefts: A population-based study. *American Journal of Public Health* 77 (5): 623-5.

Khouzami VA, JWC Johnson, NH Daikoku, et al. March 1983. Comparison of urinary estrogens, contraction stress tests and nonstress tests in the management of postterm pregnancy. *Journal of Reproductive Medicine* 28 (3): 189-94.

Kincaid-Smith P, and M Bullen. 20 February 1965. Bacteriuria in pregnancy. *Lancet* 1: 395-399.

Klebanoff MA, PH Shiono, HW Berendes, et al. 28 July 1989. Facts and artifacts about anemia and preterm delivery. *Journal of the American Medical Association* 262 (4): 511-5.

Kleinman JC, and A Kopstein. July 1987. Smoking during pregnancy, 1967-80. *American Journal of Public Health* 77 (7): 823-5.

Kleinman JC, MB Pierre, JH Madans, et al. 1988. The effects of maternal smoking on fetal and infant mortality. *American Journal of Epidemiology* 127 (2): 274-82.

Klonoff-Cohen HS, DA Savitz, RC Cefalo, et al. 8 December 1989. An epidemiologic study of contraception and preeclampsia. *Journal of the American Medical Association* 262 (22): 3143-7.

Kotelchuck M, JB Schwartz, MT Anderka, et al. October 1984. WIC participation and pregnancy outcomes: Massachusetts statewide evaluation project. *American Journal of Public Health* 74 (10): 1086-92.

Kramer MS, FH McLean, ME Boyd, et al. 9 December 1988. The validity of gestational age estimation by menstrual dating in term, preterm, and postterm gestations. *Journal of the American Medical Association* 260 (22): 3306-8.

Kremkau FW. June 1984. Safety and long-term effects of ultrasound: What to tell your patients. *Clinical Obstetrics and Gynecology* 27 (2): 269-75.

Kruse J, M Le Fevre, and S Zweig. May 1986. Changes in smoking and alcohol consumption during pregnancy: A population-based study in a rural area. *Obstetrics and Gynecology* 67 (5): 627-32.

Kumar ML, NV Dawson, AJ McCullough, et al. September 1987. Should all pregnant women be screened for hepatitis B? *Annals of Internal Medicine* 107 (2): 273-7.

Lagrew DC, and RK Freeman. 1986. Management of postdate pregnancy. *American Journal of Obstetrics and Gynecology* 154 (1): 8-13.

Langer O. 1990. Critical issues in diabetes and pregnancy: Early identification, metabolic control, and prevention of adverse outcome. In *New Perspectives on Prenatal Care*. Editors Merkatz IR, and JE Thompson, 445-59. New York, NY: Elsevier Science Publishing Co., Inc.

Layde PM, SD von Allmen, and GP Oakley Jr. June 1979. Maternal serum alpha-fetoprotein screening: A cost-benefit analysis. *American Journal of Public Health* 69 (6): 566-73.

Lieberman E, KJ Ryan, RR Monson, et al. 1988. Association of maternal hematocrit with premature labor. *American Journal of Obstetrics and Gynecology* 159 (1): 107-14.

Lindheimer MD, and AI Katz. 12 September 1985. Current concepts: Hypertension in pregnancy. *New England Journal of Medicine* 313 (11): 675-80.

Lindsay MK, HB Peterson, TI Feng, et al. September 1989. Routine antepartum human immunodeficiency virus infection screening in an inner-city population. *Obstetrics and Gynecology* 74 (No. 3, Part 1): 289-94.

Little BB, LM Snell, and LC Gilstrap III. October 1988. Methamphetamine abuse during pregnancy: Outcome and fetal effects. *Obstetrics and Gynecology* 72 (4): 541-4.

Little RE. December 1977. Moderate alcohol use during pregnancy and decreased infant birth weight. *American Journal of Public Health* 67 (12): 1154-6.

Macri JN, and RR Weiss. 1982. Prenatal serum alpha-fetoprotein screening for neural tube defects. *Obstetrics and Gynecology* 59 (5): 633-9.

Main DM, and SG Gabbe. October 1987. Risk scoring for preterm labor: Where do we go from here? *American Journal of Obstetrics and Gynecology* 157 (No. 4, Part 1): 789-93.

Malecki JM, O Guarin, A Hulbert, et al. March 1986. Prevalence of hepatitis B surface antigen among women receiving prenatal care at the Palm Beach County Health Department. *American Journal of Obstetrics and Gynecology* 154: 625-6.

Martin DH, L Koutsky, DA Eschenbach, et al. 19 March 1982. Prematurity and perinatal mortality in pregnancies complicated by maternal chlamydia trachomatis infections. *Journal of the American Medical Association* 247 (11): 1585-8.

Mayer JP, B Hawkins, and R Todd. January 1990. A randomized evaluation of smoking cessation interventions for pregnant women at a WIC clinic. *American Journal of Public Health* 80 (1): 76-8.

McIntosh ID. March 1984. Smoking and pregnancy: Attributable risk and public health implications. *Canadian Journal of Public Health* 75: 141-8.

McMillan JA, LB Weiner, HV Lamberson, et al. 1985. Efficacy of maternal screening and therapy in the prevention of chlamydia infection of the newborn. *Infection* 13: 263-66.

McQuillan GM, TR Townsend, CB Johannes, et al. 1987. Prevention of perinatal transmission of hepatitis B virus: The sensitivity, specificity, and predicitive value of the recommended screening questions to detect high-risk women in an obstetric population. *American Journal of Epidemiology* 126 (3): 484-91.

Mercado A, G Johnson Jr., D Calver, et al. 1989. Cocaine, pregnancy, and postpartum intracerebral hemorrhage. *Obstetrics and Gynecology* 73: 467-8.

Merkatz IR, MA Duchon, TS Yamashita, et al. May 1980. A pilot community-based screening program for gestational diabetes. *Diabetes Care* 3 (3): 453-7.

1990. *New Perspectives on Prenatal Care*. Editors Merkatz IR, and JE Thompson,New York, NY: Elsevier Science Publishing Co., Inc.

Metcoff J, P Costiloe, WM Crosby, et al. May 1985. Effect of food supplementation (WIC) during pregnancy on birth weight. *American Journal of Clinical Nutrition* 41: 933-47.

Miller E, JW Hare, JP Cloherty, et al. 28 May 1981. Elevated maternal hemoglobin A(1c) in early pregnancy and major congenital anomalies in infants of diabetic mothers. *New England Journal of Medicine* 304 (22): 1331-4.

Mills JL, BI Graubard, EE Harley, et al. 12 October 1984. Maternal alcohol consumption and birth weight. *Journal of the American Medical Association* 252 (14): 1875-9.

Mills JL, GG Rhoads, JL Simpson, et al. 17 August 1989. The absence of a relation between the periconceptional use of vitamins and neural-tube defects. *New England Journal of Medicine* 321 (7): 430-5.

Milunsky A, and E Alpert. 21 September 1984. Results and benefits of a maternal serum alpha-fetoprotein screening program. *Journal of the American Medical Association* 252 (11): 1438-42.

Milunsky A, H Jick, SS Jick, et al. 24 November 1989. Multivitamin/folic acid supplementation in early pregnancy reduces the prevalence of neural tube defects. *Journal of the American Medical Association* 262 (20): 2847-52.

Milunsky A, SS Jick, CL Bruell, et al. 2 1989. Predictive values, relative risks, and overall benefits of high and low maternal serum alpha-fetoprotein screening in singleton pregnancies: New epidemiologic data. *American Journal of Obstetrics and Gynecology* 161: 291-7.

Minkoff HL, and SH Landesman. 1988. The case for routinely offering prenatal testing for human immunodeficiency virus infection. *Pediatrics* 82: 941-944.

Morrow-Tlucak M, CB Ernhart, RJ Sokol, et al. May 1989. Underreporting of alcohol use in pregnancy: Relationship to alcohol problem history. *Alcoholism: Clinical and Experimental Research* 13 (3): 399-401.

Murata, PJ, EA McGlynn, AL Siu, et al. 1992. *Prenatal Care: A Literature Review and Quality Assessment Criteria*. RAND, Santa Monica, CA.

Murphy JF, J O'Riordan, RG Newcombe, et al. 3 May 1986. Relation of haemoglobin levels in first and second trimesters to outcome of pregnancy. *Lancet* 1: 992-4.

Nadel AS, JK Green, LB Holmes, et al. 30 August 1990. Absence of need for amniocentesis in patients with elevated levels of maternal serum alpha-fetoprotein and normal ultrasonographic examinations. *New England Journal of Medicine* 323 (9): 557-61.

Naeye RL. 1979. Weight gain and the outcome of pregnancy. *American Journal of Obstetrics and Gynecology* 135 (1): 3-9.

Nanda D, J Feldman, I Delke, et al. 1990. Syphilis among parturients at an inner city hospital: Association with cocaine use and implications for congenital syphilis rates. *New York State Journal of Medicine* 90 (10): 488-90.

National Institutes of Health Consensus Conference. 3 August 1984. The use of diagnostic ultrasound imaging during pregnancy. *Journal of the American Medical Association* 252 (5): 669-72.

Neilson JP, SP Munjanja, and CR Whitfield. 3 November 1984. Screening for small for dates fetuses: A controlled trial. *British Medical Journal* 289: 1179-82.

Nesheim BI, I Benson, A Braekken, et al. 1987. Ultrasound in pregnancy. *International Journal of Technology Assessment in Health Care* 3: 463-70.

O'Connor MC. 17 August 1987. Drugs of abuse in pregnancy--an overview. *Medical Journal of Australia* 147: 180-3.

Olsen J, A da Costa Pereira, and SF Olsen. January 1991. Does maternal tobacco smoking modify the effect of alcohol on fetal growth? *American Journal of Public Health* 81 (1): 69-73.

Oro AS, and SD Dixon. 1987. Perinatal cocaine and methamphetamine exposure: Maternal and neonatal correlates. *Journal of Pediatrics* 111 (4): 571-8.

Orstead C, D Arrington, SK Kamath, et al. January 1985. Efficacy of prenatal nutrition counseling: Weight gain, infant birth weight, and cost-effectiveness. *Journal of the American Dietetic Association* 85 (1): 40-5.

Osterloh JD, and BL Lee. 1989. Urine drug screening in mothers and newborns. *American Journal of Diseases in Children* 143: 791-3.

O'Sullivan JB, SS Gellis, RV Dandrow, et al. May 1966. The potential diabetic and her treatment in pregnancy. *Obstetrics and Gynecology* 27 (5): 683-9.

O'Sullivan JB, CM Mahan, D Charles, et al. 1 August 1973. Screening criteria for high-risk gestational diabetic patients. *American Journal of Obstetrics and Gynecology* 116 (7): 895-900.

Ouellette EM, HL Rosett, P Rosman, et al. 8 September 1977. Adverse effects on offspring of maternal alcohol abuse during pregnancy. *New England Journal of Medicine* 297 (10): 528-30.

Patterson TF, and VT Andriole. December 1987. Bacteriuria in pregnancy. *Infectious Disease Clinics of North America* 1 (4): 807-22.

Pels RJ, DH Bor, S Woolhandler, et al. 1 September 1989. Dipstick urinalysis screening of asymptomatic adults for urinary tract disorders. *Journal of the American Medical Association* 262 (9): 1221-4.

Persson B, M Stangenberg, U Hansson, et al. 1985. Gestational diabetes mellitus (GDM): Comparative evaluation of two treatment regimens, diet versus insulin and diet. *Diabetes* 34 (Suppl 2): 101-5.

Petitti DB, and C Coleman. 1990. Cocaine and the risk of low birth weight. *American Journal of Public Health* 80 (1): 25-8.

Poovorawan Y, S Sanpavat, W Pongpunlert, et al. 9 June 1989. Protective efficacy of a recombinant DNA hepatitis B vaccine in neonates of HBe antigen-positive mothers. *Journal of the American Medical Association* 261 (22): 3278-81.

Pritchard JA, FG Cunningham, and SA Pritchard. 1 April 1984. The Parkland Memorial Hospital protocol for treatment of eclampsia: Evaluation of 245 cases. *American Journal of Obstetrics and Gynecology* 148 (7): 951-63.

Prober CG, PA Hensleigh, FB Boucher, et al. 7 April 1988. Use of routine viral cultures at delivery to identify neonates exposed to herpes simplex virus. *New England Journal of Medicine* 318 (14): 887-91.

Pyati SP, RS Pildes, NM Jacobs, et al. 9 June 1983. Penicillin in infants weighing two kilograms or less with early-onset group B streptococcal disease. *New England Journal of Medicine* 308 (23): 1383-9.

Reading AE, and DN Cox. 1982. The effects of ultrasound examination on maternal anxiety levels. *Journal of Behavioral Medicine* 5 (2): 237-47.

Redman CWG, and M Jefferies. 9 April 1988. Revised definition of pre-eclampsia. *Lancet* 1: 809-12.

Reece J, PR Donovan, and AY Pellett. December 1987. Iron supplementation in pregnancy: Testing a new clinic protocol. *Journal of the American Dietetic Association* 87 (12): 1682-3.

Regan JA, S Chao, and LS James. 1981. Premature rupture of membranes, preterm delivery, and group B streptococcal colonization of mothers. *American Journal of Obstetrics and Gynecology* 141 (2): 184-6.

Reuwer PJH, EA Sijmons, GW Rietman, et al. 22 August 1987. Intrauterine growth retardation: Prediction of perinatal distress by Doppler ultrasound. *Lancet* 2: 415-18.

Robinson L, P Grau, and BF Crandall. July 1989. Pregnancy outcomes after increasing maternal serum alpha-fetoprotein levels. *Obstetrics and Gynecology* 74 (1): 17-20.

Robitaille Y, and MS Kramer. October 1985. Does participation in prenatal courses lead to heavier babies. *American Journal of Public Health* 75 (10): 1186-9.

Rogers MS, and PG Needham. 1985. Evaluation of fundal height measurement in antenatal care. *Australian and New Zealand Journal of Obstetrics and Gynaecology* 25: 87-90.

Romero R, E Oyarzun, M Mazor, et al. 1989. Meta-analysis of the relationship between asymptomatic bacteriuria and preterm delivery/low birth weight. *Obstetrics and Gynacology* 73 (4): 576-82.

Rosett HL, and L Weiner. 15 July 1981. Identifying and treating pregnant patients at risk from alcohol. *Canadian Medical Association Journal* 125: 149-54.

Rosett HL, L Weiner, and KC Edelin. 15 April 1983. Treatment experience with pregnant problem drinkers. *Journal of the American Medical Association* 249 (15): 2029-33.

Rosner MA, L Keith, and I Chasnoff. 1982. The Northwestern University Drug Dependence Program: The impact of intensive prenatal care on labor and delivery outcomes. *American Journal of Obstetrics and Gynecology* 144 (23): 23-7.

Rothenberg R. 1979. Ophthalmia neonatorum due to Neisseria gonorrhoeae: Prevention and treatment. *Sexually Transmitted Diseases* 6 (2, Suppl): 187-91.

Rush D. 15 September 1981. Nutritional services during pregnancy and birthweight: A retrospective matched pair analysis. *Canadian Medical Association Journal* 125: 567-76.

Rush D, JM Alvir, DA Kenny, et al. 1988. Historical study of pregnancy outcomes. *American Journal of Clinical Nutrition* 48: 412-28.

Rush D, Z Stein, and M Susser. April 1980. A randomized controlled trial of prenatal nutritional supplementation in New York City. *Pediatrics* 65 (4): 683-97.

Sadovnick AD, and PA Baird. 1983. A cost-benefit analysis of a population screening programme for neural tube defects. *Prenatal Diagnosis* 3: 117-126.

Sadovnick AD, and PA Baird. July 1982. Maternal age-specific costs of detecting down syndrome and neural tube defects. *Canadian Journal of Public Health* 73: 248-50.

Saito M, K Yazaw, A Hashiguchi, et al. 1 January 1972. Time of ovulation and prolonged pregnancy. *American Journal of Obstetrics and Gynecology* 112 (1): 31-8.

Schachter J, M Grossman, RL Sweet, et al. 27 June 1986. Prospective study of perinatal transmission of chlamydia trachomatis. *Journal of the American Medical Association* 255 (24): 3374-7.

Schachter J, RL Sweet, M Grossman, et al. 30 January 1986. Experience with the routine use of erythromycin for chlamydial infections in pregnancy. *New England Journal of Medicine* 314 (5): 276-9.

Schalm SW, JA Mazel, GC de Gast, et al. June 1989. Prevention of hepatitis B infection in newborns through mass screening and delayed vaccination of all infants of mothers with hepatitis B surface antigen. *Pediatrics* 83 (6): 1041-8.

Schiff E, E Peleg, M Goldenberg, et al. 10 August 1989. The use of aspirin to prevent pregnancy-induced hypertension and lower the ratio of thromboxane A(2) to prostacyclin in relatively high risk pregnancies. *New England Journal of Medicine* 321 (6): 351-6.

Schulz KF, W Cates Jr., and PR O'Mara. 1987. Pregnancy loss, infant death, and suffering: Legacy of syphilis and gonorrhoea in Africa. *Genitourinary Medicine* 63: 320-5.

Scott GB, C Hutto, RW Makuch, et al. 28 December 1989. Survival in children with perinatally acquired human immunodeficiency virus type 1 infection. *New England Journal of Medicine* 321 (26): 1791-6.

Seeds JW. October 1984. Impaired fetal growth: Ultrasonic evaluation and clinical management. *Obstetrics and Gynecology* 64 (4): 577-84.

Sexton M, and JR Hebel. 17 February 1984. A clinical trial of change in maternal smoking and its effect on birth weight. *Journal of the American Medical Association* 251 (7): 911-5.

Shapiro H, and E Lyons. 1989. Late maternal age and postdate pregnancy. *American Journal of Obstetrics and Gynecology* 160 (4): 909-12.

Shime J, DJ Gare, J Andrews, et al. 1984. Prolonged pregnancy: Surveillance of the fetus and the neonate and the course of labor and delivery. *American Journal of Obstetrics and Gynecology* 148 (5): 547-52.

Shiono PH, MA Klebanoff, and GG Rhoads. 3 January 1986. Smoking and drinking during pregnancy: Their effects on preterm birth. *Journal of the American Medical Association* 255 (1): 82-4.

Showstack JA, PP Budetti, and D Minkler. September 1984. Factors associated with birthweight: An exploration of the roles of prenatal care and length of gestation. *American Journal of Public Health* 74 (9): 1003-8.

Sibai BM. July 1988. Pitfalls in diagnosis and management of preeclampsia. *American Journal of Obstetrics and Gynecology* 159 (1): 1-5.

Sibai BM, AR Gonzalez, WC Mabie, et al. 1987. A comparison of labetalol plus hospitalization versus hospitalization alone in the management of preeclampsia remote from term. *Obstetrics and Gynecology* 70 (No. 3, Part 1): 323-7.

Sibai BM, JM Graham, and JH McCubbin. 1984. A comparison of intravenous and intramuscular magnesium sulfate regimens in preeclampsia. *American Journal of Obstetrics and Gynecology* 150 (6): 728-33.

Sibai BM, M Taslimi, TN Abdella, et al. 1985. Maternal and perinatal outcome of conservative management of severe preeclampsia in midtrimester. *American Journal of Obstetrics and Gynecology* 152 (1): 32-7.

Siegel JD, GH McCracken Jr., N Threlkeld, et al. 2 October 1980. Single-dose penicillin prophylaxis against neonatal group B streptococcal infections. *New Enlgna Journal of Medicine* 303 (14): 769-75.

Singer DE, JH Samet, CM Coley, et al. 15 October 1988. Screening for diabetes mellitus. *Annals of Internal Medicine* 109: 639-49.

Slater RM, FL Wilcox, WD Smith, et al. 20 June 1987. Phenytoin infusion in severe pre-eclampsia. *Lancet* 1: 1417-21.

Sokol RJ, RB Woolf, MG Rosen, et al. August 1980. Risk, antepartum care, and outcome: Impact of a maternity and infant care project. *Obstetrics and Gynecology* 56 (2): 150-6.

Steel JM, FD Johnstone, DA Hepburn, et al. 10 November 1990. Can prepregnancy care of diabetic women reduce the risk of abnormal babies? *British Medical Journal* 301: 1070-4.

Stenqvist K, I Dahlen-Nilsson, G Lidin-Janson, et al. 1989. Bacteriuria in pregnancy: Frequency and risk of acquisition. *American Journal of Epidemiology* 129 (2): 372-9.

Stevens CE, RP Beasley, J Tsui, et al. 10 April 1975. Vertical transmission of hepatitis B antigen in Taiwan. *New England Journal of Medicine* 292 (15): 771-4.

Stevens CE, PT Toy, MJ Tong, et al. 22 March 1985. Perinatal hepatitis B virus transmission in the United States: Prevention by passive-active immunization. *Journal of the American Medical Association* 253 (12): 1740-5.

Stewart PJ, and GC Dunkley. 15 November 1985. Smoking and health care patterns among pregnant women. *Canadian Medical Association Journal* 133: 989-1082.

Stockbauer JW. July 1987. WIC prenatal participation and its relation to pregnancy outcomes in Missouri: A second look. *American Journal of Public Health* 77 (7): 813-8.

Stray-Pedersen B. October 1983. Economic evaluation of maternal screening to prevent congenital syphilis. *Sexually Transmitted Diseases* 10 (4): 167-72.

Strecher VJ, MH Becker, NM Clark, et al. March 1989. Using patients' descriptions of alcohol consumption, diet, medication compliance, and cigarette smoking: The validity of self-reports in research and practice. *Journal of General Internal Medicine* 4: 160-6.

Summers PR, MK Biswas, JG Pastorek II, et al. May 1987. The pregnant hepatitis B carrier: Evidence favoring comprehensive antepartum screening. *Obstetrics and Gynecology* 69 (5): 701-4.

Susser M. April 1981. Prenatal nutrition, birthweight, and psychological development: An overview of experiments, quasi-experiments, and natural experiments in the past decade. *American Journal of Clinical Nutrition* 34: 784-803.

Sweeney C, H Smith, JC Foster, et al. May 1985. Effects of a nutrition intervention program during pregnancy: Maternal data phases 1 and 2. *Journal of Nurse-Midwifery* 30 (3): 149-58.

Sweet RL, DV Landers, C Walker, et al. 1987. Chlamydia trachomatis infection and pregnancy outcome. *American Journal of Obstetrics and Gynecology* 156 (4): 824-33.

Tejani N, and LI Mann. December 1977. Diagnosis and management of the small-for-gestation-age fetus. *Clinical Obstetrics and Gynecology* 20 (4): 943-55.

Thacker SB. May 1985. Quality of controlled clinical trials. The case of imaging ultrasound in obstetrics: A review. *British Journal of Obstetrics and Gynaecology* 92: 437-44.

Thiagarajah S, FJ Bourgeois, GM Harbert, et al. 1 September 1984. Thrombocytopenia in preeclampsia: Associated abnormalities and management principles. *American Journal of Obstetrics and Gynecology* 150 (1): 1-7.

Torrance GW, and A Zipursky. June 1984. Cost-effectiveness of antepartum prevention of Rh immunization. *Clinics in Perinatology* 11 (2): 267-81.

Tovey LAD, and JM Taverner. 18 April 1981. A case for the antenatal administration of anti-D immunoglobulin to primigravidae. *Lancet* 1: 878-81.

U.S. Department of Health and Human Services. 1991. *Healthy People 2000: National Health Promotion and Disease Prevention Objectives*. U.S. Government Printing Office, Washington, DC.

U.S. Preventive Services Task Force. 1989. *Guide to Clinical Preventive Services: An Assessment of the Effectiveness of 169 Interventions*. Baltimore, MD: Williams and Wilkins.

U.S. Public Health Service, Expert Panel on the Content of Prenatal Care. 1989. *Caring for Our Future: The Content of Prenatal Care*. Washington, DC: U.S. Department of Health and Human Services, Public Health Service.

United Kingdom Collaborative Study. 25 June 1977. Maternal serum-alpha-fetoprotein measurement in antenatal screening for anencephaly and spina bifida in early pregnancy. *Lancet* 2: 1323-32.

Vorherr H. 1 September 1975. Placental insufficiency in relation to postterm pregnancy and fetal postmaturity: Evaluation of fetoplacental function; management of the postterm gravida. *American Journal of Obstetrics and Gynecology* 123 (1): 67-103.

Wadland WC, and DA Plante. 1989. Screening for asymptomatic bacteriuria in pregnancy: A decision and cost analysis. *Journal of Family Practice* 29 (4): 372-6.

Wainright RL. 1983. Change in observed birth weight associated with change in maternal cigarette smoking. *American Journal of Epidemiology* 117 (6): 668-75.

Waldenstrom U, O Axelsson, S Nilsson, et al. September 1988. Effects of routine one-stage ultrasound screening in pregnancy: A randomised controlled trial. *Lancet* 2: 585-8.

Ward RHT, DVI Fairweather, GA Whyley, et al. 1981. Four years' experience of maternal alpha-fetoprotein screening and its effect on the pattern of antenatal care. *Prenatal Diagnosis* 1: 91-101.

Waterson EJ, and IM Murray-Lyon. 1989. Screening for alcohol related problems in the antenatal clinic: An assessment of different methods. *Alcohol and Alcoholism* 24 (1): 21-30.

Wennergren M, and K Karlsson. July 1982. A scoring system for antenatal identification of fetal growth retardation. *British Journal of Obstetrics and Gynaecology* 89: 520-4.

Williamson DF, MK Serdula, JS Kendrick, et al. 6 January 1989. Comparing the prevalence of smoking in pregnant and nonpregnant women, 1985 to 1986. *Journal of the American Medical Association* 261 (1): 70-4.

Williams K. 1985. Screening for syphilis in pregnancy: An assessment of the costs and benefits. *Community Medicine* 7 (1): 37-42.

Witter FR, and CM Weitz. July 1987. A randomized trial of induction at 42 weeks gestation versus expectant management for postdates pregnancies. *American Journal of Perinatology* 4 (3): 206-11.

Worthington-Roberts BS, and LV Klerman. 1990. Maternal Nutrition. In *New Perspectives on Prenatal Care*. Editors Merkatz IR, and JE Thompson, 235-71. New York, NY: Elsevier Science Publishing Co., Inc.

Xu Z, C Liu, DP Francis, et al. November 1985. Prevention of perinatal acquisition of hepatitis B virus carriage using vaccine: Preliminary report of a randomized, double-blind placebo-controlled and comparative trial. *Pediatrics* 76 (5): 713-8.

Yeh S, and JA Read. September 1982. Management of post-term pregnancy in a large obstetric population. *Obstetrics and Gynecology* 60 (3): 282-7.

Zuckerman B, DA Frank, R Hingson, et al. 23 March 1989. Effects of maternal marijuana and cocaine use on fetal growth. *New England Journal of Medicine* 320 (12): 762-8.

15. PRETERM LABOR, CORTICOSTEROIDS FOR FETAL MATURATION
Deidre Gifford, M.D.

This review is based primarily on the results of a National Institutes of Health (NIH) consensus development panel on the effect of corticosteroids for fetal maturation on perinatal outcomes (NIH Consensus Statement, 1994). This publication comprehensively reviews the available literature on antenatal corticosteroid administration, its risks and benefits, and makes specific treatment recommendations. It also contains a meta-analysis of available randomized trials of antenatal corticosteroid administration.

IMPORTANCE

Preterm birth (commonly defined as delivery prior to 37 weeks gestation) occurs in 7-10 percent of pregnancies and is a major cause of infant morbidity and mortality. Preterm births are associated with more than $2 billion in health care costs annually (NIH, 1994) and are the second leading cause of infant deaths in the United States. Neonatal complications such as respiratory distress syndrome (RDS), intraventricular hemorrhage (IVH) and necrotizing enterocolitis (NEC) contribute to morbidity and mortality. Multiple randomized controlled trials have demonstrated that the administration of corticosteroids to the mother prior to delivery when preterm birth is anticipated can result in significant reductions in these adverse outcomes. The NIH (1994) reports that only 12-18 percent of women who deliver preterm infants weighing 500-1500 grams actually receive this therapy.

EFFICACY AND/OR EFFECTIVENESS OF INTERVENTIONS

Data on the risks and benefits of antenatal steroid administration in preterm delivery come from two sources: meta-analysis of 15 randomized controlled trials (NIH, 1994) and a large observational data set. The observational data come from two large multi-center networks studying preterm birth, and from several randomized trials of neonatal surfactant administration after preterm delivery, in which data on antenatal steroid administration were available. Data on more than 30,000 preterm infants are available.

The meta-analysis showed a reduction in the incidence of neonatal mortality (OR 0.6, 95 percent CI 0.5-0.8) and RDS (OR 0.5, 95 percent CI 0.4-0.6) when antenatal corticosteroids were administered to mothers of infants born at 24-34 weeks gestation. Similarly, results from the meta-analysis showed a decrease in IVH (OR 0.5, 95 percent CI 0.3-0.9) with antenatal steroid administration. These findings have been confirmed in the observational studies. Although the meta-analysis of randomized trials showed a reduction in NEC, the observational data showed no reduction in this outcome. The beneficial effects of antenatal steroids are seen consistently in babies of both sexes and in both white and nonwhite infants.

Dexamethasone and betamethasone, in doses of 6 mg every 12 hours for four doses, and 12 mg every 12 hours for 2 doses, respectively, have been shown to be effective. No other antenatal corticosteroid has been extensively studied. Maximum benefit to the infant appears to begin at 24 hours after the initiation of treatment, but some benefit begins even prior to this time. No benefit has been demonstrated in infants beyond 34 weeks gestation.

One possible explanation for the low prevalence of use of this intervention, despite its demonstrated efficacy, is the concern about adverse short and long term effects on both mother and infant. Several studies have followed infants for as long as 12 years following corticosteroid administration and have shown no adverse outcomes in the areas of motor skills, language, cognition, memory, concentration, or scholastic achievement. Because of the possible increased risk of neonatal and maternal infection, the use of antenatal steroids in preterm premature rupture of the membranes (PPROM) remains controversial. The risk of maternal infection after steroid administration may be increased in the case of PPROM; however, there is no evidence that steroid administration interferes with the ability to make the diagnosis. There is also concern about an increased risk of neonatal infection. In the meta-analysis cited above, the typical OR of neonatal infection in infants with PPROM after steroid administration was 1.29, 95 percent CI 0.74-2.26. However, steroids are associated with a significant reduction in RDS in this group as well (OR 0.50, 95 percent CI 0.38-0.66). The NIH (1994) cites "...strong evidence from observational studies that even in the presence of PPROM, the incidence of neonatal mortality and IVH is reduced when antenatal corticosteroids are used. Although the risk of neonatal infection associated with antenatal corticosteroid use in the face of PPROM may be increased, the magnitude of the increase is small. Because of the effectiveness of antenatal corticosteroids in reducing mortality and IVH in fetuses of less than 30-32 weeks gestation, antenatal corticosteroid use is appropriate in the absence of chorioamnionitis." An American College of Obstetricians and Gynecologists (ACOG) committee opinion (ACOG Committee Opinion, 1994) states the support of the ACOG for all of the conclusions of the NIH panel, with the exception of the one pertaining to PPROM. The ACOG Committee (1994) feels that "...further research is needed to evaluate the risks and benefits of using corticosteroids in women who have preterm PROM" although they do not cite specific research questions to be addressed.

RECOMMENDED QUALITY INDICATORS FOR CORTICOSTEROIDS FOR FETAL MATURATION IN LABOR

The following criteria apply to all women admitted to the hospital for preterm labor or for delivery.

Treatment

	Indicator	Quality of evidence	Literature	Benefits	Comments
1.	Women admitted to the hospital with labor, between 24 and 34 weeks gestation and without ruptured membranes, should receive antenatal steroids, even if delivery is anticipated in less than 24 hours.	I	Crowley, 1994, in NIH, 1994; NIH, 1994	Reduce neonatal mortality and intraventricular hemorrhage.	Currently, less than 20% of women who deliver preterm receive antenatal steroids. The use of antenatal steroids under these conditions results in a reduction in neonatal mortality (OR=0.6), RDS (OR=0.5), IVH (OR=0.5) and NEC. Serious adverse effects on mother and infant have not been proven, but each may be at an increased risk for infection if used in PPROM. We assume that fetuses of mothers admitted to the hospital for preterm labor at these gestational ages are at risk for preterm delivery.
2.	Steroid treatment should consist of either: - Betamethasone 12 mg. IM q24h x 2, or - Dexamethasone 6 mg. IM q12h x 4.	I	NIH, 1994	Reduce neonatal mortality and intraventricular hemorrhage.	These regimens have been proven to be effective.
3.	Women admitted to the hospital at 24-32 weeks gestation with ruptured membranes should receive antenatal steroid administration.	II-2	NIH, 1994	Reduce neonatal mortality and intraventricular hemorrhage.	Reduction in infant mortality and IVH with a relatively small increase in the risk of neonatal infection. An ACOG committee feels that the available information does not provide a clear indication for the use of antenatal steroids in the presence of PPROM.

Quality of Evidence Codes:

I:	RCT
II-1:	Nonrandomized controlled trials
II-2:	Cohort or case analysis
II-3:	Multiple time series
III:	Opinions or descriptive studies

REFERENCES - CORTICOSTEROIDS FOR FETAL MATURATION IN LABOR

American College of Obstetricians and Gynecologists. December 1994. Antenatal corticosteroid therapy for fetal maturation. *ACOG Committee Opinion* 147: 1-2.

National Institutes of Health. November 1994. *Report of the Consensus Development Conference on the Effect of Corticosteroids for Fetal Maturation on Perinatal Outcomes*. U.S. Department of Health and Human Services, Public Health Service, Bethesda, MD.

16. PREVENTIVE CARE

Eve A. Kerr, M.D., M.P.H., Lisa Schmidt, M.P.H., Deidre Gifford, M.D., and Steven Asch, M.D., M.P.H.

Many observers believe that much of medicine's contribution to this century's overall increase in life expectancy is due to office-based preventive services. Clinical preventive services have also contributed to a reduction in the prevalence of many diseases that once devastated adult women. Cervical cancer mortality has declined 73 percent since 1950 in part due to the institution of regular Papanicolaou testing to detect cervical dysplasia (U.S. Preventive Services Task Force [USPSTF], 1989). Similarly, age-adjusted mortality for strokes has declined by more than half in part due to early detection and treatment of hypertension (USPSTF, 1989).

Despite these sound clinical reasons for emphasizing prevention in medicine, studies have shown that physicians often fail to provide recommended clinical preventive services (USPSTF, 1989). Explanations cited include lack of time, no reimbursement, and confusion as to which preventive services are recommended or efficacious in reducing morbidity and mortality (USPSTF, 1989). Although physician visits for preventive care services constitute a large proportion of overall physician visits, data from the 1993 National Health Interview Survey (NHIS) indicate that only 63 percent of individuals 18 to 64 years of age were asked at least one screening question (diet, physical activity, alcohol or drug use, history of sexually transmitted disease and contraceptive use) during their last routine check-up. Moreover, only 60 percent of respondents reported having their cholesterol checked in the last five years, 57 percent reported receiving a tetanus booster in the last ten years, and 78 percent of women reported receiving a Pap test in the last three years (National Center for Health Statistics [NCHS], 1994).

In deciding what constitutes necessary or appropriate preventive care, experts have recommended evaluating three areas: 1) the burden of suffering associated with the condition 2) the accuracy and acceptability of screening tests and 3) the efficacy of treatment at the preclinical state versus treatment after the disease manifests itself (Hayward et al., 1991). Several organizations have done systematic reviews of certain clinical preventive services for various age groups. The USPSTF (1989) recommends a variety of screening and counseling services for healthy adult women aged 19-50. These include: history of and counseling for tobacco, alcohol and drug use, sexual practices, dietary intake, and physical activity; measurement of blood pressure, blood cholesterol, height and weight; screening for cervical and breast cancer; and, status of tetanus-diphtheria immunizations.

Those preventive services for which there is agreement among the major review bodies are included as quality indicators for this study. Many of these preventive services can, and should be, included as part of a doctor visit for another illness or reason. Each preventive service and indicator is examined in terms of its importance and efficacy/effectiveness.

IMMUNIZATIONS
Lisa Schmidt, M.P.H., and Eve A. Kerr, M.D., M.P.H.

The primary references for this review were two *Morbidity and Mortality Weekly Reports* (Centers for Disease Control [CDC], 1991; CDC, 1994b) issued by the Advisory Committee on Immunization Practices (ACIP) and the Guide to Clinical Preventive Services of the USPSTF (1989). In addition, a review article by Gardner and Schaffner (1993), which summarizes the literature on recommended adult immunization practices, was consulted.

IMPORTANCE

Tetanus

Tetanus, an acute infectious disease of the nervous system, is caused by the bacillus *Clostridium tetani*. It is characterized by spasms of the voluntary muscles and painful convulsions and may eventually lead to death. Death occurs in 26 to 31 percent of all cases

(USPSTF, 1989). The CDC reported 31 cases of tetanus between January and October 1993 (CDC, 1994a).

Serosurveys undertaken since 1977 indicate that many U.S. adults are not protected against tetanus. It is estimated that 6 to 11 percent of adults 18-39 years of age may lack protective levels of circulating tetanus antitoxin (CDC, 1991). The protective percent increases for older adults (CDC, 1991).

Diphtheria

Diphtheria is caused by the bacterium *Corynebacterium diphtheriae*. Both toxigenic and nontoxigenic strains of *C. diphtheriae* can cause disease, but only strains that produce toxin cause myocarditis and neuritis. Toxigenic strains are more often associated with severe or fatal illness in noncutaneous (respiratory or other mucosal surface) infections (CDC, 1991). From 1980 to 1989, only 24 cases of respiratory diphtheria were reported; two cases were fatal and 18 (75 percent) occurred in persons 20 years of age or older (CDC, 1991). The CDC reported only 1 case between January and October 1994 (CDC, 1994a).

Limited serosurveys conducted since 1977 indicate that 22 to 62 percent of adults 18-39 years of age may lack protective levels of circulating antitoxin against diphtheria (CDC, 1991). A complete vaccination series substantially reduces the risk of developing diphtheria and vaccinated persons who develop disease have milder illnesses (CDC, 1991).

Influenza

Yearly influenza vaccination is recommended for those over age 65 and for persons at high risk of complications from influenza. According to the Centers for Disease Control (CDC) (CDC, 1994b), these include adults under age 65 who:

- are residents of nursing homes and other chronic-care facilities that house persons of any age with chronic medical conditions;
- have chronic disorders of the pulmonary or cardiovascular system (e.g., asthma, chronic obstructive pulmonary disease, congestive heart failure); or

- have required regular medical follow-up or hospitalization
  during the preceding year because of chronic metabolic diseases
  (including diabetes mellitus), renal dysfunction,
  hemoglobinopathies, or immunosuppression (including
  immunosuppression caused by medications).

EFFICACY AND/OR EFFECTIVENESS OF INTERVENTIONS

The ACIP recommends that all adults receive a tetanus booster at least once every ten years and that a complete series of combined tetanus-diphtheria (Td) toxoids should be given to patients who have not received a primary series (CDC, 1994a; ACP, 1994; USPSTF, 1989). In addition, pregnant women, who are not fully immunized, should complete the immunization series (Gardner and Schaffner, 1993). Td is highly effective in producing protective antibody titers; a completed primary series generally induces protective levels of serum antitoxin that persist for 10 or more years (CDC, 1991).

Local reactions (tenderness and erythema) are common after a Td injection, but severe reactions are rare. Because Arthus-type hypersensitivity reactions occur most commonly after multiple boosters, Td boosters should not be given to anyone who, within the previous five years, has either completed a primary series or received a booster dose (Gardner and Schaffner, 1993).

SEXUALLY TRANSMITTED DISEASES AND HIV PREVENTION
Eve A. Kerr, M.D., M.P.H.

Approach

The primary references for this review were the Guide to Clinical Preventive Services of the USPSTF (1989) and the *Healthy People 2000* National Health Promotion and Disease Prevention Objectives (USPHS, 1991).

IMPORTANCE

An estimated 1-1.5 million people are infected with the human immunodeficiency (HIV) virus (USPSTF, 1989). Within 10 years of infection with HIV, approximately 50 percent of persons develop AIDS and another 40 percent or more develop other clinical illnesses associated with HIV infection (USPHS, 1991). Persons with AIDS can develop severe opportunistic infections, malignancies, and multiple-system medical complications. In a study performed before the licensure of AZT, the five-year survival rate was only 15 percent (USPSTF, 1989). The economic consequences of AIDS are enormous; it is estimated that the annual cost of treating AIDS is $2.2 billion (USPSTF, 1989).

Almost 12 million cases of sexually transmitted diseases occur annually (USPHS, 1991). Each year there are about 3-4 million cases of chlamydia, 2 million cases of gonorrhea, over 35,000 cases of primary and secondary syphilis, and 270,000 primary episodes of genital herpes (USPSTF, 1989). These diseases are associated with considerable morbidity. Chlamydia and gonorrhea produce mucopurulent cervicitis and pelvic inflammatory disease (PID) in women. PID is an important risk factor for ectopic pregnancy and infertility; approximately 1 million cases of PID are reported annually in the United States (USPSTF, 1989). Syphilis produces ulcers of the genitalia, pharynx, and rectum and can progress to secondary and tertiary syphilis if left untreated (USPSTF, 1989). Genital herpes causes painful vesicular and ulcerative lesions and recurrent infections due to latent infection (USPSTF, 1989). The total societal costs of STDs is estimated to be $3.5 billion annually (USPHS, 1991).

EFFICACY AND/OR EFFECTIVENESS OF INTERVENTIONS

The most efficacious means of reducing the risk of acquiring AIDS and other STDs through sexual contact is either abstinence from sexual relations or maintenance of a mutually monogamous sexual relationship with an uninfected partner (USPSTF, 1989). In addition, the use of latex condoms and spermicides may reduce the risk of infection with HIV or other STDs (USPSTF, 1989). Intravenous drug use and unsterilized needles should be avoided to reduce the risk of HIV infection. The prevalence of HIV infection in heterosexual partners of persons in high-risk categories may be as high as 11 percent and 60 percent of heterosexual partners of HIV-infected individuals may be seropositive (USPSTF, 1989).

The primary purpose of HIV and STD counseling is to prevent further spread of infection (USPHS, 1991). Physicians can play an important role in preventing infection in asymptomatic persons by reinforcing and clarifying educational messages, providing literature and community resource references for additional information, and dispelling misconceptions about unproven modes of transmission (USPSTF, 1989). Although it has not been proven that physicians can change the sexual behavior of patients, there is evidence that the frequency of high-risk behaviors can be reduced in response to information provided through public education (USPSTF, 1989). A survey of primary care physicians found that only 10 percent asked new patients questions specific enough to identify those at risk of exposure to HIV (USPSTF, 1989).

It is recommended that clinicians take a complete sexual and drug use history on all adult patients to identify risk factors for HIV and AIDS. In addition, clinicians should counsel at-risk patients on measures to prevent STDs and HIV. Risk factors include: not being in a monogamous relationship; having more than two sexual partners in the past six months; having a history of STDs; having a history of intravenous drug abuse; having sexual relations with an infected partner; having a history of blood transfusion between 1978 and 1985; being a hemophiliac; and being born to an infected mother.

Sexually active patients should receive complete information on their risk for acquiring STDs (USPSTF, 1989). The key elements of counseling include: advising sexually active patients that abstaining from sex or maintaining a mutually faithful monogamous sexual relationship with a partner known to be uninfected are the most effective strategies to prevent infection with HIV or other sexually transmitted diseases; advising against sexual activity with individuals whose infection status is uncertain; advising patients that a nonreactive HIV test does not rule out infection if the sexual partner has not been monogamous for at least six months before the test;

advising that a condom at each sexual encounter should be used and anal
intercourse should be avoided if the patient chooses to engage in sexual
activity with multiple partners; and, advising women of the potential
risks of HIV infection during pregnancy (USPSTF, 1989).

OBESITY COUNSELING

Lisa Schmidt, M.P.H., and Eve A. Kerr, M.D., M.P.H.

The primary references for this review were the Guide to Clinical
Preventive Services of the USPSTF (1989) and the *Healthy People 2000*
National Health Promotion and Disease Prevention Objectives (USPHS,
1991).

IMPORTANCE

Obesity has been defined as being 20 percent or more overweight
(USPSTF, 1989) or a body mass index (BMI) greater than 27.3 for women
(USPHS, 1991). It is estimated that approximately 32 million American
adults aged 25-74 are overweight (USPSTF, 1989). Obesity is prevalent
in minority populations, especially among minority women. In 1976-80,
approximately 44 percent of black women aged 20 and older, 39 percent of
Mexican-American women, 34 percent of Cuban women, and 37 percent of
Puerto Rican women were overweight (USPHS, 1991). Poverty level is also
related to overweight in women. Between 1976 and 1980, 37 percent of
women with incomes below the poverty level were overweight compared with
25 percent of those above the poverty level (USPHS, 1991).

Morbid obesity, defined as being 50 to 100 percent, or 100 pounds,
above the desirable weight has been correlated with increased mortality
and morbidity. The prevalence of diabetes and hypertension is three
times higher in overweight persons than in those of normal weight
(USPSTF, 1989). There is a clear association between obesity and
hypercholesterolemia and a possible independent relationship between
obesity and coronary artery disease. In addition, obesity may influence
the risk of cancer of the colon, rectum, gallbladder, biliary tract,

breast, cervix, endometrium, and ovary (USPSTF, 1989). Finally, obesity affects the quality of life by limiting mobility, physical endurance, and other functional measures (USPSTF, 1989).

EFFICACY AND/OR EFFECTIVENESS OF INTERVENTIONS

Extremely overweight individuals can be easily identified in the clinical setting by their physical appearance. More precise methods, however, are required to identify mildly or moderately obese persons.

The most common clinical method for detecting obesity is the evaluation of body weight and height based on tables of average weights; however, this method only approximates the extent of obesity (USPSTF, 1989). The criteria for desirable body weight are a matter of controversy among experts and vary considerably in different weight-height tables (USPSTF, 1989). Another method of measuring obesity is the measurement of body fat distribution. This can be measured in the clinical setting by comparing the circumference or skinfold thickness of the trunk and limbs. A waist-hip circumference greater than 0.8 in women may be a reliable predictor of complications from obesity (USPSTF, 1989). Studies have shown that these measurements compare favorably with estimates obtained from hydrostatic weighing (USPSTF, 1989).

The purpose of screening for obesity is to convince the individual to lose weight thereby preventing the complications of obesity. Although there is little evidence from prospective studies that losing weight improves longevity, there is evidence that obesity increases mortality and that weight loss reduces important risk factors such as hypertension, elevated serum cholesterol, and impaired glucose tolerance (USPSTF, 1989).

Periodic height and weight measurements, although not proven to be effective in motivating patients to lose weight, are inexpensive, rapid and acceptable to patients. They may also be useful for the detection of medical conditions causing unintended weight loss and weight gain, such as cancer or thyroid disorders (USPSTF, 1989). The reliability of other methods of detecting obesity, such as the measurement of skinfold thickness and limb circumference, requires further study before these techniques are deemed suitable for widespread implementation in the clinical setting (USPSTF, 1989). There are inadequate data to determine the optimal frequency of obesity screening (USPSTF, 1989). The Institute of Medicine recommends height and weight measurements at five age intervals during adulthood: 18-24, 25-39, 40-59, 60-74, and over 75 (USPSTF, 1989). The American Heart Association recommends body weight measurements every five years (USPSTF, 1989). The USPHS recommends reducting the prevalence of obesity to no more that 20 percent among people age 20 and older. Special population targets include reducing obesity to 25 percent in low-income women aged 20 and older, 30 percent for Black women aged 20 and older, and 25 percent for Hispanic women aged 20 and older (USPHS, 1991).

SEAT BELT USE COUNSELING
Lisa Schmidt, M.P.H., and Eve A. Kerr, M.D., M.P.H.

The primary references for this review were the Guide to Clinical Preventive Services of the USPSTF (1989) and the *Healthy People 2000* National Health Promotion and Disease Prevention Objectives (USPHS, 1991).

IMPORTANCE

Injuries are the fourth leading cause of death in the United States and the leading cause of death in persons under age 45. Motor vehicle injuries account for about one-half of these deaths (USPSTF, 1989). In 1986, nearly 48,000 Americans died in motor vehicle crashes, and each year several million suffer nonfatal injuries (USPSTF, 1989). Although males and persons aged 15-24 account for one-third of all deaths from motor vehicle accidents (MVA), a significant number of women and children are killed or injured in MVAs each year. Many of these deaths and injuries are preventable with use of a safety restraint. However, only 46 percent of Americans used seat belts in 1988, up from 13 percent in 1978 (USPSTF, 1989).

EFFICACY AND/OR EFFECTIVENESS OF INTERVENTIONS

The effectiveness of safety belts has been demonstrated in a variety of study designs that include laboratory experiments (using human volunteers, cadavers, and anthropomorphic crash dummies), postcrash comparisons of injuries sustained by restrained and unrestrained occupants, and postcrash judgments by crash analysts regarding the probable effects of restraints had they been used (USPSTF, 1989). It has been estimated on the basis of such evidence that the proper use of lap and shoulder belts can decrease the risk of moderate to serious injury to front seat occupants by 45 to 55 percent and can reduce crash mortality by 40 to 50 percent (USPSTF, 1989). When brought to the hospital, crash victims who are wearing safety belts at the time of the crash have less severe injuries, are less likely to require admission, and have lower hospital charges (USPSTF, 1989).

The USPSTF recommends that clinicians regularly urge their patients to use safety belts whenever driving or riding in an automobile. In addition, they should be counseled regarding the dangers of operating a motor vehicle while under the influence of alcohol or other drugs, as well as on the risks of riding in a vehicle operated by someone who is under the influence of these substances (USPSTF, 1989). A number of other organizations have issued recommendations on physician counseling of patients on seat belt use, including the American Medical Association, the American College of Physicians, the American Academy of Family Physicians and the National Highway Traffic Safety Administration (USPSTF, 1989). In addition, the American College of Obstetricians and Gynecologists has issued recommendations for the use of passenger restraints by pregnant women (USPSTF, 1989). Lastly, the *Healthy People 2000* objectives includes a risk reduction objective to increase the use of occupant protection systems to at least 85 percent of motor vehicle occupants (USPHS, 1991).

It is not known, however, how effectively clinicians can alter behaviors regarding seat belt use. In one survey, patients claimed to have increased their use of safety belts as a result of a brief statement by their physician during a routine office visit, but the study lacked controls and the patients were carefully selected (USPSTF,

1989). Other measures that have proven successful in motivating people to use safety belts, such as community educational programs and intensive psychological strategies, may not be generalizable to the clinical practice setting (USPSTF, 1989).

BREAST EXAMINATION
Lisa Schmidt, M.P.H., and Eve A. Kerr, M.D., M.P.H.

The general approach to clinical breast examination was obtained from a review of the U.S. Preventive Services Task Force recommendations on breast cancer screening (USPSTF, 1989) and review articles obtained from a MEDLINE search which identified all English language review articles related to breast cancer screening between the years of 1985 and 1995.

IMPORTANCE

Breast cancer is the most commonly diagnosed cancer and the second leading cause of cancer deaths among women (CDC, 1992b). Breast cancer accounts for 32 percent of all cancers in women and 18 percent of female cancer deaths (American College of Obstetricians and Gynecologists [ACOG], 1991). In 1987, approximately 41,000 women died from breast cancer; the mortality rate was 27.1 deaths/100,000 women (CDC, 1992a). The probability that an average-risk woman will be diagnosed with breast cancer in the coming 10 years is about 130 in 10,000 for a 40 year old woman and the chance of dying from breast cancer diagnosed in the coming 10 years is about 90 in 10,000 for a 40 year old woman; these rates increase with age (Eddy, 1989).

EFFICACY AND/OR EFFECTIVENESS OF INTERVENTIONS

Three screening tests are usually considered for breast cancer: clinical breast examination (CBE); mammography; and, breast-self examination. Currently, there is controversy about the role of routine mammography in women under the age of 50. Many of the professional societies, such as the American Cancer Society, ACOG, and the National

Cancer Institute differ in their recommendations for routine mammography for women in this age group. Moreover, a meta-analysis by Kerlikowske et al. (1995) showed that screening mammography did not significantly reduce breast cancer mortality in women 40-49 years of age. The other screening technique, routine breast self-examination, has also not been shown to be an effective method of screening for breast cancer (Austoker, 1994). Therefore, only CBE will be included as a quality indicator for breast cancer screening for women under age 50.

Based on data from the 1992 National Health Interview Survey, Makuc reported that only 62 percent of women aged 40-49 received a CBE in 1992 (NCHS, 1994). Of women in this age category, only 56 percent with less than 12 years of education received a CBE, while 68 percent of women with 13 or more years education received a CBE.

Results on the effectiveness of CBE in detecting breast masses vary in the literature. According to Hindle (1990) and the USPSTF (1989), new techniques for CBE have increased clinician's sensitivity to smaller breast lesions, however the sensitivity and specificity varies with the skill and experience of the clinician and with the characteristics of the individual breast being examined. Over the five years of the Breast Cancer Detection Demonstration Project (BCDDP), the estimated sensitivity of clinical examination alone was 45 percent (USPSTF, 1989). Data from studies using manufactured breast models showed that for breast lumps 1.0 cm in diameter mean sensitivity was 65 percent among registered nurses and 87 percent among physicians; this compared to only 55 percent sensitivity for untrained women (USPSTF, 1989). Rosner and Blaird (1985) found that physical examination correctly identified only 58 percent of 66 palpable cysts. The sensitivity of CBE in the Health Insurance Plan of Greater New York (HIP) and the BCDDP was about 50 percent (Eddy, 1989).

Evidence in the literature about the effectiveness of CBE alone in reducing mortality from breast cancer indicate that CBE was responsible for approximately two-thirds of the effect of the combined strategy of mammography and clnical breast examination (Eddy, 1989). In addition, although no formal analyses on the independent contributions of CBE and mammography have been presented in the BCDDP, Eddy reports that it is likely that any increased effectiveness seen in the BCDDP is a result of improvements in the mammography technology and that CBE alone would have had only half the estimated effectiveness. Using a computer model, CAN*TROL, and data from the HIP and BCDDP, Eddy shows that, in asymptomatic women aged 40 to 50, annual CBE for ten years decreases the probability of death from breast cancer by 15 to 29 per 10,000 and increases life expectancy by 13 to 27 days. Adding mammography to the CBE decreases the probability of death by an additional 8 to 29 per 10,000 and adds an additional 7 to 29 days of life expectancy. Eddy also estimates that if 25 percent of asymptomatic women in the U.S. between ages 40 and 50 were screened annually with CBE between 1989 and the year 2000, the number of breast cancer deaths in that age group would decrease by 300 to 760. Thus, although there appears to be some benefit associated with CBE alone, these benefits must be weighed against the costs associated with the screening, including the costs of doing a work up of every breast mass detected, some of which will be false positives.

For asymptomatic women, the American Cancer Society recommends a CBE every three years for women between the ages of 20 and 40 and annual CBEs for women 40 and older (Mettlin and Smart, 1994). The USPSTF (1989) and the American College of Physicians (McGuire, 1989) also recommend annual CBEs for women aged 40 and older. The National Cancer Institute recommends regular breast examinations for all women (USPSTF, 1989). However, because the effectiveness of yearly CBE is not well documented, we recommend that the quality indicator for breast cancer screening should be at least one CBE every three years, during a routine visit for a pelvic exam. This indicator is designed to coincide with the indicator for regular cervical cancer screening which recommends a Pap smear every three years for asymptomatic women less than 50 years of age.

HYPERLIPIDEMIA SCREENING
Steven Asch, M.D., M.P.H.

IMPORTANCE

Identifying high blood cholesterol in asymptomatic patients allows modifications of an important risk factor for coronary artery disease, the leading cause of death in the United States (Reed, 1987). The MRFIT trial found that patients with a cholesterol in the highest quintile (>246 mg/dl) were 3.4 times as likely to die from coronary heart disease as those in the lowest quartile (<181) (Martin et al., 1986). Several other major observational cohorts including Framingham and Whitehall have demonstrated the same risk relationship between cholesterol (particularly low density lipoprotein subcomponent and cardiovascular mortality) and most have found a synergistic relationship between cholesterol and other cardiovascular risk factors like hypertension and smoking (Littenberg et al., 1991, in Eddy, 1991; Rose and Shipley, 1986; and Kannel et al., 1971). THough recently disputed, the relationship between serum cholesterol and *total* mortality appears to be J-shaped; most experts believe that the higher mortality rates in patients with very low cholesterol derive from occult malignancies or other serious illnesses rather than low cholesterol inducing those conditions (Littenberg et al., 1991, in Eddy, 1991). The relationship between hypertriglyceridemia and coronary artery disease is less certain, but several clinical studies have shown that an unusually large number of people with coronary artery disease have high levels of triglycerides in the blood (American Heart Association [AHA], 1993). The AHA estimates that cardiovascular disease costs the U.S. about $80 billion each year (AHA, 1993).

EFFICACY AND/OR EFFECTIVENESS OF INTERVENTIONS

Screening

The tests for total cholesterol, HDL cholesterol and LDL cholesterol, and triglycerides are inexpensive and safe. The accuracy of the tests varies somewhat by laboratory. The American College of Pathology found a range of 197 to 379 mg/dl in 5000 samples with a known concentration of 262 mg/dl mailed to labs throughout the country (Laboratory Standardization Panel of the National Cholesterol Education Program, 1988). The same study found similar problems with the measurement of triglycerides, HDL and LDL. Serum cholesterol varies somewhat with recent dietary fat intake; serum triglycerides also vary greatly with a number of other noncardiac conditions including liver disease, pancreatitis and hyperthyroidism. Despite this, there is no strong evidence that fasting lipids are more predictive of coronary artery disease than nonfasting lipids. Perhaps more importantly for the current study of predominantly young women, cholesterol measurements in younger patients are highly predictive of elevations later in life (Gillum et al., 1982). Like in hypertension, while the screening test itself poses little risk to the patient's health, incorrectly labeling a patient as having high cholesterol may impose some risk of unnecessary side effects from pharmacologic therapy.

Efficacy of Early Treatment

No clinical studies have directly assessed whether early detection of hyperlipidemia prevents heart disease, though there is widespread agreement that early treatment should be more efficacious than treatment after the development of atherosclerosis (Littenberg et al., 1991, in Eddy, 1991). However, several randomized controlled trials of lipid lowering treatment in hypercholesterolemic patients have shown modest reductions in mortality, though the study populations have in general been middle aged men. The WHO Cooperative Trial (Report from the Committee of Principal Investigators, 1978, 1980, 1984) divided 15,000 men into two groups, those taking clofibrate and a control group receiving placebo capsules. Those receiving medication experienced a 20 percent reduction in fatal myocardial infarction and a 25 percent reduction in nonfatal myocardial infarction. The Helsinki Heart Study, a trial of over 4000 asymptomatic men, found the incidence of cardiac events to be 34 percent lower among those receiving gemfibrozil (Frick et al., 1987). The Lipid Research Clinic's (LRC) Coronary Primary

Prevention Trial compared cholestyramine and placebo in almost 4000 men
and found a 19 percent reduction in cardiovascular events (LRC, 1979;
LRC, 1983a; LRC, 1983b; LRC, 1984a; LRC, 1984b). There was no
difference in overall mortality in this study due to an excess of cancer
and trauma deaths in the control group. Two of three studies testing
dietary and other nonpharmacologic interventions, MRFIT, Oslo, and
Wadsworth, found decreased cardiovascular mortality in the intervention
group (Report from the Committee of Principal Investigators, 1984;
Dayton, 1969; Hjermann et al., 1981). More recently, the Scandinavian
Simvastatin Survival Study (SSSS) found that, among patients age 35 to
69 of both genders with known coronary artery disease and mild to
moderate hypercholesterolemia, Simvastatin (a cholesterol-lowering drug)
significantly reduced the overall risk of death when compared to placebo
(RR=0.70; 95 percent CI 0.58-0.85, p=0.0003). The study demonstrated
benefits among women as well as men (SSSS, 1994).

The cost effectiveness of screening for and treating hyperlipidemia
has been the subject of some controversy. Estimates have varied from
$11,000 to $56,000 per year of life saved, but most authors have
concluded that screening younger patients is more cost effective than
screening older patients (Littenberg et al., 1991, in Eddy, 1991; and
Taylor et al., 1987).

RECOMMENDATIONS

The USPSTF recommends that all adults undergo blood cholesterol
measurement every five years and more often for patients with known
cardiac risk factors. The American College of Physicians recommends
that cholesterol be measured once in early adulthood to identify those
with severe or familial hypercholesterolemia. The Canadian Task Force
(CTF) on Periodic Health Examination concluded that insufficient
evidence existed for screening all asymptomatic patients. It is
recommended that physicians use their clinical judgment in deciding
whether to screen and suggested that men aged 30-59 would benefit most
(USPSTF, 1989; Littenberg et al., 1991, in Eddy, 1991; CTF, 1993).

HYPERTENSION SCREENING

See Chapter 12 for discussion of hypertension screening.

CERVICAL CANCER SCREENING
Deidre Gifford, M.D.

The following guidelines are based primarily on the U.S. Preventive Services Task Force's review of "Screening for Cervical Cancer" (U.S. Preventive Services Task Force [USPSTF], 1989). In addition, we performed a review of the English language literature between 1990 and 1995. Articles were obtained using a MEDLINE search with the search terms cervix dysplasia, cervix neoplasms, and vaginal smears. This document addresses the questions of which populations should be screened and at what interval, as well as management of women with abnormal tests. This review does not address treatment of confirmed cervical cancer.

IMPORTANCE

There are approximately 13,000 new cases of cervical cancer diagnosed each year in the United States, and about 7,000 deaths annually from the disease. The annual incidence of invasive cervical cancer is estimated to be 20 per 100,000, and the lifetime probability of developing cervical cancer was estimated in 1985 to be 0.7 percent (Eddy, 1990). Five-year survival for women with advanced disease is about 40 percent, whereas it is about 90 percent for women with localized cancer (USPSTF, 1989). Cervical cancer is a good candidate for screening programs because it has a long preinvasive stage during which the disease can be detected and cured.

EFFECTIVENESS OF INTERVENTIONS

Screening

The Pap smear is the primary method of screening for cervical cancer. Pap smears can detect early cell changes which are precursors to invasive disease. Women in whom such abnormalities are detected can then have further diagnostic testing and treatment with interventions such as colposcopy and biopsy, cervical conization, and local excision, which can prevent further progression of the disease.

Evidence of the effectiveness of screening programs comes from observational studies showing decreases in cervical cancer mortality following the introduction of population screening programs. Such decreases have been observed in the United States and Canada, as well as in several European countries (USPSTF, 1989). For example, data from Iceland demonstrated a rising cervical cancer mortality rate during the 1960s. Screening was introduced in 1964, and by 1970 the annual mortality rate began to decline. By 1974, it had fallen significantly, decreasing from 23 per 100,000 in 1965-1969 to about 15 per 100,000 in 1970-74 (Johannesson et al., 1978). Further evidence comes from Canada, where the reduction in cervical cancer mortality has been noted to correlate with the proportion of the population screened with Pap tests (Eddy, 1990). In addition to this evidence, several case control studies have noted a marked decrease in risk of developing cervical cancer in women screened with pap smears when compared to unscreened women. Such studies indicate that screening for cervical cancer with Pap smears is highly effective, decreasing the occurrence of invasive cancer by 60-90 percent (Eddy, 1990).

The effectiveness of cervical cancer screening appears to increase with decreasing screening intervals. This evidence also comes from case control studies, which demonstrated decreased relative risks of invasive disease in women with shorter screening intervals (Eddy, 1990). However, there is also evidence that annual screening may produce only a minimally lower risk of invasive disease than screening every two to three years (USPSTF, 1989; Eddy, 1990). According to one study of eight cervical cancer screening programs in Europe and Canada, the incidence of cervical cancer can be reduced by 64.1 percent with a screening interval of ten years, by 83.6 percent with a five-year interval, and by 90.8 percent, 92.5 percent and 93.5 percent with intervals of three, two and one years, respectively (IARC Working Group, 1986).

Several important risk factors have been identified for cervical cancer (Eddy, 1990). These include:

1) race/ethnicity, with blacks and Hispanics having a two-fold increased risk;

2) early age at first sexual intercourse;

3) number of sexual partners;

4) smoking;

5) human immunodeficiency virus (HIV) infection; and

6) human papillomavirus (HPV) infection.

There is also some evidence that long-term use of oral contraceptives may predispose a woman to cervical neoplasia. There has been debate in the literature about whether or not women with such risk factors should be screened more frequently than the general population of women. Published recommendations leave room for physician discretion in screening such women. Consensus has been reached by the American Cancer Society, the National Cancer Institute, the American College of Obstetricians and Gynecologists (ACOG), the American Medical Association, the American Nurses Association, the American Academy of Family Physicians and the American Medical Women's Association (Fink, 1988) on a guideline that recommends annual Pap smears for all women who are or have been sexually active, or who are at least 18 years of age. After three normal annual smears, and *if recommended by the physician*, less frequent testing is permitted.

The USPSTF (1989) makes similar recommendations about the onset of testing and about annual testing until three normal tests have been obtained. They add that "...pap tests are appropriately performed at an interval of one to three years, to be recommended by the physician on the basis of risk factors (e.g., early onset of sexual intercourse, history of multiple sexual partners, low socioeconomic status). Women who have never been sexually active or who have had a total hysterectomy

for benign indications with previously normal screening do not need
regular Pap smears because they are not at risk for cervical cancer.

Management of Women with Abnormal Pap Smears

Although there is generally less consensus about appropriate
treatment and follow-up of abnormal pap smears than there is about their
effectiveness as a screening technique, reductions in cervical cancer
mortality are dependent on follow-up and treatment of women who have
positive screening exams.

The classification of abnormal smears is variable, with different
systems for reporting abnormalities (Table 16.1).

Table 16.1

Cytopathology Reporting Systems for Pap Smears

Class system	World Health Organization System	Cervical Intraepithelial Neoplasia System	Bethesda System
I	Normal	Normal	Within normal limits
II	Inflammation		Other Infection Reactive and reparative
III	Dysplasia Mild Moderate Severe	CIN-1 CIN-2	Squamous intraepi thelial lesions Low grade High grade
IV	Carcinoma in situ	CIN-3	
V	Invasive squamous cell carcinoma Adenocarcinoma	Invasive squamous cell carcinoma Adenocarcinoma	Squamous cell carcinoma Adenocarcinoma

Source: Miller et al., 1992

The Bethesda system was introduced to replace the previous Pap
classifications and to facilitate precise communication between
cytopathologists and clinicians. There is not universal agreement that

it is superior to the CIN designations (Kurman et al., 1991), nor is there any evidence that it has been widely adopted.

Recommendations for follow-up of abnormal smears have been summarized by the report of a Canadian National workshop on screening for cancer of the cervix (Miller et al., 1991). First, they stress that screening recommendations (as summarized above) apply only to women with normal screening exams, and that women with abnormal smears should be screened and treated differently. This group recommends that women with so-called "benign atypia," mild dysplasia (CIN I, low grade SIL) or HPV infection without dysplasia should be rescreened at intervals of 6-12 months, and referred for colposcopy if the abnormality persists at 24 months past the original smear. This is based on the finding that many of these lesions will regress spontaneously without intervention (Montz et al., 1992); however, some have argued that the inconvenience, distress, and possibly the cost of this strategy are excessive, and that all women with abnormal smears should be referred immediately for colposcopic evaluation (Soutter, 1992; Wright et al., 1995). ACOG suggests that women with these low grade lesions may either be followed at six-month intervals or referred for colposcopy. They recommend colposcopic evaluation eventually for all women with "persistent" lesions.

There is agreement about management of women with more dysplastic lesions on pap smear. Women with Pap smears read as "moderate dysplasia," "severe dysplasia," "carcinoma in-situ," CIN II or greater, high grade squamous intraepithelial lesions, squamous cell carcinoma or adenocarcinoma should be referred for colposcopic evaluation. Further, the presence of a visible cervical lesion, even with a normal Pap smear, requires colposcopy because of the possibility of a false negative screening test (Miller et al., 1991; ACOG Technical Bulletin, 1993).

RECOMMENDED QUALITY INDICATORS FOR ROUTINE PREVENTIVE CARE

The following criteria apply to nonpregnant, healthy, adult women under 50 years of age.

Screening

Indicator	Quality of evidence	Literature	Benefits	Comments
Immunizations				
1. Notation of date that a patient received a tetanus/diphtheria booster within the last ten years should be included in the medical record.	III	USPSTF, 1989; ACIP, 1994	Prevention of tetanus and diphtheria infection, which can lead to respiratory compromise and death.	A completed primary immunization series generally induces protective serum antitoxin levels that lasts for approximately 10 years. Td boosters are necessary to maintain immunized status in adults.
2. Women with any of the following conditions should receive receive a yearly influenza vaccine: a. asthma, b. chronic obstructive pulmonary disease, c. chronic cardiovascular disorders, d. diabetes mellitus, e. renal failure, f. hemoglobinopathies (e.g., sickle cell disease), or g. immunosuppresssion.	I-III	CDC, 1994c	Prevent pneumonia. Prevent mortality from influenza.	The influenza vaccine has been shown to prevent influenza. Patients at risk for developing complications from influenza should be vaccinated.
Sexually Transmitted Diseases and HIV Prevention				
3. Patients should be asked if they have ever been sexually active.	III	USPSTF, 1989	Prevent HIV; Prevent STDs.**	Patients who have ever been sexually active may be at risk of HIV or STD infections.
4. Patients who have ever been sexually active should be asked the following questions: if they currently have a single sexual partner; if they have had more than 2 sexual partners in the past 6 months; and if they have had a history of any STDs.	III	USPSTF, 1989	Prevent HIV; Prevent STDs.**	Non-monogamous relationships, more than 2 sexual partners in the past 6 months and past history of STDs are risk factors for HIV and/or other STDs.
5. Patients should be asked about current or past use of intravenous drugs at least once.	III	USPSTF, 1989	Prevent HIV; Prevent STDs.**	Intravenous drug use is a risk factor for HIV infection.
6. Patients who are sexually active and not in a monogamous relationship, have had more than 2 sexual partners in the past six months, have a history of STDs, or have used intravenous drugs, should be counseled regarding the prevention and transmission of HIV and other STDs.	III	USPSTF, 1989	Prevent HIV; Prevent STDs.**	Persons with risk factors for HIV or other STDs should receive appropriate counseling
Obesity Counseling				

#	Description	Grade	Source	Objective	Comment
7.	The medical record should include measurements of height and weight at least once.	III	USPSTF, 1989; USDHHS, 1991	Prevention of complications of obesity, including hypertension, high serum cholesterol and impaired glucose tolerance.	This will serve to identify individuals who are obese. However, it is debatable whether physician counseling for obesity is effective in adults.
Seat Belt Use Counseling					
8.	Patients should receive counseling regarding the use of seat belts on at least one occasion.	III	USPSTF, 1989	Prevention of motor vehicle injuries and fatalities.	Clinician suggestion may affect this behavior.
Breast Examination					
9.	A clinical breast exam should be performed on women aged 40 to 50 at least once every three years during a routine visit for a pelvic exam.	III	USPSTF, 1989; McGuire, 1990; Mettlin and Smart, 1994	Prevent late-stage breast cancer; Decrease mortality from breast cancer.	This coincides with the recommended screening interval for cervical cancer for women aged 40 to 50.
Hyperlipidemia Screening					
10.	As a screen for familial hypercholesterolemia, the medical record should indicate that adult women have undergone a cholesterol measurement at sometime in their lives.		USPSTF, 1989	Prevent morbidity and mortality of coronary artery disease.	Early identification may enhance treatment of outcomes.
11.	In women with known cardiac risk factors including hypertension, smoking, diabetes, family history of myocardial infarction or familial hypercholesterolemia in a first degree relative, the medical record should indicate a serum cholesterol and triglycerides level in the last 5 years.		USPSTF, 1989; SSSS, 1994	Prevent morbidity and mortality of coronary artery disease.	These patients are not at increased risk of serious complications. Cholesterol-lowering drugs can reduce morbidity and mortality.
Cervical Cancer Screening					
12.	The medical record should contain the date and result of the last Pap smear.	II-2	USPSTF, 1989	Prevent cervical cancer morbidity and mortality.* Prevent cervical cancer.	The appropriate timing of the next Pap smear is determined by the time elapsed since the last smear, and the result of the last smear.
13.	Women who have not had a Pap smear within the last 3 years should have one performed (unless never sexually active or have had a hysterectomy).	II-2	USPSTF, 1989	Prevent cervical cancer morbidity and mortality.* Prevent cervical cancer.	The maximum interval for women with intact uteri is every three years. The incidence of cervical cancer is increased when screening intervals exceed 3 years.
14.	Women who have not had 3 consecutive normal smears and who have not had a Pap smear within the last year should have one performed.	III	ACOG, 1993	Prevent cervical cancer morbidity and mortality.* Prevent cervical cancer.	A normal Pap smear is defined as one without atypia, dysplasia, CIS or invasive carcinoma. If there is no documentation of the actual pathology/cytology reports (i.e., because previous Pap smears were done at another facility) but there is documentation that all previous Paps were normal in the history, then the appropriate screening interval may be regarded as three years.
15.	Women with a history of cervical dysplasia or carcinoma-in-situ who have not had a Pap smear within the last year should have one performed.	III	Miller et al., 1991; ACOG, 1993	Prevent cervical cancer morbidity and mortality.* Prevent cervical cancer.	These women are at increased risk for cervical disease, and should not be returned to the usual screening intervals.

#	Recommendation	Source	Quality of Evidence	Goal	Comments
16.	Women with severely abnormal Pap smear should have colposcopy performed.***	Miller et al., 1991	III	Prevent cervical cancer morbidity and mortality.*	Appropriate follow-up for abnormal findings is key in preventing progression to cervical cancer or disease progression.
17.	If a woman has a Pap smear that is not normal but is not severely abnormal,*** then one of the following should occur within 1 year of the initial Pap: 1) repeat Pap smear; or 2) colposcopy.	Miller et al., 1991	III	Prevent cervical cancer morbidity and mortality.*	Patients with intermediate findings should be monitored closely. In many cases, abnormal findings resolve spontaneously, so follow-up with Pap smears or immediate colposcopy are both appropriate.
18.	Women with a Pap smear that is not "normal" but is not severely abnormal*** and who have had the abnormality documented on at least 2 Pap smears in a 2-year period should have colposcopy performed.	Miller et al., 1991	III	Prevent cervical cancer morbidity and mortality.*	Patients with intermediate findings should be monitored closely since some portion of these may represent preinvasive disease, or progress to a high-grade SIL. If findings persist, colposcopy should be performed. This may be difficult to operationalize for women who have not been enrolled in the same plan for two years or more.

*Morbidity of cervical cancer includes postsurgical and chemotherapeutic complications, infertility, incontinence, and pain from metastases.

**HIV causes fatigue, diarrhea, neuropathic symptoms, fevers, and opportunistic infections (OIs). OIs cause a wide variety of symptoms, including cough, shortness of breath, and vomiting. Average life expectancy after HIV infection is less than 10 years. Other STDs include gonorrhea, syphilis, and chlamydia. They cause a wide variety of symptoms, including dysuria, genital ulcers, infertility, rashes, neurologic and cardiac problems and rarely contribute to mortality. Preventing HIV and STDs has the added benefit of interrupting the spread of disease and preventing morbidity and mortality in those who thus avoid infection.

***Severely abnormal Pap smear: "moderate dysplasia," "severe dysplasia," "carcinoma in situ," CIS, CIN II, CIN III, "high grade SIL," squamous cell carcinoma, or adenocarcinoma.

Quality of Evidence Codes:

I:	RCT
II-1:	Nonrandomized controlled trials
II-2:	Cohort or case analysis
II-3:	Multiple time series
III:	Opinions or descriptive studies

288

REFERENCES - ROUTINE PREVENTIVE CARE

American College of Obstetricians and Gynecologists. August 1993. Cervical cytology: Evaluation and management of abnormalities. *ACOG Technical Bulletin* 183: 1-8.

American College of Physicians. 1994. *Guide for Adult Immunization*, Third ed. Philadelphia, PA: American College of Physicians.

American College of Obstetricians and Gynecologists. June 1991. Nonmalignant conditions of the breast. *ACOG Technical Bulletin* 156: 1-6.

American Heart Association. 1993. *Heart and Stroke Facts*. Dallas, TX: American Heart Association.

Austoker J. 16 July 1994. Cancer prevention in primary care: Screening and self examination for breast cancer. *British Medical Journal* 309: 168-74.

Canadian Task Force on the Periodic Health Examination. 15 February 1993. The periodic health examination, 1993 update: 2. Lowering the blood total cholesterol level to prevent coronary heart disease. *Canadian Medical Association Journal* 148 (4): 521-38.

Centers for Disease Control. 24 April 1992. Breast and cervical cancer surveillance, United States, 1973-1987. *Morbidity and Mortality Weekly Report* 41 (SS-2): 1-16.

Centers for Disease Control. 24 April 1992. Cancer screening behaviors among U.S. women: Breast cancer, 1987-1989, and cervical cancer, 1988-1989. *Morbidity and Mortality Weekly Report* 41 (SS-2): 17-34.

Centers for Disease Control. 8 August 1991. Diphtheria, tetanus, and pertussis: Recommendations for vaccine use and other preventive measures: Recommendations of the Immunization Practices Advisory Committee (ACIP). *Morbidity and Mortality Weekly Report* 40 (RR-10): 1-28.

Centers for Disease Control. 28 January 1994. General recommendations on immunization: Recommendations of the Advisory Committee on Immunization Practices (ACIP). *Morbidity and Mortality Weekly Report* 43 (RR-1): 1-38.

Centers for Disease Control. 2 December 1994. Monthly immunization table. *Morbidity and Mortality Weekly Report* 43 (47): 878.

Dayton S, ML Pearce, S Hashimoto, et al. July 1969. A controlled clinical trial of a diet high in unsaturated fat in preventing complications of atherosclerosis. *Circulation* 40 (1-Suppl. II): II1-II63.

Eddy DM. 1 September 1989. Screening for breast cancer. *Annals of Internal Medicine* 111 (5): 389-99.

Eddy DM. 1 August 1990. Screening for cervical cancer. *Annals of Internal Medicine* 113 (3): 214-26.

Fink DJ. March 1988. Change in American Cancer Society checkup guidelines for detection of cervical cancer. *Cancer Journal for Clinicians* 38 (2): 127-128.

Frick MH, O Elo, K Haapa, et al. 1987. Helsinki heart study: Primary prevention trial with Gemfibrozil in middle-aged men with dyslipidemia. Safety of treatment, changes in risk factors, and incidence of coronary heart disease. *New England Journal of Medicine* 317 (20): 1237-45.

Gardner P, and W Schaffner. 29 April 1993. Immunization of adults. *New England Journal of Medicine* 328 (17): 1252-8.

Gillum RF, HL Taylor, J Brozek, et al. 1982. Blood lipids in young men followed 32 years. *Journal of Chronic Diseases* 35: 635-41.

Hayward RSA, EP Steinberg, DE Ford, et al. 1 May 1991. Preventive care guidelines: 1991. *Annals of Internal Medicine* 114 (9): 758-83.

Hindle WH. August 1990. Breast masses: In-office evaluation with diagnostic triad. *Postgraduate Medicine* 88 (2): 85-94.

Hjermann I, K Velve Byre, I Holme, et al. 12 December 1981. Effect of diet and smoking intervention on the incidence of coronary heart disease. *Lancet* 2: 1303-1310.

IARC Working Group on Evaluation of Cervical Cancer Screening Programmes. 13 September 1986. Screening for squamous cervical cancer: Duration of low risk after negative results of cervical cytology and its implication for screening policies. *British Medical Journal* 293: 659-64.

Johannesson G, G Geirsson, and N Day. 1978. The effect of mass screening in Iceland, 1965-74, on the incidence and mortality of cervical carcinoma. *International Journal of Cancer* 21: 418-25.

Kannel WB, WP Castelli, T Gordon, et al. January 1971. Serum cholesterol, lipoproteins, and the risk of coronary heart disease: The Framingham study. *Annals of Internal Medicine* 74 (1): 1-12.

Kerlikowske K, D Grady, SM Rubin, et al. 11 January 1995. Efficacy of screening mammography: A meta-analysis. *Journal of the American Medical Association* 273 (2): 149-54.

Kurman RJ, GD Malkasian, A Sedlis, et al. May 1991. From Papanicolaou to Bethesda: The rationale for a new cervical cytologic classification. *Obstetrics and Gynecology* 77 (5): 779-82.

Laboratory Standardization Panel of the National Cholesterol Education Program. 1988. Current status of blood cholesterol measurement in clinical laboratories in the United States: A report from the Laboratory Standardization Panel of the National Cholesterol Education Program. *Clinical Chemistry* 34 (1): 193-201.

The Lipid Research Clinics Program. 1979. The Coronary Primary Prevention Trial: Design and implementation. *Journal of Chronic Diseases* 32: 609-31.

The Lipid Research Clinics Program. 20 January 1984. The Lipid Research Clinics Coronary Primary Prevention Trial results. I: Reduction in incidence of coronary heart disease. *Journal of the American Medical Association* 251 (3): 351-74.

The Lipid Research Clinics Program. 20 January 1984. The Lipid Research Clinics Coronary Primary Prevention Trial results. II: The relationship of reduction in incidence of coronary heart disease to cholesterol lowering. *Journal of the American Medical Association* 251 (3): 365-74.

The Lipid Research Clinics Program. 1 1983. Participant recruitment to the Coronary Primary Prevention Trial. *Journal of Chronic Diseases* 36 (6): 451-65.

The Lipid Research Clinics Program. 2 1983. Pre-entry characteristics of participants in the Lipid Research Clinics' Coronary Primary Prevention Trial. *Journal of Chronic Diseases* 36 (6): 467-79.

Littenberg B, AM Garber, and HC Sox. 1991. Screening for hypertension. In *Common Screening Tests*. Editor Eddy DM, 22-47 &397. Philadelphia, PA: American College of Physicians.

Martin MJ, SB Hulley, WS Browner, et al. 25 October 1986. Serum cholesterol, blood pressure, and mortality: Implictions from a cohort of 361,662 men. *Lancet* 2: 933-936.

McGuire LB. 15 November 1989. Screening for breast cancer. *Annals of Internal Medicine* 111 (10): 858-9.

Mettlin C, and CR Smart. August 1994. Breast cancer detection guidelines for women aged 40-49 years: Rationale for the American Cancer Society reaffirmation of recommendations. *Cancer Journal for Clinicians* 44 (4): 248-55.

Miller AB, G Anderson, J Brisson, et al. 15 November 1991. Report of a national workshop on screening for cancer for the cervix. *Canadian Medical Association Journal* 145 (10): 1301-25.

Miller KE, DP Losh, and A Folley. January 1992. Evaluation and follow-up of abnormal pap smears. *American Family Physician* 45: 143-50.

Montz F, BJ Monk, JM Fowler, et al. September 1992. Natural history of the minimally abnormal papanicolaou smear. *Obstetrics and Gynecology* 80 (3): 385-8.

National Center for Health Statistics. December 1994. *Current estimates from the National Health Interview Survey, 1993*. U.S. Department of Health and Human Services, Hyattsville, MD.

National Center for Health Statistics. 3 August 1994. *Health insurance and cancer screening among women*. U.S. Department of Health and Human Services, Hyattsville, MD.

Reed DM, CJ MacLean, and T Hayashi. 1987. Predictors of atherosclerosis in the Honolulu heart program. *American Journal of Epidemiology* 126 (2): 214-25.

Report from the Committee of Principal Investigators. 1978. A co-operative trial in the primary prevention of ischaemic heart disease using clofibrate. *British Heart Journal* 40: 1069-1118.

Report of the Committee of Principal Investigators. 23 August 1980. W.H.O. cooperative trial on primary prevention of ischaemic heart disease using clofibrate to lower serum cholesterol: Mortality follow-up. *Lancet* 2: 379-85.

Report of the Committee of Principal Investigators. 15 September 1984. W.H.O. cooperative trial on primary prevention of ischaemic heart disease with clofibrate to lower serum cholesterol: Final mortality follow-up. *Lancet* 2: 600-4.

Rose G, and M Shipley. 2 August 1986. Plasma cholesterol concentration and death from coronary heart disease: 10 year results of the Whitehall study. *British Medical Journal* 293: 306-7.

Rosner D, and D Blaird. 1985. What ultrasonography can tell in breast masses that mammography and physical examination cannot. *Journal of Surgical Oncology* 28: 308-13.

Scandinavian Simvastatin Survival Study Group. 19 November 1994. Randomised trial of cholesterol lowering in 4444 patients with coronary heart disease: The Scandinavian Simvastatin Survival Study (4S). *Lancet* 344: 1383-9.

Soutter WP. 23 May 1992. Conservative treatment of mild/moderate cervical dyskaryosis. *Lancet* 339: 1293.

Taylor WC, TM Pass, DS Shepard, et al. April 1987. Cholesterol reduction and life expectancy: A model incorporating multiple risk factors. *Annals of Internal Medicine* 106 (4): 605-14.

U.S. Department of Health and Human Services. 1991. *Healthy People 2000: National Health Promotion and Disease Prevention Objectives*. U.S. Government Printing Office, Washington, DC.

U.S. Preventive Services Task Force. 1989. *Guide to Clinical Preventive Services: An Assessment of the Effectiveness of 169 Interventions*. Baltimore, MD: Williams and Wilkins.

Wright TC, XW Sun, and J Koulos. February 1995. Comparison of management algorithms for the evaluation of women with low-grade cytologic abnormalities. *Obstetrics and Gynecology* 85: 2.

17. UPPER RESPIRATORY INFECTIONS
Eve A. Kerr, M.D., M.P.H.

We conducted a MEDLINE search of the medical literature for all English-language review articles published between 1990 and 1995 for the following topics: pharyngitis, common cold, influenza, rhinovirus, bronchitis- acute, cough, and rhinitis. We selected articles from the MEDLINE results and references from the review articles were obtained in areas of controversy. In addition, we consulted two medical texts (Panzer et al., 1991; Barker et al., 1991) for general clinical approaches to respiratory infections. This section first outlines our findings on the general importance of URIs and then discusses five common clinical subcategories: pharyngitis, bronchitis, influenza, nasal congestion, and sinusitis.

IMPORTANCE

Respiratory tract infections account for more than 10 percent of all office visits to the primary care physician (Perlman and Ginn, 1990). According to the 1993 National Health Interview Survey (NHIS), over 250 million cases of respiratory infections occur in the U.S. yearly (National Center for Health Statistics [NCHS], 1994b). Respiratory infections include the common cold, influenza, pharyngitis, sinusitis, bronchitis, and pneumonia. Influenza and the common cold account for the majority of cases. Women aged 18-44 reported 394.2 restricted activity days per 100 persons per year due to acute respiratory conditions; this represents 47 percent of all restricted activity days for acute conditions for women in this age category (NCHS, 1994b).

PHARYNGITIS, ACUTE

EFFICACY AND/OR EFFECTIVENESS OF INTERVENTIONS

Diagnosis

Multiple bacterial and viral organisms may cause acute pharyngitis (Barker et al., 1991). In evaluating acute pharyngitis, the critical clinical decision is whether or not to use antibiotics, or to culture, for group A streptococcal infection. Group A streptococcus is the causative agent of rheumatic fever, which can result in serious renal and cardiac disease. The incidence of rheumatic fever is currently low, and has been decreasing independent of antibiotic use (Little and Williamson, 1994). In fact, over 78,000 persons would be required in an RCT to show convincingly a 50 percent reduction in the attack rate of rheumatic fever with antibiotics (Shvartzman, 1994). The benefit of prescribing antibiotics for pharyngitis must be weighed against the costs. Little and Williamson (1994) estimate that if every case of pharyngitis were treated with antibiotics, the average general practitioner in the United Kingdom would have roughly a 1-in-3 chance of having a patient die from anaphylaxis after treatment for sore throat. This is slightly higher than the chances of nephritis or rheumatic fever developing post-pharyngitis, neither of which have a high death rate.

Komaroff (1986) has helped define pretest probabilities and diagnostic strategies for pharyngitis (Panzer et al., 1991). Based on prospective studies estimating sensitivity and specificity of clinical findings with respect to confirmed diagnosis of Group A streptococcal infection, Komaroff has determined that in adult patients who have a sore throat, but do not have a fever, tonsillar exudate, or anterior cervical adenopathy, the probability of streptococcal pharyngitis is less than 3 percent. On the other hand, when all three of these findings are present, the probability of streptococcal pharyngitis is at least 40 percent.

Diagnostic tests that are useful to determine the presence of group A streptococcus include throat culture and rapid streptococcal antigen tests. Throat cultures are shown to be falsely negative in approximately 10 percent of patients (Panzer et al., 1991). Rapid antigen tests are highly specific, but variably sensitive (80-95 percent) (Panzer et al., 1991).

According to Komaroff (1986) and based on the prospective studies of persons with sore throat, a reasonable diagnostic strategy is as follows:

1) Patients with pharyngitis who have a low probability of streptococcal infection (lack of fever, cervical adenopathy, and tonsillar exudate) do not require a throat culture or treatment with antibiotics. The exceptions to this are: persons with a history of rheumatic fever, documented streptococcal exposure in the past week, and residence in a community in which there is a current streptococcal epidemic.

2) Persons with an intermediate probability of streptococcal infection (presence of one or two of the following: fever, cervical adenopathy, or tonsillar exudate) should receive a throat culture. Whether to treat immediately or await culture results is left to the discretion of the clinician.

3) Persons with a high probability of streptococcal pharyngitis (presence of all three of the following: fever, cervical adenopathy, and tonsillar exudate) should be treated immediately with antibiotics. Throat culture is not required for confirmation.

4) In young persons, the diagnosis of mononucleosis, especially for pharyngitis of greater than one week's duration (Wood et al., 1980), should also be entertained.

Treatment

For documented or presumed group A streptococcus, treatment with penicillin or erythromycin is appropriate. Treatment should be for 10 days with penicillin V or erythromycin, or with a single intramuscular injection of 1.2 million units of penicillin B benzathine (Perlman and Ginn, 1990; Barker et al., 1991).

Follow-up

Follow-up cultures are indicated if there is a history of rheumatic fever in the patient or a household contact (Barker et al., 1991).

BRONCHITIS, ACUTE

IMPORTANCE

Acute bronchitis is an inflammatory disorder of the tracheobronchial tree that results in acute cough without signs of pneumonia (Billas, 1990). An estimated 12 million physician visits per year are made for acute bronchitis, with annual costs upward of $300 million for physician visits and prescription costs (Billas, 1990).

EFFICACY AND/OR EFFECTIVENESS OF INTERVENTIONS

Diagnosis

The causative organism of acute bronchitis is usually viral, but a variety of bacterial organisms may cause or contribute to bronchitis (e.g., *Streptococcus pneumoniae, Mycoplasma pneumoniae, Chlamydia pneumoniae, B. catarrhalis, and Bordetella pertussis*) (Billas, 1990; Barker et al., 1991). Cough may be nonproductive initially but generally becomes mucopurulent. The duration of cough is two weeks or less. Sputum characteristics are not helpful in distinguishing etiology of cough (Barker et al., 1991). Pharyngitis, fatigue and headache often precede onset of cough. Examination of the chest is usually normal, but may reveal rhonchi or rales without any evidence of consolidation. A detailed history must be obtained to rule in or out other possible causes for acute cough. Acute cough is defined as lasting less than three weeks (Pratter et al., 1993). Bronchitis, sinusitis, and the common cold are probably the most common causes of acute cough. Cough secondary to irritants (e.g., tobacco smoke) and allergies (e.g., from allergic rhinitis) are the next most common causes of cough (Zervanos and Shute, 1994).

Treatment

Most authorities agree that treatment with antibiotics in patients who are otherwise healthy and free of systemic symptoms is not useful (Barker et al., 1991; Billas, 1990). Orr et al. (1993) conducted a review of all randomized placebo-controlled trials of antibiotics for acute bronchitis published in the English language between 1980 and 1992. Four studies showed no significant benefit of using antibiotics, while two studies (one using erythromycin and the other using trimethoprim sulfa) did show benefit in decrease of subjective symptoms.

INFLUENZA

IMPORTANCE

Data from the 1981 NHIS indicated that there are approximately 112 million episodes of influenza-like illness annually in the United States, with an attack rate of 49.7 episodes per 100 persons per year (Garibaldi, 1985). Most influenza symptoms are cause by influenza A virus, which is dispersed by sneezing, coughing, or talking. While generally a self-limited disease, pandemics of influenza have caused heavy death tolls (Wiselka, 1994). Influenza causes between 10,000 and 20,000 deaths in the United States annually, especially among the elderly and those with chronic medical conditions (Fiebach and Beckett, 1994). In addition, influenza can cause complications such as pneumonitis, secondary pneumonia, Reye's syndrome, myositis and myoglobinuria, myocarditis, and neurologic sequelae (Wiselka, 1994; Barker et al., 1991). While most women under age 50 are at low risk of complications, influenza takes its toll in restricted activity days, amounting to over 420 million restricted activity days per year, or 1.9 per person per year (Garibaldi, 1985).

EFFICACY AND/OR EFFECTIVENESS OF INTERVENTIONS

Diagnosis

Uncomplicated influenza has an abrupt onset of systemic symptoms including fever, chills, headache and myalgias. The fever generally persists 3-4 days, but may persist up to 7 days. Respiratory symptoms (e.g., cough, hoarseness, nasal discharge, pharyngitis) begin when systemic symptoms begin to resolve. Physical findings include toxic appearance, cervical lymphadenopathy, hot skin, watery eyes and, rarely, localized chest findings (e.g., rales).

Treatment

Treatment for uncomplicated influenza is generally symptomatic, with rest, fluid intake, and aspirin or acetaminophen. Dyspnea, hemoptysis, wheezing, purulent sputum, fever persisting more than 7 days, severe muscle pain, and dark urine, may indicate onset of influenza complications (Barker et al., 1991). Amantadine has been shown to decrease virus shedding and shorten duration of influenza symptoms if treatment was started within 48 hours of symptom onset. Common side-effects include headache, light headedness, dizziness and insomnia. Amantadine should be considered for use in patients at high risk (see Section C: Influenza, of Chapter 16) who develop symptoms of a flu-like illness during an influenza outbreak (Delker et al., 1980).[4] According to a 1979 National Institutes of Health (NIH) consensus development conference, adults who should be considered for prophylaxis include those with chronic diseases, those whose activities are vital to community function and who have not been vaccinated, and persons in semi-closed institutional environments (NIH, 1979).

---

[4]Rimantadine is also an appropriate form of treatment.

NASAL CONGESTION AND RHINORRHEA

IMPORTANCE

Over 8 million visits for nasal congestion as the principal reason for patient visit occurred in 1989 across all age groups in the United States (NCHS, 1992). Nasal congestion may be due to a variety of causes, the principal of these being acute viral infection (i.e., common cold), allergic rhinitis and infectious sinusitis (acute or chronic) (Canadian Rhinitis Symposium, 1994). Other common causes include vasomotor rhinitis and rhinitis medicomentosa. Appropriate treatment rests in making distinctions among these causes. Other less common reasons for rhinitis include atrophic rhinitis, hormonal rhinitis and mechanical/obstructive rhinitis. For a more detailed discussion of allergic rhinitis, see Chapter 3.

The Canadian Rhinitis Symposium convened in January of 1994 to develop a guide for assessing and treating rhinitis (Canadian Rhinitis Symposium, 1994). The guidebook is extensive, but essential elements for diagnosis and treatment are discussed below.

EFFICACY AND/OR EFFECTIVENESS OF INTERVENTIONS

Diagnosis and Treatment

The following may serve to differentiate between (1) allergic rhinitis, (2) infectious viral rhinitis (common cold) and (3) sinusitis.

Allergic Rhinitis

Symptoms: Nasal congestion, sneezing, palatal itching, rhinorrhea with or without allergic conjunctivitis. Symptoms are seasonal or perennial and may be triggered by allergens such as pollens, mites, molds, and animal danders.

Physical exam: nasal mucosa is pale or hyperemic; edema with or without watery secretions are frequently present.

Treatment: Treatment of allergic rhinitis should include antihistamines, nasal cromolyn and/or nasal glucocorticoid sprays. Oral decongestants may be used for symptomatic relief. If prescribed, topical nasal decongestants are indicated for short term use only.

Infectious Viral Rhinitis

<u>Symptoms</u>: Nasal congestion and rhinorrhea. Other symptoms of viral infectious rhinitis included mild malaise, sneezing, scratchy throat, and variable loss of taste and smell. Colds due to rhinoviruses typically last one week, and rarely as long as two weeks (Barker et al., 1991). Symptoms are generally of acute onset, unless chronic sinusitis is present (see below - chronic sinusitis). Symptoms of coexisting acute sinusitis may also be present (see below - acute sinusitis).

<u>Physical exam</u>: Mucosa hyperemic and edematous with or without purulent secretions; physical exam should include nasal cavity and sinuses (for presence of sinusitis) and ears (for presence of otitis media) (Barker et al., 1991). Sinus tenderness and fever may be present with sinusitis

<u>Treatment</u>: Treatment of infectious viral rhinitis without sinusitis is symptomatic. Use of oral decongestants or short term nasal decongestants is appropriate but not necessary. For coexisting sinusitis, treatment should be with antibiotics in addition to decongestants (see acute sinusitis below).

Sinusitis

<u>Symptoms/Physical Exam/Treatment</u>: See discussions below on acute and chronic sinusitis.

SINUSITIS

IMPORTANCE—ACUTE AND CHRONIC SINUSITIS

According to the 1991 National Ambulatory Medical Care Survey, chronic sinusitis was the eighth most common diagnosis rendered by physicians for office visits in 1991 (NCHS, 1994c). This translates to 1.7 percent of all visits among children and adults. Patients frequently mentioned symptoms which could be attributable to sinusitis--

headache in 1.5 percent of visits and nasal congestion in 1.3 percent of visits. In adults 25-44 years of age, sinusitis accounted for 2.3 percent of visits and allergic rhinitis for 2.3 percent. Among women of all ages, chronic sinusitis accounted for 1.8 percent of all visits (NCHS, 1994c). While little data exists on the incidence of acute sinusitis, chronic sinusitis was reported by over 30 million persons in the 1986-1988 NHIS (NCHS, 1993).

EFFICACY AND/OR EFFECTIVENESS OF INTERVENTIONS

Acute Sinusitis

Diagnosis

Acute sinusitis is defined as a sinus infection that lasts less than 3 weeks. Acute sinusitis is a complication in about 0.5 percent of viral upper respiratory tract infections (Barker, 1991). By definition, acute sinusitis has a duration of less than three weeks (Stafford, 1992). Symptoms that may increase the likelihood of acute sinusitis being present include fever, malaise, cough, nasal congestion, toothache, purulent nasal discharge, little improvement with nasal decongestants, and headache or facial pain exacerbated by bending forward (Williams and Simel, 1993). Transillumination may improve the accuracy of diagnosis for maxillary sinusitis, but its usefulness is operator sensitive (Williams and Simel, 1993).

Treatment

Treatment is based on controlling infection and reducing tissue edema. Ten to fourteen days of antibiotics should be instituted for treatment of acute sinusitis, although there is some recent evidence that 3 days may suffice (Williams et al., 1995). In addition, oral or topical decongestants should be used. If a topical nasal decongestant is prescribed, treatment should be limited to no more than 4 days (Barker et al., 1991; Stafford, 1992). Antihistamines, because of their drying action on the nasal mucosa, have no role in the treatment of most patients with acute sinusitis, except when patients also manifest symptoms of allergic rhinitis (thin, watery rhinorrhea, and sneezing) (Stafford, 1992).

Follow-up

If symptoms fail to improve after 7 days, a 10-14 day course of
therapy with another antibiotic should be prescribed (Stafford, 1992).
If symptoms persist after 2 courses of antibiotics, referral to an
otolaryngologist and/or more definitive diagnostic studies (e.g., x-ray,
sinus CT, nasal endoscopy) are indicated (Stafford, 1992).

Chronic Sinusitis

Diagnosis

Sinusitis that has continued for 3 months or more is considered
chronic (Stafford, 1992). Chronic sinusitis appears to result from
episodes of prolonged, repeated, or inadequately treated acute
sinusitis. Chronic sinusitis generally presents with dull ache or
pressure across the midface, which patients characterize as a headache.
The headache may be worse in the morning and with head movement. In
addition, patients may also complain of nasal congestion and thick
pharyngeal secretions, blocked or popping ears, dental pain, chronic
cough, mild facial swelling, and eye pain (Godley, 1992).

Conditions that commonly predispose to chronic sinusitis include
previous acute sinusitis, allergic rhinitis, environmental irritants,
nasal polyposis, and viral infection (Godley, 1992).

Diagnosis rests on history, evaluation by nasal endoscopy, and CT
scanning (Bolger and Kennedy, 1992). In general, if the history is
strongly suggestive of chronic sinusitis, one should treat first with
antibiotics (see below). If medical therapy is unsuccessful or if the
disease recurs repeatedly, referral to an otolaryngologist for
endoscopic examination is indicated (Bolger and Kennedy, 1992).
Endoscopic examination is more specific for chronic sinusitis than is CT
scanning. If endoscopic findings are equivocal, a CT scan may
demonstrate underlying sinus disease. However, a CT is best performed
four to six weeks after optimal medical therapy is instituted to
optimize specificity (Bolger and Kennedy, 1992).

Treatment

Medical treatment should be attempted first. First-line therapy
for chronic disease is amoxicillin and clavulonic acid (Augmentin),
three times daily for 21 to 28 days (Bolger and Kennedy, 1992), or

trimethoprim-sulfamethoxazole, cefaclor, cefuroxime, and cefixime (Godley, 1992). Other medications that may be used include oral decongestants, nasal steroids, and antihistamines for patients with an allergic component.

Surgical treatment is reserved for cases when medical therapy fails. Currently, endoscopic surgery is the method of choice (Bolger and Kennedy, 1992). Endoscopic examination and debridement of the operative cavity are required once or twice weekly for four to six weeks to promote healing and prevent stenosis of the sinus ostia. Complications of surgery include CSF rhinorrhea, diplopia, blindness and meningitis. However, the rates of complications are very low among experienced surgeons. In studies reporting success rates of surgery in consecutive patients, up to 93 percent of patients reported substantial symptomatic improvement in a two-year follow-up, and subsequent revision surgery is reported in 7-10 percent (Bolger and Kennedy, 1992). It should be noted that no randomized controlled trials or case-controlled studies for endoscopic surgery have been performed.

RECOMMENDED QUALITY INDICATORS FOR UPPER RESPIRATORY INFECTIONS

These indicators apply to women age 18-50.

Diagnosis

	Indicator	Quality of evidence	Literature	Benefits	Comments
Pharyngitis					
1.	If a patient presents with a complaint of sore throat, the medical history should document presence or absence of previous episodes of rheumatic fever.	III	Barker et al., 1991	Prevent rheumatic heart disease.	In patients with previous rheumatic fever, one would be more inclined to obtain a culture and treat with antibiotics, since these patients are at higher risk for complications.
2.	History/physical exam should document presence or absence of fever, tonsillar exudate and anterior cervical adenopathy.	II	Komaroff, 1986	Alleviate sore throat. Prevent rheumatic heart disease. Prevent rheumatic fever.	If all three are present, the probability of streptococcal infections is greater than 40% and one would be inclined to treat empirically without culture.
Bronchitis/Cough					
3.	The history of patients presenting with cough of less than 3 weeks' duration should document: presence or absence of preceding viral infection (e.g., common cold, influenza that started 2 weeks or less prior to onset of cough).	III	Zervanos and Shute, 1994	Decrease cough. Prevent allergic reactions from antibiotics.	If preceding viral infection were present and the patient has no other complications (e.g., fever, shortness of breath), a diagnosis of viral bronchitis is likely. This diagnosis is self-limited and antibiotics are not necessary. No preceding viral infection would lead one to search for non-viral causes of bronchitis.
4.	The history of patients presenting with cough of less than 3 weeks' duration should document presence or absence of fever and shortness of breath (dyspnea).	III	Barker et al., 1991	Decrease cough. Decrease shortness of breath. Prevent development of emphysema. Prevent development of sepsis.	These symptoms are consistent with possible pneumonia, which would require antibiotic treatment.
5.	Patients presenting with acute cough should receive a physical examination of the chest for evidence of pneumonia.	III	Barker et al., 1991	Decrease cough. Decrease shortness of breath. Prevent development of emphysema. Prevent development of sepsis.	Signs of consolidation would lead one on a different diagnostic and treatment path.
6.	Patients presenting with acute cough and with evidence of consolidation on physical exam of the chest (dullness to percussion, egophony, etc.) should receive a chest x-ray to look for evidence of pneumonia.	III	Barker et al., 1991	Decrease cough. Decrease shortness of breath. Prevent development of emphysema. Prevent development of sepsis.	Presence of pneumonia would necessitate different treatment and follow-up plans.

	Indicator		Literature	Benefits	Comments
Nasal Congestion					
7.	If a patient presents with the complaint of nasal congestion and/or rhinorrhea not attributed to the common cold, the history should include: seasonality of symptoms, presence or absence of sneezing, facial pain, fever, specific irritants, use of topical or systemic nasal decongestants.	III	Payton, 1994	Decrease nasal congestion. Decrease rhinorrhea.	Nasal congestion can result from multiple causes in addition to the common cold. The most important of these, because of availability of treatment, are allergic rhinitis, sinusitis, and topical nasal decongestant abuse (rhinitis medicamentosa). If the practitioner does not attribute symptoms to the common cold, symptoms specific to these alternate diagnoses should be elicited.
Acute Sinusitis					
8.	If the diagnosis of acute sinusitis is made, symptoms should be present for a duration of less than 3 weeks (e.g., fever, malaise, cough, nasal congestion, purulent nasal discharge, ear pain or blockage, post-nasal drip, dental pain, headache, or facial pain).	III	Barker et al., 1991; Williams & Simel, 1993	Decrease nasal congestion, fever, post-nasal drip, headache and facial pain.	Acute sinusitis is defined as lasting less than 3 weeks. If symptoms last longer, the patient may have chronic sinusitis, which is more difficult to treat and requires longer duration of antibiotic therapy.

Treatment

	Indicator	Quality of evidence	Literature	Benefits	Comments
Pharyngitis					
9.	Patients with sore throat and fever, tonsillar exudate and anterior cervical adenopathy should receive immediate treatment for presumed streptococcal infection.	II	Komaroff, 1986; Panzer, 1991	Decrease sore throat. Prevent rheumatic fever.	Since throat cultures and rapid antigen tests vary in their sensitivity and specificity, this combination of symptoms is sufficient to warrant antibiotic treatment without further laboratory testing.
10.	Treatment of streptococcal throat infection should be with penicillin V or erythromycin for 10 days; or with a single injection of benzathine penicillin.	III	Barker et al., 1991	Decrease sore throat. Prevent rheumatic fever.	This is the current standard of care, although other antibiotics (e.g., ampicillin) are also effective.
11.	If an antibiotic is NOT prescribed with the diagnosis of sore throat, a throat culture or rapid antigen test should be obtained if any of the following are present: a) fever; b) tonsillar exudate; c) anterior cervical adenopathy.	II	Komaroff, 1986	Prevent rheumatic fever.	Each finding increases the probability of streptococcal infection.
12.	If an antibiotic is prescribed, documentation of presence or absence of drug allergies should be in the chart.	III	Barker et al., 1991	Avoid allergic reactions.	Allergy to antibiotics is relatively common. Approximately 2% of persons treated with penicillin derivatives develop an allergic reaction. Since alternative antibiotic regimens usually exist, it is wise to be aware of patients' allergy status before prescribing antibiotic.

Bronchitis/Cough

#	Indicator	Level	Reference	Benefits	Comments
13.	If an antibiotic is prescribed for acute cough, documentation of drug allergies should be in the chart.	III	Barker et al., 1991	Avoid allergic reactions.	Allergy to antibiotics is relatively common. Approximately 2% of persons treated with penicillin derivatives develop an allergic reaction. Since alternative antibiotic regimens usually exist, it is wise to be aware of patients' allergy status before prescribing antibiotic.
14.	If the history documents cigarette smoking in a patient with acute cough, encouragement to stop smoking should be documented.	III	Barker et al., 1991	Prevent future bronchitic episodes. Prevent smoking-related morbidity and mortality.	Smokers are predisposed to bronchitis. Symptomatic patients present a window of opportunity to counsel regarding smoking cessation.

Influenza

#	Indicator	Level	Reference	Benefits	Comments
15.	Women with asthma, chronic obstructive pulmonary disease, chronic cardiovascular disorders, diabetes mellitus, renal failure, hemoglobinopathies (e.g., sickle cell disease) or immunosuppresssion, who present with symptoms of influenza within the first 48 hours should be considered for treatment with amantadine.	I-III	NIH Consensus Development Conference, 1980	Decrease pneumonia. Decrease mortality.	Amantadine decreases duration of symptoms and perhaps severity of disease. Patients at risk for developing complications from influenza should be treated with amantadine. Complications of influenza include pneumonia and death.

Nasal Congestion

#	Indicator	Level	Reference	Benefits	Comments
16.	If topical or systemic nasal decongestants are prescribed, duration of treatment should be for no longer than 4 days.	III	Stafford et al., 1992; Barker et al., 1991	Prevent rhinitis medicamentosa.	Long-term treatment with topical decongestants can cause rebound congestion (rhinitis medicamentosa).

Acute Sinusitis

#	Indicator	Level	Reference	Benefits	Comments
17.	Treatment for acute sinusitis should be with antibiotics for at least 10 days.	I-III	Williams et al., 1995	Decrease nasal congestion. Decrease fever. Decrease facial pain. Prevent development of chronic sinusitis.	Antibiotics have proven benefit but the length of treatment is somewhat controversial.
18.	Treament for acute sinusitis should include a systemic or topical nasal decongestant.	III	Stafford et al., 1992	Decrease nasal congestion. Decrease fever. Decrease facial pain. Prevent development of chronic sinusitis.	The purpose is to decrease mucosal edema.
19.	If topical or systemic nasal decongestants are prescribed, duration of treatment should be for no longer than 4 days	III	Stafford et al., 1992; Barker et al., 1991	Prevent rhinitis medicamentosa.	Long term treatment with topical decongestants can cause rebound congestions (rhinitis medicamentosa).
20.	If an antibiotic is prescribed for acute sinusitis, documentation of presence or absence of drug allergies should be in the chart.	III	Stafford et al., 1992	Avoid allergic reactions.	Allergy to antibiotics is relatively common. Approximately 2% of persons treated with penicillin derivatives develop an allergic reaction. Since alternative antibiotic regimens usually exist, it is wise to be aware of patients' allergy status before prescribing antibiotic.
21.	In the absence of symptoms of allergic rhinitis (thin, watery rhinorrhea, and sneezing), antihistamines should not be prescribed for acute sinusitis.	III	Stafford et al., 1992	Prevent antihistamine side effects.	Antihistamines should only be used if allergic symptoms are present. No RCTs have been done in this area.

22.	If symptoms fail to improve after one week of antibiotic treatment, therapy with another antibiotic for at least 10 days should be instituted.	III	Stafford et al., 1992	Decrease nasal congestion. Decrease fever. Decrease facial pain. Prevent development of chronic sinusitis.	A trial with another antibiotic is in order if symptom relief does not occur within 10 days..
23.	If the patient does not improve after two courses of antibiotics, referral to an otolaryngologist for a diagnostic test (CT, x-ray, ultrasound of the sinuses) is indicated.	III	Stafford et al., 1992	Decrease nasal congestion. Prevent development of chronic sinusitis.	Reevaluation of diagnosis and/or surgical treatment may be indicated.
	Chronic Sinusitis				
24.	If a diagnosis of chronic sinusitis is made, the patient should be treated with at least 3 weeks of antibiotics.	III	Stafford et al., 1992	Decrease nasal congestion and other symptoms of chronic sinusitis.* Prevent recurrence of sinusitis.	It is generally agreed that a longer duration of treatment for chronic sinusitis is necessary than for acute sinusitis. However, the exact number of days has not been defined in RCTs. The literature cites 3 weeks as standard of care.
25.	If patient has repeated symptoms after 2 separate 3 week trials of antibiotics, a referral to an otolaryngologist is indicated.	III	Bolger and Kennedy, 1992	Decrease nasal congestion and other symptoms of chronic sinusitis.* Prevent recurrence of sinusitis.	While medical treatment is still first-line therapy, surgical treatment may be indicated if two courses of antibiotics fail to relieve symptoms.
26.	If topical or systemic nasal decongestants are prescribed, duration of treatment should be for no longer than 4 days.	III	Stafford et al., 1992; Barker et al., 1991	Prevent rhinitis medicamentosa.	Long-term treatment with topical decongestants can cause rebound congestion (rhinitis medicamentosa).
27.	In the absence of symptoms of allergic rhinitis (thin, watery rhinorrhea, and sneezing), antihistamines should not be prescribed.	III	Stafford et al., 1992	Prevent antihistamine side effects.	Antihistamines may be detrimental to treatment secondary to drying properties. Therefore, they should only be used if allergic symptoms are present. No RCTs have been done in this area.

*Symptoms of chronic sinusitis include nasal congestions, fever, headache, facial pain, toothache, rhinorrhea, and purulent nasal discharge.

Quality of Evidence Codes:

I: RCT
II-1:   Nonrandomized controlled trials
II-2:   Cohort or case analysis
II-3:   Multiple time series
III: Opinions or descriptive studies

REFERENCES - UPPER RESPIRATORY INFECTIONS

Barker LR, JR Burton, and PD Zieve, Editors. 1991. *Principles of Ambulatory Medicine*, Third ed.Baltimore, MD: Williams and Wilkins.

Billas A. December 1990. Lower respiratory tract infections. *Primary Care* 17 (4): 811-24.

Bolger WE, and DW Kennedy. 30 September 1992. Changing concepts in chronic sinusitis. *Hospital Practice* 27 (9A): 20-2, 26-8.

Canadian Rhinitis Symposium. 1994. Assessing and treating rhinitis: A practical guide for Canadian physicians. Proceedings of the Canadian Rhinitis Symposium; Toronto, Ontario; January 14-15, 1994. *Canadian Medical Journal* 15 (Suppl. 4): 1-27.

Centers for Disease Control. 27 May 1994. Prevention and control of influenza: Part I, vaccines. *Morbidity and Mortality Weekly Report* 43 (RR-9): 1-13.

Delker LL, L Moser, H Robert, et al. 1980. Amantadine: Does it have a role in prevention and treatment of influenza? *Annals of Internal Medicine* 92 (Part 1): 256-8.

Fiebach N, and W Beckett. 28 November 1994. Prevention of respiratory infections in adults: Influenza and pneumococcal vaccines. *Archives of Internal Medicine* 154: 2545-57.

Garibaldi RA. 28 June 1985. Epidemiology of community-acquired respiratory tract infections in adults: Incidence, etiology, and impact. *American Journal of Medicine* 78 (Suppl. 6B): 32-7.

Godley FA. May 1992. Chronic Sinusitis: An Update. *American Family Physician* 45 (5): 2190-9.

Komaroff A, TM Pass, MD Aronson, et al. January 1986. The prediction of streptococcal pharyngitis in adults. *Journal of General Internal Medicine* 1: 1-7.

Little PS, and I Williamson. 15 October 1994. Are antibiotics appropriate for sore throats? *British Medical Journal* 309: 1010-11.

National Center for Health Statistics. December 1994. *Current estimates from the National Health Interview Survey, 1993*. U.S. Department of Health and Human Services, Hyattsville, MD.

National Center for Health Statistics. April 1992. *National Ambulatory Medical Care Survey: 1989 summary*. U.S. Department of Health and Human Services, Hyattsville, MD.

National Center for Health Statistics. 1994. *National Ambulatory Medical Care Survey: 1991 summary*. U.S. Department of Health and Human Services, Hyattsville, MD.

National Center for Health Statistics. February 1993. *Prevalence of selected chronic conditions: United States, 1986-88*. U.S. Department of Health and Human Services, Hyattsville, MD.

National Institutes of Health Consensus Development Conference Summaries. *Amantadine: Does it have a role in the prevention and treatment of influenza?*, 51-6. Sponsored by the National Institute of Allergy and Infectious Diseases, October 15-16, 1979.

Orr PH, K Scherer, A Macdonald, et al. 1993. Randomized placebo-controlled trials of antibiotics for acute bronchitis: A critical review of the literature. *Journal of Family Practice* 36 (5): 507-12.

Panzer RJ, ER Black, and PF Griner, Editors. 1991. *Diagnostic Strategies for Common Medical Problems*. Philadelphia, PA: American College of Physicians.

Perlman PE, and DR Ginn. January 1990. Respiratory infections in ambulatory adults: Choosing the best treatment. *Postgraduate Medicine* 87 (1): 175-84.

Pratter MR, T Bartter, S Akers, et al. 15 November 1993. An algorithmic approach to chronic cough. *Annals of Internal Medicine* 119 (10): 977-83.

Shvartzman P. 15 October 1994. Careful prescribing is beneficial. *British Medical Journal* 309: 1011-12.

Stafford CT. November 1990. The clinician's view of sinusitis. *Otolaryngology-Head and Neck Surgery* 103 (Volume 5, Part 2): 870-5.

Williams JW, DR Holleman Jr., GP Samsa, et al. 5 April 1995. Randomized controlled trial of 3 vs 10 days of trimethoprim/sulfamethoxazole for acute maxillary sinusitis. *Journal of the American Medical Association* 273 (13): 1015-21.

Williams JW, and DL Simel. 8 September 1993. Does this patient have sinusitis? Diagnosing acute sinusitis by history and physical examination. *Journal of the American Medical Association* 270 (10): 1242-6.

Wiselka M. 21 May 1994. Influenza: Diagnosis, management, and prophylaxis. *British Medical Journal* 308: 1341-5.

Wood RW, RK Tompkins, and BW Wolcott. November 1980. An efficient strategy for managing acute respiratory illness in adults. *Annals of Internal Medicine* 93 (5): 757-63.

Zervanos NJ, and KM Shute. March 1994. Acute, disruptive cough: Symptomatic therapy for a nagging problem. *Postgraduate Medicine* 95 (4): 153-68.

18. URINARY TRACT INFECTION
Eve A. Kerr, M.D., M.P.H.

The general approach to urinary tract infections (UTIs) was obtained from one ambulatory medical text chapter (Barker et al., 1991), a textbook of diagnostic strategies (Panzer et al., 1991), and review articles which dealt with diagnosis and management of urinary tract infections. The review articles were chosen from a MEDLINE search which identified all English language review articles on urinary tract infection between the years of 1990 and 1995. Further, since the main controversy in UTIs concerns laboratory testing and therapy, we selected and reviewed references from the review articles which related to laboratory testing and antibiotic therapy. Finally, we performed another MEDLINE search (1990-1995) to identify any randomized controlled trials (RCTs) regarding treatment of UTIs.

IMPORTANCE

UTIs are among the most common bacterial infections seen by physicians and are the most common bacterial infection in women (Winickoff et al., 1981). They affect 10-20 percent of women in the United States annually and account for over 5 million office visits per year. Outpatient expenditures for patients with UTIs in the United States approach $1 billion (Powers, 1991).

EFFICACY AND/OR EFFECTIVENESS OF INTERVENTIONS

Screening

There is no role for screening for UTIs for bacteriuria in otherwise healthy non-pregnant women under age 50 (Pels et al., 1989).

Diagnosis

The diagnosis of UTI is suggested by the history. An uncomplicated UTI is suggested by symptoms of bladder irritation and occasionally hematuria. An upper tract infection is suggested by the concomitant presence of fever, chills, and/or back pain. In addition, vaginal

infections (due to candida and trichomonas) and urethritis (due to
Chlamydia trachomatis, Neisseria gonorrhoeae, or herpes simplex virus)
could present with UTI-type symptoms. Therefore, a history of vaginal
discharge and sexual activity should be sought. Since pregnant patients
and those with diabetes and immunosuppression are treated differently,
the history should specifically include these questions (Barker et al.,
1991).

The urinalysis is the most important initial study in the
evaluation of a patient suspected of having a UTI by history. A
negative urinalysis makes the diagnosis of UTI extremely unlikely
(Barker et al., 1991). A specimen should be collected by the "clean-
catch" method to minimize likelihood of contamination (Barker et al.,
1991), or by catheterization when the "clean-catch" method is
impossible. A finding by microscopic examination using a high-power
lens of bacteria of more than seven white cells/mm^3 in unspun urine or
more than two white cells per high-power field in spun urine is
consistent with an UTI. The leukocyte esterase test has a sensitivity
for defining UTI (if the test is positive) of between 62 and 68 percent,
with a positive predictive value of only 46-55 percent and a negative
predictive value of 88-92 percent (Pfaller and Koontz, 1985). A nitrite
test has a sensitivity of 35-85 percent and specificity of 92-100
percent for the presence of bacteria (Pappas, 1991). The leukocyte-
esterase nitrite combination has a sensitivity of 79.2 percent, a
specificity of 81 percent and a negative predictive value of 94.5
percent for specimens with $\geq10^5$ CFU/ml (Pfaller and Koontz, 1985).

A combination of findings (i.e., bacteriuria, pyuria and a positive
nitrite test) is more highly predictive for UTI (Bailey, 1995).

The criteria for appropriate use of a culture are shown in Table
18.1

Table 18.1

Criteria for Appropriate Use of Culture

A culture should be obtained in women who have:

- "several" (three or more) infections in the past year
- diabetes or immunocompromised state
- fever, chills and/or flank pain
- acute pyelonephritis
- structural or functional anomalies of the urinary tract
- symptoms for more than 7 days before presentation
- pregnancy
- uncertain clinical or urinalysis features
- a relapse of symptoms after initial treatment
- age older than 65
- had a recent hospitalization or invasive procedure

Sources: Powers, 1991; Barker et al., 1991; Panzer et al., 1991.

Treatment

Treatment currently rests with the appropriate use of antibiotics. A single-dose or a three-day course of an oral antimicrobial has been shown to eradicate approximately 90-95 percent of cases of uncomplicated UTI in young women. However, therapy for three days or longer was more effective than single-dose therapy in most trials and in a meta-analysis (Stamm and Hooton, 1993; Elder, 1992; Johnson and Stamm, 1989; Norrby, 1990). Seven-day regimens should be reserved for patients with "complicated lower tract infections" (See Table 18.2).

Table 18.2

Definition of Complicated Lower Tract Infections

Diabetes or immunocompromised state

Functional or structural anomaly of the urinary tract

Symptoms for longer than 7 days

Recent urinary tract infection

Acute pyelonephritis or more than 3 urinary tract
  infections in past year

Use of diaphragm

Age older than 65

Pregnancy

Sources: Stamm and Hooton, 1993; Johnson and Stamm, 1989.

Patients with mild to moderate acute uncomplicated pyelonephritis should be treated for 10-14 days as outpatients (Stamm et al., 1987). Severe pyelonephritis, with nausea and vomiting, or possible urosepsis, may require hospitalization, as does pyelonephritis in pregnancy.

In general, trimethoprim/sulfamethoxazole double strength (160 mg/800 mg) is the most effective first-line agent, with resistance in 5-15 percent of cases. It should be used unless there is documented resistance, allergy, or pregnancy. Amoxicillin and nitrofurantoin have higher rates of failure (Stamm and Hooton, 1993; Johnson and Stamm, 1989; Elder, 1992; Norrby, 1990). The use of quinolones, while effective (Stein et al., 1987; Hooton et al., 1991), should be reserved for patients with known resistance or allergy to other first-line agents to avoid unnecessary expense and the promotion of resistant strains (Sable and Scheld, 1993).

Follow-up

Experts disagree on necessity for follow-up. Some feel a follow-up culture is unnecessary if symptoms of uncomplicated UTI have resolved within 3 days of starting treatment (Stamm and Hooton, 1993; Patton et al., 1991; Winickoff et al., 1981; Schultz et al., 1984). Barker et al. (1991) stipulate that the urinalysis should be re-evaluated within 7 days if a single-dose regimen was utilized or within 4 weeks if a 7-10 days course was used even if symptoms have cleared. Most experts agree, however, that follow-up culture is indicated within 2 weeks of complicated cystitis or pyelonephritis (Stamm and Hooton, 1993).

RECOMMENDED QUALITY INDICATORS FOR URINARY TRACT INFECTIONS

The following criteria apply to women under age 50 without diabetes or immunocompromise.

Diagnosis

	Indicator	Quality of evidence	Literature	Benefits	Comments
1.	In women presenting with dysuria, presence or absence of fever and flank pain should be elicited.	III	Barker et al., 1991; Powers, 1991	Alleviate pain and fever. Prevent sepsis. Prevent abscess formation.	Fever and flank pain increase probability of upper tract infection (pyelonephritis).
2.	In women presenting with dysuria, a history of vaginal discharge should be elicited.	III	Panzer et al., 1991; Barker et al., 1991	Alleviate dysuria. Prevent allergic reactions from antibiotics. Prevent antibiotic associated diarrhea and yeast vaginitis.	Dysuria may be caused by vaginitis (and rarely cervicitis) as well as UTI. By evaluating cause for dysuria, treatment for vaginitis may be initiated and avoidance of antibiotics for non-UTI causes can be accomplished.
3.	If a woman presents with dysuria and a complaint of vaginal discharge, a speculum exam and microscopic examination of discharge (if any) should be performed (e.g., KOH and saline wet mount).	III	Panzer et al., 1991	Alleviate dysuria. Prevent allergic reactions to antibiotics. Prevent antibiotic associated diarrhea and yeast vaginitis.	Dysuria may be caused by vaginitis (and rarely cervicitis) as well as UTI. By evaluating cause for dysuria, treatment for vaginitis may be initiated and avoidance of antibiotics for non-UTI causes can be accomplished. This is implied from recommendation regarding treatment.
4.	Women presenting with dysuria should be asked about the possibility of concurrent pregnancy (e.g., date of LMP) or be given a pregnancy test.	III	Panzer et al., 1991; Barker et al., 1991	Avoid spontaneous abortion.	Women who are pregnant and have UTI are at risk for spontaneous abortion. Treatment needs to be for a longer period of time and follow-up cultures are necessary to document eradication of infection.
5.	A urinalysis should be performed on women in whom urinary tract infection is suspected.	III	Johnson and Stamm, 1989; Panzer et al., 1991	Prevent allergic reactions from antibiotics. Prevent antibiotic-associated diarrhea and yeast vaginitis.	Urinalysis, if negative for white blood cells, rules out UTI and antibiotics do not need to be used.
6.	A urine culture should be obtained for women who have dysuria and any one of the following: a. "several" (three or more) infections in the past year b. diabetes or immunocompromised state c. fever, chills and/or flank pain d. diagnosis of pyelonephritis e. structural or functional anomalies of the urinary tract f. pregnancy g. a relapse of symptoms, or h. a recent hospitalization or invasive procedure.	III	Powers, 1991; Barker et al., 1991; Panzer et al., 1991	Alleviate dysuria. Prevent pyelonephritis. Prevent uti recurrence.	Appropriate and prompt treatment in these instances can prevent complications and recurrences. However, there is little empiric evidence to support the timing for obtaining a urine culture.

318

	Indicator	Quality of evidence	Literature	Benefits	Comments
7.	If the patient has dysuria and a urinalysis shows more than 5 WBC per high-power field, the patient should receive treatment with antimicrobials.	II-2 III	Panzer et al., 1991; Barker et al., 1991	Prevent complications of untreated infection (including pyelonephritis from lower tract UTI, and PID, ectopic pregnancy and infertility from cervicitis).	Patients with pyuria and dysuria almost always have an infection that will respond to antimicrobial agents. This infection may not always be a UTI (for example, chlamydia urethritis can present with dysuria and pyuria). Treatment of UTI can prevent complications of upper tract infection and sepsis. Treatment of chlamydial infection can prevent future PID, ectopic pregnancies, and infertility. The number of WBC per high power field indicative of a UTI in centrifuged urine is usually given as 2-5. We have chosen the upper range.
8.	If a diagnosis of UTI (upper or lower tract) has been made, the patient should be treated with antimicrobial therapy.	III; II-2	Stamm and Hooton, 1993; Johnson and Stamm, 1989; Powers, 1991	Prevent complications of untreated infection.	Both upper and lower tract infections respond to a number of antimicrobial agents. Trimethoprim-sulfa is usually chosen as a first line agent. While no RCTs have shown benefits of treatment, it is recognized that treatment of both lower and upper tract infections is beneficial (see above).
9.	Trimethoprim-sulfamethoxazole should be used as a first-line agent in outpatients with uncomplicated lower tract infection unless there is: 1) documented history of allergy; 2) suspected drug resistance; or 3) pregnancy.	II-2; III	Johnson and Stamm, 1989; Carlson, 1985; Sable, 1993	Decrease dysuria. Prevent drug resistance.	This recommendation is based on studies of susceptibility of urinary tract infections to various antibiotics and costs, primarily reviewed in the Johnson and Stamm article. TMP-SMZ is the most effective antibiotic (least resistance, lower rates of recurrence). Flouroquinolones, while equally effective, have a broader spectrum and casual use promotes resistance in the individual and population.

319

#	Indicator	Quality of Evidence	References	Objectives	Literature Review/Comments
10.	Treatment with antimicrobials for uncomplicated lower tract infection should not exceed 7 days.	I; III	Stamm and Hooton, 1993; Johnson and Stamm, 1989; Elder, 1992; Fihn et al., 1988	Decrease dysuria. Prevent antibiotic allergic reactions. Prevent antibiotic associated diarrhea. Prevent antibiotic associated superinfections.	Several studies, summarized in the review articles cited, have shown that one day therapy is effective but that it may increase relapse. A well conducted RCT by Fihn et al using TMP-Sulfa showed that although a 10 day tx yielded superior cure rate at 2 weeks, by 6 weeks the advantage had diminished. The adverse effects were higher in the 10 day group. Therefore, several experts advocate the 3-day regimen in absence of RCT data on the 3-day regimen. There is no evidence that the benefit of prolonged therapy outweighs the risk of antibiotic allergies, superinfection, diarrhea and constitutional symptoms.
11.	At least 10 days of antimicrobial therapy should be prescribed for a suspected upper tract infection (pyelonephritis).	III	Johnson and Stamm, 1989; Stamm and Hooton, 1993; Stamm et al., 1991	Decrease pain. Decrease fever. Prevent recurrence of UTI. Prevent complications (such as sepsis and abscess).	In general, it is agreed that a longer duration of treatment is necessary for upper tract than lower tract infections. Untreated infections can lead to recurrence and abscess. There is some controversy about the need for 10 versus 14 days of treatment and studies have reached varying conclusions. The review by Johnson and Stamm indicates that there is not enough evidence to warrant treatment for less than 14 days, based on recurrence of infection. However, as this is an area of controversy, we have proposed at least 10 days of treatment.
12.	A patient with known or suspected upper tract infection who has uncontrolled vomiting in the office or ER should be hospitalized.	III	Stamm and Hooton, 1993	Decrease pain. Decrease fever. Prevent sepsis.	If vomiting cannot be controlled in the office or ED, it is unlikely that the patient will be able to take oral medications at home. Some hospitals have provisions to administer IV antibiotics in the home.
13.	A pregnant patient with pyelonephritis should be hospitalized.	III	Stamm and Hooton, 1993	Prevent spontaneous abortion.	Patients who are pregnant and have pyelonephritis are at risk for spontaneous abortion and need IV therapy.
14.	Regimens of at least 7 days should be used for patients with complicated lower tract infections: those with: a. diabetes, b. functional or structural anomaly of the urinary tract, c. symptoms for longer than 7 days, d. recent urinary tract infection, e. use of diaphragm, and f. pregnancy.	III	Stamm and Hooton, 1993	Prevent recurrence of UTI. Prevent sepsis. Prevent abscess formation. Prevent spontaneous abortion.	While there are no RCTs that demonstrate the optimal duration of treatment in these situations, a longer duration of treatment than for an uncomplicated lower tract infection is recommended because eradication is more difficult (i.e., in structural anomalies) and/or potential complications secondary to incomplete eradication are more serious (i.e, diabetes, pregnancy).

Follow-up

	Indicator	Quality of evidence	Literature	Benefits	Comments
15.	For upper tract infection or complicated lower tract infection, a repeat culture should be obtained within 2 weeks of finishing treatment.	III	Barker et al., 1991; Stamm and Hooton, 1993	Prevent recurrence of UTI.	Since eradication of organism is sometimes difficult in pyelonephritis and complicated lower tract infections, and incomplete eradication may lead to complications, a repeat culture is indicated.

Quality of Evidence Codes:

I: RCT
II-1:   Nonrandomized controlled trials
II-2:   Cohort or case analysis
II-3:   Multiple time series
III: Opinions or descriptive studies

321

REFERENCES - URINARY TRACT INFECTION

Bailey BL. January 1995. Urinalysis predictive of urine culture results. *Journal of Family Practice* 40 (1): 45-50.

Barker LR, JR Burton, and PD Zieve, Editors. 1991. *Principles of Ambulatory Medicine*, Third ed.Baltimore, MD: Williams and Wilkins.

Carlson KJ, and AG Mulley. 1985. Management of acute dysuria. *Annals of Internal Medicine* 102 (2): 244-9.

Elder NC. 1 November 1992. Acute urinary tract infection in women: What kind of antibiotic therapy is optimal. *Postgraduate Medicine* 92 (6): 159-72.

Fihn SD, C Johnson, PL Roberts, et al. March 1988. Trimethoprim-sulfamethoxazole for acute dysuria in women: A single-dose or 10-day course. *Annals of Internal Medicine* 108 (3): 350-7.

Hooton TM, C Johnson, C Winter, et al. 1991. Single-dose and three-day regimens of ofloxacin versus trimethoprim-sulfamethoxazole for acute cystitis in women. *Antimicrobial Agents and Chemotherapy* 35 (7): 1479-83.

Johnson JR, and W Stamm. 1 December 1989. Urinary tract infections in women: Diagnosis and treatment. *Annals of Internal Medicine* 111 (11): 906-17.

Norrby SR. May 1990. Short-term treatment of uncomplicated lower urinary tract infections in women. *Reviews of Infectious Diseases* 12 (3): 458-67.

Panzer RJ, ER Black, and PF Griner, Editors. 1991. *Diagnostic Strategies for Common Medical Problems*.Philadelphia, PA: American College of Physicians.

Pappas PG. March 1991. Laboratory in the diagnosis and management of urinary tract infections. *Medical Clinics of North America* 75 (2): 313-25.

Patton JP, DB Nash, and E Abrutyn. March 1991. Urinary tract infection: Economic considerations. *Medical Clinics of North America* 75 (2): 495-513.

Pels RJ, DH Bor, S Woolhandler, et al. 1 September 1989. Dipstick urinalysis screening of asymptomatic adults for urinary tract disorders. *Journal of the American Medical Association* 262 (9): 1221-4.

Pfaller MA, and FP Koontz. May 1985. Laboratory evaluation of leukocyte esterase and nitrite tests for the detection of bacteriuria. *Journal of Clinical Microbiology* 21 (5): 840-2.

Powers RD. May 1991. New directions in the diagnosis and therapy of urinary tract infections. *American Journal of Obstetrics and Gynecology* 164 (Volume 5, Part 2): 1387-9.

Sable CA, and WM Scheld. June 1993. Fluoroquinolones: How to use (but not overuse) these antibiotics. *Geriatrics* 48 (6): 41-51.

Schultz HJ, LA McCaffrey, TF Keys, et al. June 1984. Acute cystitis: A prospective study of laboratory tests and duration of therapy. *Mayo Clinic Proceedings* 59: 391-7.

Stamm WE, and TM Hooton. 28 October 1993. Management of urinary tract infections in adults. *New England Journal of Medicine* 329 (18): 1328-34.

Stamm WE, M McKevitt, and GW Counts. May 1987. Acute renal infection in women: Treatment with trimethoprim-sulfamethoxazole or ampicillin for two or six weeks. *Annals of Internal Medicine* 106 (3): 341-5.

Stein GE, N Mummaw, EJ Goldstein, et al. October 1987. A multicenter comparative trial of three-day norfloxacin vs ten-day sulfamethoxazole and trimethoprim for the treatment of uncomplicated urinary tract infections. *Archives of Internal Medicine* 147: 1760-2.

Winickoff RN, SI Wilner, G Gall, et al. February 1981. Urine culture after treatment of uncomplicated cystitis in women. *Southern Medical Journal* 74 (2): 165-9.

19. VAGINITIS AND SEXUALLY TRANSMITTED DISEASES, DIAGNOSIS AND TREATMENT
Eve A. Kerr, M.D., M.P.H.

The general approach to reviewing vulvovaginitis and sexually transmitted diseases (STDs) was obtained from a general text on ambulatory medicine (Barker et al., 1991) and a text of diagnostic strategies for common medical problems (Panzer et al., 1991). Specific treatment recommendations were derived from the Centers for Disease Control (CDC) 1993 Treatment Guidelines to Sexually Transmitted Diseases (CDC, 1993). The guidelines were based on systematic literature reviews by CDC staff and consensus opinions by experts. The literature reviews are summarized, in part, in the April 1995 Supplement to *Clinical Infectious Diseases*, which we reviewed to add greater detail to treatment controversies. The following review and recommendations pertain to non-pregnant, non-HIV infected women.

VULVOVAGINITIS

IMPORTANCE

The most common causes of vulvovaginal infections are: *Gardnerella vaginalis, Candida albicans,* and *Trichomonas vaginalis.* An estimated 75 percent of women will experience at least one episode of vulvovaginal candidiasis in their lifetimes, and 40-45 percent will experience two or more episodes (CDC, 1993). There are an estimated 10 million visits to physicians' offices each year for vaginitis (Reef et al., 1995). *Vulvovaginal candidiasis* and bacterial vaginosis (*G. vaginalis*) are not considered sexually transmitted diseases, although women who are not sexually active are rarely affected by bacterial vaginosis (CDC, 1993). *T. vaginalis* is transmitted through sexual activity. Gonorrhea and chlamydial infections, although not causative of vulvovaginitis, sometimes present with an abnormal discharge. In fact, as many as 25 percent of women with a discharge have cervical infections (Panzer et al., 1991).

Candidal vaginitis does not have important medical sequlea but does cause discomfort that may impair the patient's quality of life. Bacterial vaginosis may be associated with pelvic inflammatory disease (PID) (Joesoef and Schmid, 1995). A recent randomized controlled trial (RCT) found that women with bacterial vaginosis who were treated with metronidazole prior to their abortion had a threefold decrease in PID following the abortion compared to untreated women (Joesoef and Schmid, 1995).

EFFICACY AND/OR EFFECTIVENESS OF INTERVENTIONS

Screening

There is no indication for general population screening for vaginitis.

Diagnosis

The approach to diagnosis is well summarized in Panzer et al. (1991). The history and physical examination have poor predictive value. For example, approximately 35 percent of symptomatic patients had no infection, 32 percent of asymptomatic patients had infection, and approximately 15 percent of infected patients had normal pelvic examinations. Risk factors for sexually transmitted diseases (STDs)--such as the number of sexual partners in the past month, history of sexually transmitted disease, presence of genitourinary symptoms, and sexual contact with an infected partner--increase the prior probability of a sexually transmitted cause for vaginal discharge.

It is difficult to determine fully the operating characteristics of diagnostic tests for vaginitis. See Table 19.1 for details.

Table 19.1

Operating Characteristics of Common Diagnostic Tests for Vaginal and Cervical Infection

Test	Sensitivity %	Specificity %
Vaginal infection		
Trichomonas vaginalis		
Saline wet mount	50-75	70-98
Direct fluorescent antibody	80-86	98
Vaginal candidiasis		
Potassium hydroxide preparation	30-84	90-99
Bacterial vaginosis		
Vaginal pH	81-97	...
Clue cells	85-90	80
"Whiff" test	38-84	...
Thin homogeneous discharge	80	...
Gram stain of vaginal wash	97	79
Abnormal amines by chromatography	98	...
Cervical infection		
Chlamydia trachomatis		
Direct fluorescent antibody	70-87	97-99
Enzyme immunoassay	80-85	98
Culture (single cervical swab)	70-80	98
Neisseria gonorrhoeae		
Cervix gram stain	50-79	98
Culture (single cervical swab)	85-90	98
Herpes simplex virus		
Tzanck smear: vesicular; pustular; crusted	67; 54; 17	85
Culture: vesicular; pustular; crusted	70; 67; 17	...

Source: Panzer et al., 1991.

Trichomonas vaginalis

The wet mount is highly specific (70-98 percent) but not particularly sensitive (50-75 percent).

Candida albicans

The potassium hydroxide preparation has varied sensitivity (30-84 percent) compared with culture, but is highly specific (90-99 percent).

Bacterial vaginosis/Gardnerella vaginalis.

Amsel et al. (1983) have developed criteria for diagnosis that are widely accepted (Panzer et al., 1991; Joesoef and Schmid, 1995). The diagnosis in a symptomatic patient is usually based on the presence of at least three of the four following criteria:

1) pH greater than 4.5;

2) positive whiff test;

3) clue cells on wet mount; and

4) thin homogeneous discharge.

Diagnostic strategy in the evaluation of acute vulvovaginitis is often governed by the need to institute antimicrobial therapy. The first decision point lies in determining the source of infection (i.e., whether the infection is cervical or vaginal). An assessment of risk factors for sexually transmitted disease and a careful pelvic examination will help determine this. If the discharge is thought to be vaginal in origin, then a saline wet mount, potassium hydroxide wet mount, and the application of Amsel's criteria should be used to determine the cause of vaginitis.

A small proportion of women have recurrent vulvovaginal candidiasis (i.e., three or more episodes of symptomatic vulvovaginal candidiasis annually). These women should be evaluated for predisposing conditions, such as diabetes, immunosuppression, broad spectrum antibiotic use, corticosteroid use, and HIV infection. However, the majority of women with recurrent vulvovaginal candidiasis have no identifiable risk factors (Reef et al., 1995).

Treatment

Bacterial Vaginosis/Gardnerella vaginalis

These recommendations are based, in part, on randomized controlled studies and meta-analyses reviewed by the CDC (Joesoef and Schmid, 1995). Based on the CDC review, a 7-day treatment regimen is preferred over the single-dose regimen of metronidazole. The CDC notes that topical formulations require further study. However, any of the following are considered to be appropriate treatments for non-pregnant women (CDC, 1993):

- Metronidazole 500 mg orally 2 times per day for 7 days (95 percent overall cure rate);
- Metronidazole 2 g orally in a single dose (84 percent overall cure rate);
- Clindamycin cream at night for 7 days;
- Metronidazole cream twice a day for 5 days; or
- Clindamycin 300 mg orally twice a day for 7 days.

These treatment recommendations are endorsed by the CDC and have been found effective in randomized controlled trials.[5]

T. Vaginalis

For *T. Vaginalis,* it is necessary to treat both the patient and sex partner(s) with:

- Metronidazole 2 g orally in a single dose; or
- Metronidazole 500 mg twice daily for 7 days.

Both regimens have been found to be equally effective in RCTs and result in a cure rate of approximately 95 percent (CDC, 1993).

Candida albicans

A number of topical formulations of the azole class (e.g., butoconazole, clotrimazole, miconazole, tioconazole, terconazole) provide effective treatment for vulvovaginal candidiasis with relief of symptoms and negative cultures among about 90 percent of patients after therapy is completed (CDC, 1993). These recommendations are based on clinical trials reviewed by the CDC (Reef et al., 1995).

In addition, several trials have demonstrated that oral azole drugs (e.g., fluconazole, ketoconazole, and itraconazole) may be as effective as topical agents. The FDA has approved single-dose fluconazole for the treatment of vulvovaginal candidiasis (*Wall Street Journal,* 1994). Practicing physicians report this therapy to be an effective treatment (Inman et al., 1994). Use of fluconazole is contraindicated for treatment of vaginal candidiasis in pregnancy. Optimal treatment for

---

[5]The individual randomized controlled trials were not reviewed.

recurrent vulvovaginal candidiasis is not well established, but a role
for oral agents is being investigated (Reef et al., 1995).

Follow-up Care

Follow-up is unnecessary for women whose symptoms resolve after
treatment (CDC, 1993).

DISEASES CHARACTERIZED BY CERVICITIS

IMPORTANCE

Mucopurulent cervicitis is most often caused by *N. Gonorrhoea* and
C. trachomatis--two sexually transmitted infections. *C. trachomatis* is
the most common cause of cervical infection, with a prevalence ranging
from about 5-15 percent in asymptomatic women and 20-30 percent in women
treated in sexually transmitted disease clinics. The incidence of
chlamydial infection in 1988 was 215 per 100,000 (USDHHS, 1990).
Approximately 13 percent of women with chlamydial infection have
concurrent gonococcal infection and approximately 30 percent of women
with gonococcal infection have chlamydial infection (Panzer et al.,
1991). Transmission of gonorrhea from infected men to uninfected women
occurs in 90 percent of exposures. The incidence of gonorrhea infection
among women age 15-44 in 1989 was 501 per 100,000 (USDHHS, 1990).
Initially, both gonococcal and chlamydial infections may be
asymptomatic, or present with vaginal symptoms (e.g., mucopurulent
vaginal discharge, vaginal itching, dyspareunia, dysuria, vague lower
abdominal pain), anorectal symptoms, and pharyngeal symptoms. However,
both have the potential to cause pelvic inflammatory disease, the
sequelae of which include ectopic pregnancy and infertility.

EFFICACY AND/OR EFFECTIVENESS OF INTERVENTIONS

Screening

Screening for both *N. gonorrhoea* and *C. trachomatis* should be performed with the yearly pelvic examination for all women with multiple male sexual partners or with other sexually transmitted diseases (Barker, 1991), and perhaps of all sexually active women age 24 or younger (CDC, 1993).

Diagnosis

The presence of symptoms (mucopurulent vaginal discharge, vaginal itching, dyspareunia, dysuria, vague lower abdominal pain) in the right clinical context (sexually active woman) would lead one to suspect cervicitis. Physical exam may reveal red, edematous and friable cervix with mucopurulent cervical discharge.

C. Trachomatis

Diagnosis in patients with symptoms of cervicitis is confirmed by direct fluorescent antibody testing (sensitivity 70-87 percent, specificity 97-99 percent; Panzer et al., 1991) or enzyme immunoassay (sensitivity 80-85 percent, specificity 98 percent; Panzer et al., 1991).

N. Gonorrhoea

Suspected gonococcal infection may be initially confirmed by gram stain (sensitivity 50-79 percent, specificity 98 percent; Panzer et al., 1991) and subsequently by culture (sensitivity 85-90 percent, specificity 98 percent; Panzer et al., 1991).

Treatment

In patients with inconclusive symptoms and/or physical exam, one must take into account the pre-test probabilities of infection when determining the need for treatment. Therefore, in populations with a high prevalence of sexually transmitted diseases, and in women with known or suspected exposures, or if the patient is unlikely to return for treatment, one should treat without waiting for confirmatory cultures. Otherwise, results of tests should dictate the need for treatment (CDC, 1993).

According to the CDC, treatment for mucopurulent cervicitis should include the following:

- Treatment for gonorrhea and chlamydia in patient populations with high prevalence of both infections, such as patients seen at many STD clinics;

- Treatment for chlamydia only, if the prevalence of *N. gonorrhoea* is low but the likelihood of chlamydia is substantial;

- Await test results if the prevalence of both infections are low and if compliance with a recommendation for a return visit is likely.

Specific treatments

C. trachomatis

The CDC, based on its review of RCTs (Weber and Johnson, 1995) recommends either of the following treatment regimens:

- Doxycylcine 100 mg orally twice a day for 7 days; or
- Azithromycin 1 g orally in a single dose.

Other effective treatments include: ofloxacin, erythromycin, or sulfisoxazole. The partner(s) should also be referred for therapy.

N. gonorrhoea

The treatment for gonorrhea follows the recommendations of the CDC based on its review of RCTs (Moran and Levine, 1995). All women treated for gonorrhea should also be treated for chlamydia (see regimens for chlamydia).

Any of the following regimens are considered to be appropriate:

- Ceftriaxone 125 mg IM in single dose;
- Cefixime 400 mg orally in a single dose;
- Ciprofloxacin 500 mg orally in a single dose; or
- Ofloxacin 400 mg orally in a single dose.

Other effective antimicrobials may be used (e.g., spectinomycin, other cephalosporins, other quinolones).

Follow-up Care

For chlamydia, follow-up cultures are not necessary for women completing treatment with doxycycline or azithromycin unless symptoms persist or re-infection is suspected (CDC, 1993). For other antibiotic regimens, testing may be considered three weeks after completion of treatment. Similarly, women who are symptom free after treatment for gonorrhea with any recommended antibiotic do not need follow-up cultures (CDC, 1993).

PELVIC INFLAMMATORY DISEASE (PID)

IMPORTANCE

PID represents a spectrum of upper genital tract inflammatory disorders, including endometritis, salpingitis, tubo-ovarian abscess, and pelvic peritonitis. More than one million cases of PID are diagnosed and treated each year in the U.S. (USDHHS, 1990). The cost of PID and associated ectopic pregnancy and infertility exceed $2.7 billion (Walker et al., 1993). If one takes into account the medical consequences of PID, including infertility, ectopic pregnancy, and chronic pelvic pain, the direct and indirect costs of PID exceed $4.2 billion annually (Walker et al., 1993).

EFFICACY/EFFECTIVENESS OF INTERVENTIONS

Diagnosis

The diagnosis of PID is usually made on the basis of clinical findings. In some cases, women may have atypical PID, with abnormal bleeding, dyspareunia, or vaginal discharge. The CDC suggests that empiric treatment of PID should be instituted on the basis of the presence of all of the following clinical criteria for pelvic inflammation and in the absence of an established cause other than PID (e.g., ectopic pregnancy, acute appendicitis) (CDC, 1993):

- Lower abdominal tenderness;

- Adnexal tenderness; and
- Cervical motion tenderness.

The specificity of the diagnosis can be increased if the following signs are also present (CDC, 1993):
- Oral temperature above 38.3° Centigrade;
- Abnormal cervical or vaginal discharge;
- Elevated erythrocyte sedimentation rate;
- Elevated C-reactive protein;
- Laboratory documentation of cervical infection with *N. gonorrhoea* or *C. Trachomatis*.

However, algorithms based only on clinical criteria fail to identify some women with PID and misclassify others (Walker et al., 1993). Assessment by endometrial biopsy, laparoscopy, or both is more specific but less sensitive (Walker et al., 1993).

Treatment

Hospitalization for antimicrobial treatment of PID is recommended by the CDC (based primarily on expert opinion) under any of the following circumstances (CDC, 1993; CDC, 1991a):
- The diagnosis is uncertain and surgical emergencies such as appendicitis and ectopic pregnancy, cannot be excluded;
- Pelvic abscess is suspected;
- The patient is pregnant;
- The patient is an adolescent;
- The patient has HIV infection;
- Severe illness or nausea and vomiting preclude outpatient management; or
- Clinical follow-up within 72 hours of starting antibiotic treatment cannot be arranged .

Treatment with antibiotics has been well studied for inpatient regimens (Walker et al., 1993). Based on RCTs, the CDC supports the use of two antibiotic regimens for inpatient treatment of PID, both with cure rates above 90 percent (CDC, 1993; Walker et al., 1993). Either of the following regimens is acceptable:

Regimen 1

- Cefoxitin 2 g IV every 6 hours or cefotetan 2 g IV every 12 hours (for at least 48 hours) and
- Doxycycline 100 mg IV or orally every 12 hours (for 14 days).

Regimen 2

- Clindamycin 900 mg IV every 8 hours, and
- Gentamicin.

The above regimen should be continued for a least 48 hours, followed by oral doxycyline or clindamycin

There is limited experience from clinical trials with outpatient regimens for PID (Walker et al., 1993). Further, no specific comparisons of outpatient versus inpatient treatment have been done. The second regimen noted below provides broader coverage against anaerobic organisms (because of the addition of clindamycin or metronidazole), but is more expensive. Patients who do not respond to outpatient therapy within 72 hours should be hospitalized, since by 72 hours patients should have improvement of subjective complaints and be afebrile (Peterson et al., 1990) Either of the following regimens is acceptable:

Regimen 1

- Cefoxitin 2 g IM plus probenecid, 1 g orally in a single dose concurrently, or ceftriaxone 250 mg IM or other parenteral third-generation cephalosporin, and
- Doxycycline 100 mg orally 2 times a day for 14 days

Regimen 2

- Ofloxacin 400 mg orally 2 times a day for 14 days, and
- Either clindamycin 450 mg orally 4 times a day, or metronidazole 500 mg orally 2 times a day for 14 days

Further research must be done before the use of limited spectrum antibiotics (such as quinolone alone) can be recommended (Walker et al., 1993).

Follow-up Care

Patients receiving outpatient therapy should receive follow up within 72 hours to document clinical improvement and should have a microbiologic re-examination 7-10 days after completing therapy.

Patients receiving inpatient therapy should have a microbiologic re-examination 7-10 days after completing therapy to determine cure. Some experts advocate another microbiologic evaluation in 4-6 levels (CDC, 1991b).

Sex partners should be empirically treated for *C. trachomatis* and *N. gonorrhoea*.

DISEASES CHARACTERIZED BY GENITAL ULCERS

IMPORTANCE

In the United States, most persons with genital ulcers have genital herpes, syphilis or chancroid; genital herpes is the most common. More than one of these diseases may be present among at least 3-10 percent of patients with genital ulcers. Each of the conditions is associated with an increased risk for HIV infection (CDC, 1993).

EFFICACY AND/OR EFFECTIVENESS OF INTERVENTIONS

Genital Herpes Simplex Infection
Screening

There is no literature that suggests a useful role for screening for herpes.

Diagnosis

On the basis of serologic studies, approximately 30 million persons in the United States may have genital herpes simplex virus (HSV) infection (CDC, 1993). Diagnosis is most often made on the basis of history and physical exam and confirmed by HSV culture or antigen test. The sensitivity of the culture decreases with the age of the lesion (sensitivities for vesicular, pustular and crusted lesions are 70 percent, 67 percent, and 17 percent respectively) (Panzer et al., 1991). Further, specimens from primary lesions and cutaneous lesions are more likely to grow herpes simplex virus.

Treatment

As summarized by the CDC, RCTs demonstrate that acyclovir is effective in decreasing symptoms and signs of HSV in first clinical episodes and when used as a suppressive (daily) therapy (CDC, 1993; Stone and Whittington, 1990). The CDC does not generally recommend acyclovir treatment for recurrent episodes because early therapy can rarely be instituted. The CDC also recommends that after one year of continuous suppressive therapy, acyclovir should be discontinued to allow assessment of the patient's rate of recurrent episodes. If recurrence rate is low, suppressive treatment may be discontinued permanently or temporarily.

Other Management Issues

Patient education is important in preventing the transmission of HSV. Patients should abstain from sexual activity while lesions are present and use condoms during all sexual exposures.

All patients with genital ulcers should receive a serologic test for syphilis. HIV testing should be considered in the management of patients with known or suspected HSV.

Chancroid

Screening

Screening for chancroid is not indicated.

Diagnosis

Chancroid is caused by the bacterium *Haemophilus ducreyi*. As many as 10 percent of patients with chancroid may be coinfected with *T. pallidum* or HSV (CDC, 1993). With lack of readily available means to

culture for *H. ducreyi,* the diagnosis rests on clinical grounds. The
CDC states that a probable diagnosis can be made if the patients has one
or more painful genital ulcers and

1) no evidence of *T. Pallidum* infection by dark-field exam or by a
   serologic test for syphilis performed at least 7 days after
   onset of ulcers; and

2) the clinical presentation of the ulcer(s) is either not typical
   of HSV or the HSV test results are negative.

Treatment

The CDC recommends treatment with single-dose Azithromycin or IM
Ceftriaxone or a 7-day course of Erythromycin.

Patients with chancroid should be tested for HIV and syphilis, and
retested three months later if initial results are negative (CDC, 1993).

Sexual partners (anyone with whom the patient has had sexual
contact within 10 days before onset of the patient's symptoms) should be
examined and treated.

Follow-up Care

Patients should be re-examined 3-7 days after initiation of
treatment to assess clinical improvement.

Primary and Secondary Syphilis

Syphilis is a systemic disease caused by *T. pallidum.* The
incidence of primary and secondary syphilis in the United States has
been steadily rising, with 118 cases per 100,000 reported in 1989
(USDHHS, 1990). In addition, there is an association between genital
ulcer disease and sexual HIV spread.

Screening

Screening of the general population is not indicated (except in
pregnancy). At-risk populations (i.e., with other sexually transmitted
diseases) should be screened using a non-treponemal test, as discussed
below (CDC, 1993).

Diagnosis

Primary syphilis should be diagnosed on the basis of presence of
(usually nonpainful) genital ulcer (or recent history of same), and
laboratory testing for syphilis. Twenty percent of patients will have a

negative non-treponemal test (VDRL or RPR) at the time of presentation, but direct examination of the chancer (dark-field microscopy or direct fluorescence antibody) will be positive (Panzer et al., 1991). Secondary syphilis is a systemic illness with a prominent rash, beginning six weeks to several months after exposure. Persons sexually exposed to a patient with syphilis in any stage should be evaluated clinically and serologically according the CDC recommendations.

Treatment

Treatment for primary and secondary syphilis should be initiated with benzathine penicillin G (2.4 units IM in single dose) in absence of allergy. One should not wait for test results to initiate treatment.

Follow-up Care

Treatment failures occur in approximately 5 percent of cases treated with penicillin regimens and more frequently with other regimens (Rofls, 1995). According to the CDC, patients should be re-examined clinically and serologically at three months and again at six months for evidence of successful treatment (CDC, 1993).

RECOMMENDED QUALITY INDICATORS FOR VAGINITIS AND SEXUALLY TRANSMITTED DISEASES

The following criteria apply to nonpregnant, non-HIV-infected women aged 18-50.

Diagnosis

	Indicator	Quality of evidence	Literature	Benefits	Comments
	Vaginitis				
1.	In women presenting with complaint of vaginal discharge, the practitioner should perform a speculum exam to determine if the discharge has a cervical or vaginal source.	III	Panzer et al., 1991	Decrease discharge, itching and dysuria.	Since implications of and treatment for cervicitis and vaginitis differ substantially, physical exam must be performed.
2.	At a minimum, the following tests should be performed on the vaginal discharge: normal saline wet mount for clue cells and trichomads; KOH wet mount for yeast hyphae.	III	Panzer et al., 1991	Decrease discharge, itching and dysuria.	pH determination is also sensitive, but its specificity is unknown. Therefore, at a minimum, the two wet mounts should be performed.
3.	A sexual history should be obtained from women presenting with a vaginal discharge. The history should include: a. No. of sexual partners in previous 6 months; b. Absence or presence of symptoms in partners; c. Use of condoms; and d. Prior history of sexually transmitted diseases.	III	Panzer et al., 1991; CDC, 1993	Decrease discharge, itching and dysuria. Decrease PID and abdominal pain. Decrease infertility. Decrease mortality from ectopic pregnancy.	In patients with one or more risk factors, prior probability for a STD (i.e., chlamydia or gonorrhea) as a cause of discharge is increased and culture for the causative organisms may be appropriate. This is important because cervicitis has more significant long-term consequences than vaginitis, such as PID, infertility and ectopic pregnancy.
4.	If three of the following four criteria are met, a diagnosis of bacterial vaginosis or gardnerella vaginosis should be made: pH greater than 4.5; positive whiff test; clue cells on wet mount; thin homogenous discharge.	III	Panzer et al., 1991; Amsel et al., 1983	Decrease discharge, itching and dysuria.	Based on Amsel et al., the presence of three criteria is highly sensitive and specific for bacterial vaginosis.
	Cervicitis				
5.	Routine testing for gonorrhea and chlamydia trachomatis (culture and antigen detection, respectively) should be performed with the routine pelvic exam for women with multiple sexual partners (more than 1 in previous 6 months).	III	CDC, 1993; ACOG, 1993 (The Obstetrician Gynecologist Primary Preventive Healthcare)	Alleviate pain. Alleviate fever. Decrease infertility. Decrease mortality from ectopic pregnancy.	This recommendation is based upon epidemiologic studies of transmission and prevalence, as summarized by the CDC. Women with multiple sexual partners are at higher risk for STDs, and these may be asymptomatic.
	Pelvic Inflammatory Disease (PID)				
6.	If a patient is given the diagnosis of PID, a speculum and bimanual pelvic exam should have been performed.	III	CDC, 1993	Alleviate pain. Alleviate fever. Decrease infertility. Decrease mortality from ectopic pregnancy.	The diagnosis of PID is based primarily on physical exam. In addition, one should obtain cervical specimens for culture. Therefore, a physical exam is mandatory before treatment can be initiated.

7.	If a patient is given the diagnosis of PID, at least 2 of the following signs should be present on physical exam: - lower abdominal tenderness - adnexal tenderness - cervical motion tenderness.	III	CDC, 1993	Alleviate pain. Alleviate fever. Decrease infertility. Decrease mortality from ectopic pregnancy.	It is important to correctly identify PID since symptoms may mimic appendicitis and ovarian torsion. The CDC states that all three signs should be present. We have stated that at least two must be present and documented.
	Genital Ulcers				
8.	If a patient presents with genital ulcer(s) of any cause, HIV testing should be recommended.	III	CDC, 1993	Delay progression to AIDS. Prevention of HIV spread.*	Based on this observation, it is particularly important to recommend testing in patients with genital ulcers, although testing could be recommended to persons with any STD.
	STDs—General				
9.	If a patient presents with any sexually transmitted disease (gonorrhea, chlamydia, trachomatis, herpes, chancroid, syphilis) a non-treponemal test (VDRL or RPR) for syphilis should be obtained.	III	CDC, 1993	Prevention of late complications of syphilis.**	Persons with one STD are at high risk for another. Since there is effective treatment to prevent late complications of syphilis, testing is recommended.

341

Treatment

	Indicator	Quality of evidence	Literature	Benefits	Comments
	Vaginitis				
10.	Treatment for bacterial vaginosis should be with metronidazole (orally or vaginally) or clindamycin (orally or vaginally).	I	CDC, 1993	Decrease discharge, itching and dysuria.	These are the only proven effective regimens. RCTs reviewed by the CDC show that the evidence for efficacy of oral treatment is better than for topical treatment.
11.	Treatment for *T. vaginalis* should be with oral metronidazole in the absence of allergy to metronidazole.	I	CDC, 1993	Decrease discharge, itching and dysuria.	Based on RCTs reviewed by the CDC, this is the only known effective treatment.
12.	Treatment for non-recurrent (three or fewer episodes in previous year) yeast vaginitis should be with topical "azole" preparations (e.g., clotrimazole, butoconazole, etc.) or fluconazole.	I	CDC, 1993;	Decrease discharge, itching and dysuria.	Based on RCTs reviewed by the CDC. These regimens are approved by the FDA.
	Cervicitis				
13.	Women treated for gonorrhea should also be treated for chlamydia.	II-2; III	CDC, 1993	Prevent PID. Decrease infertility. Decrease mortality from ectopic pregnancy.	Women with gonorrhea are likely to be coinfected with chlamydia. Since the sensitivity of chlamydia essays is variable, concurrent treatment is recommended.
	Pelvic Inflammatory Disease (PID)				
14.	Patients with PID and any of the following conditions should be hospitalized: a. appendicitis b. ectopic pregnancy c. Pelvic abscess is present or suspected d. The patient is pregnant e. The patient is an adolescent (under age 18) f. The patient has HIV infection g. Uncontrolled nausea and vomiting h. Clinical follow-up within 72 hours of starting antibiotic treatment cannot be arranged, or i. The patient does not improve within 72 hours of starting therapy.	III	CDC, 1993	Alleviate pain. Alleviate fever. Prevent sepsis. Decrease infertility. Decrease mortality from ectopic pregnancy.	While other reasons for hospitalization may exist (i.e., cannot rule out appendicitis), these have been recommended by the CDC and should be discernable by chart review. The purpose of hospitalization is to ensure effective treatment in persons at risk of complications (e.g., HIV infection) or poor follow-up (e.g., adolescents).
15.	Total antibiotic therapy for PID should be for no less than 10 days (inpatient, if applicable, plus outpatient)	III	CDC, 1993; Peterson et al., 1991	Alleviate pain. Alleviate fever. Prevent sepsis. Decrease infertility. Decrease mortality from ectopic pregnancy.	The standard of care is 10-14 days, although RCTs have not specifically addressed duration of treatment. Shorter treatment periods may results in lower cure rates.
	Genital Ulcers				
16.	Patients with genital herpes should be counseled regarding reducing the risk of transmission to sexual partners.	III	CDC, 1993	Prevent spread of genital herpes.	Genital herpes is transmissible even in the absence of current outbreak. Unlike most other STDs, there is not effective cure for herpes. Therefore, prevention of transmission is of prime importance.

#	Indicator	Quality of evidence	Literature	Benefits	Comments
17.	In the absence of allergy, patients with chancroid should be treated with azithromycin, ceftriaxone, or erythromycin.	I	CDC, 1993	Decrease pain. Heal ulcer. Limit transmission of chancroid.	These have been shown in RCTs reviewed by the CDC to be effective.
18.	In the absence of allergy, patients with primary and secondary syphilis should be treated with benzathine penicillin G (IM).	I	CDC, 1993	Prevention of late complications of syphilis.**	Penicillin is the best studied of all regimens and known to be effective through single IM administration. This recommendation is based on RCTs reviewed by the CDC.
19.	If a patient has a primary ulcer consistent with syphilis, treatment for syphilis should be initiated before laboratory testing is back.	III	CDC, 1993	Prevention of late complications of syphilis.**	Not all patients will return for follow-up. Because effective treatment exists and consequences of untreated syphilis are serious, treatment should be initiated at the time of first presentation.
	STDs—General				
20.	Sexual partners of patients with new diagnoses of gonorrhea, chlamydia, chancroid and primary or secondary syphilis should be referred for treatment.	III	CDC, 1993	Effective treatment and prevention of complications of STDs in partners. Prevention of STD spread.*	Patients with STDs have either contracted them from their current sexual partner or may have infected their current sexual partner. In either case, the most recent sexual partner should be referred for therapy. While there are specific guidelines for which partners should be referred, based on the time period from last sexual activity with the partner and infection, at least some indication that the patient was told to refer her sexual partner(s) for treatment should be in the chart.

Follow-up

	Indicator	Quality of evidence	Literature	Benefits	Comments
	Pelvic Inflammatory Disease (PID)				
21.	Patients receiving outpatient therapy for PID should receive a follow-up visit within 72 hours of diagnosis.	III	CDC, 1993; Peterson et al., 1991	Alleviate pain. Alleviate fever. Prevent sepsis. Decrease infertility. Decrease mortality from ectopic pregnancy.	Early effective treatment is important in preventing complications.
22.	Patients being treated for PID should have a microbiological re-examination (e.g., cultures) within 10 days of completing therapy.	III	CDC, 1993	Decrease infertility. Decrease mortality from ectopic pregnancy.	A small percentage of patients may not have complete resolution even after treatment (successes with various regimens vary, ranging from 80-99%).
	Genital Ulcers				
23.	Patients receiving treatment for chancroid should be re-examined within 7 days of treatment initiation to assess clinical improvement.	III	CDC, 1993	Prevention of complications of untreated syphilis.** Prevent transmission of chancroid, syphilis, and herpes.	Most patients will have improved by 7 days.

24.	Patients with primary or secondary syphilis should be re-examined clinically and serologically within 6 months after treatment.	III	CDC, 1993	Prevention of complications of untreated syphilis.**	If a treatment failure has occurred, the patient requires re-treatment.

*HIV causes fatigue, diarrhea, neuropathic symptoms, fevers, and opportunistic infections (OIs). OIs cause a wide variety of symptoms, including cough, shortness of breath, and vomiting. Average life expectancy after HIV infection is less than 10 years. Other STDs include gonorrhea, syphilis, and chlamydia. They cause a wide variety of symptoms, including dysuria, genital ulcers, infertility, rashes, neurologic and cardiac problems and rarely contribute to mortality. Preventing HIV and STDs has the added benefit of interrupting the spread of disease and preventing morbidity and mortality in those who thus avoid infection.

**Untreated syphilis infection can lead to tertiary syphilis (neurosyphilis and cardiovascular syphilis) and congential syphilis among babies born to infected mothers.

Quality of Evidence Codes:

I:	RCT
II-1:	Nonrandomized controlled trials
II-2:	Cohort or case analysis
II-3:	Multiple time series
III:	Opinions or descriptive studies

REFERENCES - VAGINITIS AND SEXUALLY TRANSMITTED DISEASES

Amsel R, PA Totten, CA Spiegel, et al. January 1983. Nonspecific vaginitis: Diagnostic criteria and microbial and epidemiologic associations. *American Journal of Medicine* 74: 14-22.

Barker LR, JR Burton, and PD Zieve, Editors. 1991. *Principles of Ambulatory Medicine*, Third ed.Baltimore, MD: Williams and Wilkins.

Centers for Disease Control. 24 September 1993. 1993 sexually transmitted diseases treatment guidelines. *Morbidity and Mortality Weekly Report* 42 (RR-14): 1-102.

Centers for Disease Control. 26 April 1991. Pelvic inflammatory disease: Guidelines for prevention and management. *Morbidity and Mortality Weekly Report* 40 (RR-5): 1-25.

Centers for Disease Control. May 1991. *Sexually Transmitted Diseases: Clinical Practice Guidelines*. Atlanta, GA: U.S. Department of Health and Human Services.

Inman W, G Pearce, and L Wilton. 1994. Safety of fluconazole in the treatment of vaginal candidiasis: A prescription-event monitoring study, with special reference to the outcome of pregnancy. *European Journal of Clinical Pharmacology* 46: 115-8.

Joesoef MR, and GP Schmid. 1995. Bacterial vaginosis: Review of treatment options and potential clinical indications for therapy. *Clinical Infectious Diseases* 20 (Suppl. 1): S72-9.

Moran JS, and WC Levine. 1995. Drugs of choice for the treatment of uncomplicated gonococcal infections. *Clinical Infectious Diseases* 20 (Suppl. 1): S47-65.

Panzer RJ, ER Black, and PF Griner, Editors. 1991. *Diagnostic Strategies for Common Medical Problems*.Philadelphia, PA: American College of Physicians.

Peterson HB, EI Galaid, and JM Zenilman. July 1990. Pelvic inflammatory disease: Review of treatment options. *Reviews of Infectious Diseases* 12 (Suppl. 6): S656-64.

Peterson HB, CK Walker, JG Kahn, et al. 13 November 1991. Pelvic inflammatory disease: Key treatment issues and options. *Journal of the American Medical Association* 266 (18): 2605-2611.

Reef SE, WC Levine, MM McNeil, et al. 1995. Treatment options for vulvovaginal candidiasis, 1993. *Clinical Infectious Diseases* 20 (Suppl. 1): S80-90.

Rolfs RT. 1995. Treatment of syphilis, 1993. *Clinical Infectious Diseases* 20 (Suppl. 1): S23-38.

Stone KM, and WL Whittington. July 1990. Treatment of genital herpes. *Reviews of Infectious Diseases* 12 (Suppl. 6): S610-9.

U.S. Department of Health and Human Services. 1991. *Healthy People 2000: National Health Promotion and Disease Prevention Objectives*. U.S. Government Printing Office, Washington, DC.

Walker CK, JG Kahn, EA Washington, et al. October 1993. Pelvic inflammatory disease: Metaanalysis of antimicrobial regimen efficacy. *The Journal of Infectious Diseases* 168: 969-78.

Wall Street Journal. 1994. Pfizer one-dose drug for yeast infections gets FDA approval. (Food and Drug Administration approves Diflucan). *Wall Street Journal*, B, 4:6.

Weber JT, and RE Johnson. 1995. New treatments for chlamydia trachomatis genital infection. *Clinical Infectious Diseases* 20 (Suppl. 1): S66-71.

APPENDIX A: DEFINITIONS FOR INDICATOR TABLES

DEFINITIONS FOR ACNE (CHAPTER 1)

Moderate acne: Red papules and many pustules present.

Severe acne: Red papules, pustules, cysts and nodules present.

DEFINITIONS FOR ALCOHOL DEPENDENCE (CHAPTER 2)

Alcohol-associated pathology: Pathology caused by alcohol abuse. We intend to operationalize this definition. Although the following list is not intended to be exhaustive, examples include: cirrhosis, pancreatitis, gastrointestinal bleeding, cardiomyopathy, assault, suicide and motor vehicle accidents. Cirrhosis, cardiomyopathy and pancreatitis may cause chronic decreases in health related quality of life due to vomiting, ascites, abdominal pain, bleeding, shortness of breath and may eventually result in mortality. Gastrointestinal bleeding has a short-term mortality risk as well as a chronic impact on health-related quality of life due to anemia and other complications. Motor vehicle accidents and assaults may result in chronic disability from injuries and death. The health related quality of life of persons other than the patient may also be affected. Liver disease and alcohol related trauma are more common in women.

Regular or binge drinkers: Patient drinks more than 2 drinks each day, more than 11 drinks in a week or more than 5 drinks in a day in the last month.

CAGE: Self-administered alcohol abuse screening instrument. The Cut down, Annoyed, Guilty, Eye-Opener (CAGE) questionnaire is a 4-question test that focuses on drinking history.

MAST: Self-administered alcohol abuse screening instrument. Michigan Alcohol Screening Test (MAST) is a 25-question instrument on lifetime alcohol abuse.

HSS: Self-administered alcohol abuse screening instrument. The Health Screening Survey (HSS) is a 9-item lifestyle questionnaire that asks parallel questions on exercise, weight control, smoking and alcohol use during the past 3 months.

AUDIT: Self-administered alcohol abuse screening instrument. The Alcohol Use Disorders Inventory Test (AUDIT) is a 10-question instrument designed for the WHO that assesses alcohol use and problems in the last 12 months.

SAAST: Self-administered Alcohol Screening Test (SAAST). 35 item questionnaire that focuses on detection of dependence.

SMAST: Short MAST (see above).

DEFINITIONS FOR ALLERGIC RHINITIS (CHAPTER 3)

There are no definitions for this chapter.

DEFINITIONS FOR ASTHMA (CHAPTER 4)

Theophylline toxicity: Toxicities include tremulousness and agitation, nausea, vomiting, and cardiac arrhythmia.

Trial of inhaled steroids: Prescription of at least the minimum dose of inhaled steroids for no less than one month

Chronic oral corticosteroids: Three or more corticosteroid tapers for exacerbations in the past year; or continuous treatment with any dose prednisone; or three or more administrations of intra-muscular corticosteroids in the past year.

DEFINITIONS FOR BREAST MASS (CHAPTER 5)

Breast mass: A palpable lump or nodule which is referred to in the medical record as a mass, lump, or nodule. Other indications of irregularity, such as "thickening," "density," or "irregularity" do not fit definition of mass.

DEFINITIONS FOR CESAREAN DELIVERY (CHAPTER 6)

Trial of labor: This term implies that vaginal delivery is intended. Labor is allowed to proceed until delivery, or until some indication for cesarean (such as fetal distress of failure to progress in labor) intervenes.

Failure to progress (FTP) in labor: Also known as "dystocia." Labor (as measured by cervical dilation and descent of the presenting part) has either stopped progressing or progresses at a rate below accepted norms. Accepted norms for cervical dilation range from 0.5 to 1.5 cm of cervical change per hour.

Electronic fetal monitoring (EFM): A method by which the fetal heart rate can be monitored continuously during labor. External EFM uses a Doppler device strapped to the mother's abdomen. Internal EFM uses a clip attached to the fetal scalp to detect electrocardiographic impulses from the fetus. Certain patterns of EFM tracing may be indicative of fetal hypoxia.

DEFINITIONS FOR CIGARETTE USE COUNSELING (CHAPTER 7)

Smoking-related morbidity and mortality: We intend to operationalize this definition. Although not intended to be exhaustive, examples include coronary heart disease, cerebrovascular disease, chronic obstructive pulmonary disease, and obstetrical complications as well as carcinoma of the lung, trachea, bronchus, esophagus, kidney, bladder, pancreas and stomach.

Counseling: We plan a broad operationalization of counseling to include everything from pamphlets and brief advice in the primary care setting to specialized structure programs.

DEFINITIONS FOR DEPRESSION (CHAPTER 8)

Medical complications of substance abuse: There are numerous medical complications of substance abuse. For alcohol, this includes: blackouts, seizures, delirium, liver failure. For IV drugs of any kind, this includes: local infection, endocarditis, hepatitis and HIV, death from overdose. For cocaine and amphetamines, this includes: seizures, myocardial infarction, and hypertensive crises.

Depressive symptoms: Included are: depressed mood, diminished interest or pleasure in activities, weight loss/gain, impaired concentration, suicidality, fatigue, feelings of worthlessness and guilt, and psychomotor agitation/retardation.

General medical disorders that contribute to depression: Included are: severe arthritis, low back pain, coronary artery disease, congestive heart failure, renal failure.

DEFINITIONS FOR DIABETES MELLITUS (CHAPTER 9)

Diabetic complications: Although the following list is not intended to be exhaustive, examples include visual loss, dysfunction of the heart, peripheral vasculature, peripheral nerves, and kidneys. We intend to operationalize this term.

Failed dietary therapy: Adherence to ADA diet fails to improve glycemic control, as glycosylated hemoglobin measure remains above 6.05 mg/dl percent for 3 months. There is no accepted definition of timeframe; we chose a conservative estimate of 3 months.

Failed oral hypoglycemics: Oral hypoglycemics at maximum recommended dose fail to bring glycosylated hemoglobin measure of glycemic control below 6.05 mg/dL percent for 3 months. There is no accepted definition of timeframe; we chose a conservative estimate of 3 months.

Failure of preferred agents: Failure to achieve glycemic control or reduce diabetic complications.

DEFINITIONS FOR FAMILY PLANNING/CONTRACEPTION (CHAPTER 10)

There are no definitions for this chapter.

DEFINITIONS FOR HEADACHE (CHAPTER 11)

New patients: Patients who present for the first time to the physician, practice or health plan. In other words, patient for whom a history and physical has been performed and is available to the physician.

New onset headache: Patient has no prior history of presenting with headache complaint.

Abnormal neurological examination: We intend to operationalize this term. Includes examination of the cranial nerves, including pupils and eye movements, examination of the deep tendon reflexes and of the fundi.

Constant headache: Unrelieved, persistent headache that may range from low-level to severe and last for 1 week. Experts contend that such headaches are more indicative of intracranial neoplasm than intermittent headaches. There is no accepted definition for timeframe; we chose a conservative estimate of 1 week.

Severe headache: Headache of a severity that prohibits daily activities.

Acute headache: Headache lasting less than one week.

Moderate or severe headaches: Headache of a severity that inhibits or prohibits daily activities.

Tension headaches: Tension headaches are likely to be described as dull, nagging and persistent, with tight and constricting pain, and are also referred to as contraction, stress or ordinary headaches. The pain of these headaches may be either unilateral or bilateral and may involve the frontal region. Pain is likely to be most severe in the neck, shoulders and occipital region.

Uncontrolled hypertension: Failure to control blood pressure to normal or stage 1 levels (systolic less than 160, diastolic less than 100).

Atypical chest pain: Chest discomfort not suggestive of coronary heart disease

Side effects of migraine therapeutic agents: Although not exhaustive, examples of side effects include the following:

Ergotamines: vasoconstriction, exacerbation of coronary artery disease, nausea, abdominal pain, somnolence;

Opiates: dependence, somnolence, withdrawal;

Phenothiazines: dystonic reactions, anticholinergic reactions, insomnia.

Migraine symptoms and headaches: Migraines typically last 4 to 72 hours, with the vast majority lasting less than 24 hours and involving headache-free periods between prostrating attacks. Migraine pain can occur anywhere in the head or face, but seems to occur most often in the temple. Common migraine symptoms include unilateral location, pulsating quality, moderate or severe intensity (inhibits or prohibits daily activities), aggravation by walking stairs or similar activity, nausea and/or vomiting, and/or photophobia and phonophobia. Classic migraine symptoms include homonymous visual disturbance, unilateral paresthesias, unilateral weakness and aphasia or unclassifiable speech difficulty.

First line therapy: Medication that should be used prior to trial of any other medication.

DEFINITIONS FOR HYPERTENSION (CHAPTER 12)

Stage 1-4 hypertension: A high blood pressure diagnostic staging system involving the following ranges of elevated cuff measurements in mm of HG: Stage 1 is mild (systolic 140-159, diastolic 90-99), Stage 2 is moderate (systolic 160-179, diastolic 100-109) and Stage 3 is severe (systolic 180-209, diastolic 110-119), Stage 4 is very severe (systolic > 209, diastolic > 120)

Premature CAD: Coronary artery disease for patients under age 55.

Tobacco abuse: Any use of tobacco products.

Medications known to cause hypertension: We are planning to operationalize this definition. Although the following list of medications is not intended to be exhaustive, examples include steroids, nasal decongestants, appetite suppressants, cyclosporine, monamine oxidase inhibitors, tricyclic antidepressants and erythropoietin.

Temporary (discontinuation of drug therapy): Interruption of therapy involving drugs known to cause hypertension to see if blood pressure normalizes, indicating the drug(s) is the cause of the patient's hypertension.

Failure on (first-line pharmacotherapy): Uncontrolled hypertension, or failure to control blood pressure to normal or stage 1 levels (systolic less than 160, diastolic less than 100)

Contraindication (for first-line pharmacotherapy): Beta blockers and/or thiazide diuretics are not recommended as first line pharmacotherapy for patients with certain concomitant diseases, such as hyperlipidemia, diabetes, asthma, gout (see text).

Persistent elevations: Elevations persisting for at least 6 months.

Hypertensive complications: Target organ damage, including cardiovascular disease, cerebrovascular disease, retinopathy and nephropathy. Cardiovascular disease can result in chest pain, shortness of breath, claudication, fatigue, and death. Cerebrovascular disease can result in neurologic symptoms (e.g., aphasia, paralysis) and death. Retinopathy can result in visual field defects and blindness. Nephropathy can result in edema, arrythmias, nausea, vomiting, fatigue, dialysis, and death.

DEFINITIONS FOR ACUTE LOW BACK PAIN (CHAPTER 13)

Acute low back pain: Less than 3 months' duration of activity intolerance due to low back pain and/or back-related leg symptoms.

Significant trauma: An injury caused by rough contact with a physical object that may have resulted in spinal fracture.

Prolonged use of steroids: Patient is receiving long-term corticosteroid therapy (greater than 3 weeks).

Unexplained weight loss: Loss of 10 percent or more of body weight if patient is not trying to lose weight.

Neurologic screening: Includes ankle and knee reflexes, ankle and great toe dorsiflexion strength, and distribution of sensory complaints.

Diagnostic testing: EMG, SEPs, ESR, CBC, UA, bone scan, pain myelography, MRI, CT, CT-myelography, discography, CT-discography.

Prolonged bed rest: Greater than 4 days.

Immunosuppression: Suppression of immunologic response. Includes immune disorders such as hematologic and solid tumors, congenital immunodeficiency, HIV and long-term immunosuppressive therapy.

DEFINITIONS FOR PRENATAL CARE (CHAPTER 14)

Screened for anemia: A hemoglobin or hematocrit (blood test)

Smoking history: Interview asking the patient whether or not she smokes

or has smoked during the pregnancy, and if so how much.

Drug history: Interview asking the patient whether or not she has used

illicit drugs during the pregnancy or prior to pregnancy, and if so which

drugs, how much and how often.

Alcohol history: Interview asking the patient whether she has used alcohol during the pregnancy, and if so how much and how often.

Quickening: First movements of the fetus felt in utero; generally occur between the 18th and 20th week of pregnancy, although they have been felt as early as 10 weeks.

Stages of labor: The first stage of labor begins with the initial contractions and continues up to the point the woman reaches 10 mm of cervical dilatation. The second stage begins when 10 cm of cervical dilatation and ends with the delivery of the infant. The third stage begins with delivery of the infant and ends with delivery of the placenta.

Pregnancy induced hypertension: The diagnosis includes: elevated blood pressure (SBP > 140 mm Hg, or DBP > 90 mm Hg, or SBP increase > 30 mm Hg or DBP increase > 15 mm Hg; AND either proteinuria 1+ or more OR edema > trace.

Intrauterine growth retardation: 4 cm less than indicated by gestational age.

DEFINITIONS FOR CORTICOSTEROIDS FOR FETAL MATURATION IN PRETERM LABOR (CHAPTER 15)

There are no definitions for this chapter.

DEFINITIONS FOR PREVENTIVE CARE (CHAPTER 16)

HIV and STD prevention counseling: Ideally, counseling will include discussion of high-risk behaviors, use of barrier contraceptives, and abstinence. However, we will accept any notation that counseling occurred as meeting this indicator.

DEFINITIONS FOR UPPER RESPIRATORY INFECTIONS (CHAPTER 17)

Preceding viral infection: Viral infection two weeks or less prior to onset of cough. Viral infection examples include common cold and influenza.

DEFINITIONS FOR URINARY TRACT INFECTION (CHAPTER 18)

Suspected upper tract infection: Concomitant presence of such symptoms as fever, chills, and/or back pain suggest an upper tract infection.

Complicated lower tract infection: Patients with diabetes, functional or structural anomalies of the urinary tract, symptoms lasting more than 7 days, recent previous urinary tract infection, use of diaphragm, pregnancy.

DEFINITIONS FOR VAGINITIS AND SEXUALLY TRANSMITTED DISEASES (CHAPTER 19)

There are no definitions for this chapter.

APPENDIX B: PANEL RATINGS SHEETS BY CONDITION

Chapter 1
QUALITY INDICATORS FOR ACNE

(DIAGNOSIS)

1. For patients presenting with a chief complaint of acne, the following history should be documented in their chart:

	Validity	Feasibility
a. Location of lesions (back, face, neck, chest).	1 2 3 4 5 6 7 8 9 (7.0, 0.6, A)	1 2 3 4 5 6 7 8 9 (7.0, 0.6, A)
b. Aggravating factors (stress, seasons, cosmetics, creams).	1 2 3 4 5 6 7 8 9 (5.0, 1.0, I)	1 2 3 4 5 6 7 8 9 (4.0, 1.6, D)
c. Menstrual history and premenstrual worsening of acne.	1 2 3 4 5 6 7 8 9 (5.0, 1.1, I)	1 2 3 4 5 6 7 8 9 (6.0, 1.4, I)
d. Previous treatments.	1 2 3 4 5 6 7 8 9 (8.0, 0.7, A)	1 2 3 4 5 6 7 8 9 (7.0, 0.8, A)
e. Medications and drug use.	1 2 3 4 5 6 7 8 9 (8.0, 0.2, A)	1 2 3 4 5 6 7 8 9 (8.0, 0.2, A)

(TREATMENT)

	Validity	Feasibility
2. If oral antibiotics are prescribed, papules and pustules must be present.	1 2 3 4 5 6 7 8 9 (8.0, 0.6, A)	1 2 3 4 5 6 7 8 9 (8.0, 0.8, A)
4. If isotretinoin is prescribed, there must be documentation of cysts and nodules.	1 2 3 4 5 6 7 8 9 (8.0, 0.2, A)	1 2 3 4 5 6 7 8 9 (8.0, 0.4, A)
5. If isotretinoin is prescribed, a negative pregnancy test should be obtained within two weeks of start of therapy.	1 2 3 4 5 6 7 8 9 (8.0, 1.4, A)	1 2 3 4 5 6 7 8 9 (8.0, 1.2, A)
6. If isotretinoin is prescribed, there should be documentation that counseling regarding the necessity of use of effective means of contraception (including abstinence) was provided.	1 2 3 4 5 6 7 8 9 (9.0, 0.3, A)	1 2 3 4 5 6 7 8 9 (8.0, 1.2, A)

(FOLLOW-UP)

	Validity	Feasibility
7. If isotretinoin is prescribed, monthly pregnancy tests should be performed.	1 2 3 4 5 6 7 8 9 (5.0, 1.7, I)	1 2 3 4 5 6 7 8 9 (6.0, 1.3, I)
8. If isotretinoin is prescribed, monthly q3 liver function tests should be performed.	1 2 3 4 5 6 7 8 9 (7.0, 1.1, I)	1 2 3 4 5 6 7 8 9 (7.0, 0.9, I)
9. If isotretinoin is prescribed, monthly q3 triglyceride levels should be performed.	1 2 3 4 5 6 7 8 9 (5.0, 1.6, I)	1 2 3 4 5 6 7 8 9 (6.0, 0.9, I)

Scales: 1 = low validity or feasibility; 9 = high validity or feasibility.

Chapter 2
QUALITY INDICATORS FOR ALCOHOL DEPENDENCE

	Validity	Feasibility

(DIAGNOSIS)

1. New patients should be screened for problem drinking. This should include an assessment of at least one of the following:

a. Quantity (e.g., drinks per day and/or frequency).

	Validity	Feasibility
	1 1 7	1 1 5 2
	1 2 3 4 5 6 7 8 9	1 2 3 4 5 6 7 8 9
	(8.0, 0.4, A)	(7.0, 0.6, A)

b. Binge drinking (e.g., more than 5 drinks in a day in the last month).

	1 2 4 2	2 2 2 1
	2	2
	1 2 3 4 5 6 7 8 9	1 2 3 4 5 6 7 8 9
	(7.0, 0.7, I)	(6.0, 1.3, I)

2. The record should indicate more detailed screening for dependence, tolerance of psychoactive effects, loss of control and consequences of use (examples include but are not confined to the following questionnaires: CAGE, MAST, HSS, AUDIT, SAAST, and SMAST), if the medical record indicates any of the following:

a. Patient drinks more than 2 drinks each day.

	1 2 6	1 3 5
	1 2 3 4 5 6 7 8 9	1 2 3 4 5 6 7 8 9
	(8.0, 0.6, A)	(7.0, 1.0, I)

b. Patient drinks more than 11 drinks per week.

	1 2 3 3	2 1 3 1 2
	1 2 3 4 5 6 7 8 9	1 2 3 4 5 6 7 8 9
	(7.0, 0.8, I)	(5.0, 1.1, I)

c. Patient drinks more than 5 drinks in a day in the last month.

	1 3 5	1 1 1 5 1
	1 2 3 4 5 6 7 8 9	1 2 3 4 5 6 7 8 9
	(8.0, 1.0, I)	(5.0, 0.9, I)

(TREATMENT)

3. Patients diagnosed with alcohol dependence should be referred for further treatment to at least one of the following:
- inpatient rehabilitation program,
- outpatient rehabilitation program,
- mutual help group (e.g., AA),
- substance abuse counseling, or
- aversion therapy.

	1 4 4	1 1 4 2 1
	1 2 3 4 5 6 7 8 9	1 2 3 4 5 6 7 8 9
	(7.0, 0.6, A)	(7.0, 0.8, A)

(FOLLOW-UP)

4. Regular or binge drinkers (as defined above) should be advised to decrease their drinking.

	2 6 1	1 1 4 2 1
	1 2 3 4 5 6 7 8 9	1 2 3 4 5 6 7 8 9
	(8.0, 0.8, A)	(7.0, 0.8, A)

5. Providers should reassess the alcohol intake of patients who report regular or binge drinking at the next routine health visit.

	1 3 5	1 2 3 2
	1 2 3 4 5 6 7 8 9	1 2 3 4 5 6 7 8 9
	(8.0, 0.8, A)	(7.0, 1.2, I)

Scales: 1 = low validity or feasibility; 9 = high validity or feasibility.

Chapter 3
QUALITY INDICATORS FOR ALLERGIC RHINITIS

	Validity	Feasibility
(DIAGNOSIS)		
1. If a diagnosis of allergic rhinitis is made, the search for a specific allergen by history should be documented in the chart (for initial history).	4 4 1 2 3 4 5 6 7 8 9 (7.0, 1.0, A)	1 2 2 3 1 2 3 4 5 6 7 8 9 (7.0, 1.4, I)
2. If a diagnosis of allergic rhinitis is made, history should include whether the patient uses any topical or nasal decongestants.	1 8 1 2 3 4 5 6 7 8 9 (8.0, 0.1, A)	4 3 2 1 2 3 4 5 6 7 8 9 (7.0, 0.7, I)
(TREATMENT)		
3. Treatment for allergic rhinitis should include at least one of the following: allergen avoidance, antihistamine, nasal steroids, nasal cromolyn.	1 6 2 1 2 3 4 5 6 7 8 9 (8.0, 0.3, A)	3 6 1 2 3 4 5 6 7 8 9 (8.0, 0.3, A)
4. If topical nasal decongestants are prescribed, duration of treatment should be for no longer than 4 days.	3 6 1 2 3 4 5 6 7 8 9 (8.0, 0.3, A)	4 3 2 1 2 3 4 5 6 7 8 9 (5.0, 0.7, A)

Scales: 1 = low validity or feasibility; 9 = high validity or feasibility.

Chapter 4
QUALITY INDICATORS FOR PERSONS WITH MODERATE TO SEVERE ASTHMA

(DIAGNOSIS)

1. Patients with the diagnosis of asthma should have had some historical evaluation of asthma precipitants (environmental exposures, exercise, allergens) within six months (before or after) of diagnosis.

Validity:
```
              1 2 6
1 2 3 4 5 6 7 8 9
(8.0, 0.4, A)
```
Feasibility:
```
              3 5 1
1 2 3 4 5 6 7 8 9
(7.0, 0.4, I)
```

2. Patients with the diagnosis of asthma should have baseline spirometry or peak flow performed within six months of diagnosis.

Validity:
```
          1   2 6
1 2 3 4 5 6 7 8 9
(8.0, 0.7, A)
```
Feasibility:
```
                4 5
1 2 3 4 5 6 7 8 9
(8.0, 0.4, A)
```

3. Peak expiratory flow rate (PEFR) or FEV1 should be measured in patients with chronic asthma (except those with only exercise-induced asthma) at least annually.

Validity:
```
            6 2
1 2 3 4 5 6 7 8 9
(7.0, 0.7, A)
```
Feasibility:
```
          1   4 3
1 2 3 4 5 6 7 8 9
(7.0, 0.9, A)
```

(THERAPY)

4. Patients with the diagnosis of asthma should have been prescribed a beta2-agonist inhaler for symptomatic relief of exacerbations to use as needed.

Validity:
```
        1 3 4 1
1 2 3 4 5 6 7 8 9
(8.0, 0.7, A)
```
Feasibility:
```
            4 4 1
1 2 3 4 5 6 7 8 9
(8.0, 0.6, A)
```

5. Patients who report using a beta2-agonist inhaler more than 3 times per day on a daily basis (not only during an exacerbation) should be prescribed a longer acting bronchodilator (theophylline) and/or an anti-inflammatory agent (inhaled corticosteroids, cromolyn).

Validity:
```
            3 6
1 2 3 4 5 6 7 8 9
(8.0, 0.3, A)
```
Feasibility:
```
        1   3 1 4
1 2 3 4 5 6 7 8 9
(7.0, 1.1, I)
```

6. Patients with asthma should not receive beta-blocker medications (e.g., atenolol, propanalol).

Validity:
```
        1 4 4
1 2 3 4 5 6 7 8 9
(8.0, 0.6, A)
```
Feasibility:
```
            2 4 3
1 2 3 4 5 6 7 8 9
(8.0, 0.6, A)
```

7. Asthmatic patients who have been treated with oral corticosteroids in the past should have documented a current or past trial of inhaled corticosteroids (prescription of at least the minimum dose of inhaled steroids for no less than 1 month).

Validity:
```
            6 3
1 2 3 4 5 6 7 8 9
(7.0, 0.6, A)
```
Feasibility:
```
        1   3 5
1 2 3 4 5 6 7 8 9
(8.0, 0.6, A)
```

8. Patients on chronic theophylline [dose > 600 mg/day] should have at least one serum theophylline level determination per year.

Validity:
```
        1 5 2 1
1 2 3 4 5 6 7 8 9
(7.0, 0.6, A)
```
Feasibility:
```
        1 5 1 2
1 2 3 4 5 6 7 8 9
(7.0, 0.7, A)
```

9. Patients with the diagnosis of asthma should have a documented flu vaccination in the fall/winter of the previous year (September - January).

Validity:
```
      2 1 5 1
1 2 3 4 5 6 7 8 9
(8.0, 0.9, A)
```
Feasibility:
```
      1 3 1 3
1 2 3 4 5 6 7 8 9
(7.0, 1.3, A)
```

10. Patients with the diagnosis of asthma should have a pneumococcal vaccination documented in the chart.

Validity:
```
    1 1 4 1 2
1 2 3 4 5 6 7 8 9
(7.0, 0.9, A)
```
Feasibility:
```
    1 1 4 1 1
1 2 3 4 5 6 7 8 9
(7.0, 1.1, I)
```

(TREATMENT OF EXACERBATIONS)

11. Patients presenting to the physician's office with an asthma exacerbation or historical worsening of asthma symptoms should be evaluated with PEFR or forced expiratory volume at 1 second (FEV1).

Validity:
```
        1 4 4
1 2 3 4 5 6 7 8 9
(7.0, 0.6, A)
```
Feasibility:
```
        3 2 4
1 2 3 4 5 6 7 8 9
(7.0, 0.8, I)
```

Scales: 1 = low validity or feasibility; 9 = high validity or feasibility.

Chapter 4
QUALITY INDICATORS FOR PERSONS WITH MODERATE TO SEVERE ASTHMA

Indicator	Validity	Feasibility
12. At the time of an exacerbation, patients on theophylline should have theophylline level measured.	2 7 9 1 2 3 4 5 6 7 8 9 (8.0, 0.2, A)	1 2 5 1 1 2 3 4 5 6 7 8 9 1 (8.0, 0.6, A)
13. A physical exam of the chest should be performed in patients presenting with an asthma exacerbation.	1 8 1 2 3 4 5 6 7 8 9 (9.0, 0.1, A)	3 6 1 2 3 4 5 6 7 8 9 (9.0, 0.3, A)
14. Patients presenting to the physician's office or ER with an FEV1 or PEFR <= 70% of baseline (or predicted) should be treated with beta2-agonists before discharge.	3 5 1 1 2 3 4 5 6 7 8 9 (8.0, 0.4, A)	1 2 5 1 1 2 3 4 5 6 7 8 9 (8.0, 0.7, A)
15. Patients who receive treatment with beta2-agonists in the physician's office or ER for FEV1 < 70% of baseline (or predicted) should have an FEV1 or PEFR repeated prior to discharge.	2 3 3 1 1 2 3 4 5 6 7 8 9 (7.0, 0.8, A)	3 4 2 1 2 3 4 5 6 7 8 9 (8.0, 0.6, A)
16. Patients with an FEV1 or PEFR <= 70% of baseline (or predicted) after treatment for asthma exacerbation in the physician's office should be placed on an oral corticosteroid taper.	1 3 5 1 2 3 4 5 6 7 8 9 (8.0, 0.7, A)	1 4 1 3 1 2 3 4 5 6 7 8 9 (7.0, 1.0, A)
17. Patients who have a PEFR or FEV1 <= 40% of baseline (or predicted) after treatment with beta2-agonists should not be discharged from ER.	1 5 3 1 2 3 4 5 6 7 8 9 (8.0, 0.4, A)	8 1 1 2 3 4 5 6 7 8 9 (8.0, 0.1, A)

(HOSPITAL TREATMENT)

Indicator	Validity	Feasibility
18. Patients admitted to the hospital for asthma exacerbation should have oxygen saturation measured.	4 5 1 2 3 4 5 6 7 8 9 (9.0, 0.4, A)	3 6 1 2 3 4 5 6 7 8 9 (9.0, 0.3, A)
19. Hospitalized patients with PEFR or FEV1 less than 25 percent of predicted or personal best should receive arterial blood gas measurement.	2 2 5 1 2 3 4 5 6 7 8 9 (9.0, 0.7, A)	4 5 1 2 3 4 5 6 7 8 9 (9.0, 0.4, A)
20. Hospitalized patients should receive systemic steroids (either PO or IV).	4 5 1 2 3 4 5 6 7 8 9 (9.0, 0.4, A)	3 6 1 2 3 4 5 6 7 8 9 (9.0, 0.3, A)
21. Hospitalized patients should receive treatment with beta2-agonists.	2 6 1 1 2 3 4 5 6 7 8 9 (8.0, 0.3, A)	1 4 4 1 2 3 4 5 6 7 8 9 (8.0, 0.6, A)
22. Hospitalized patients should receive treatment with methylxanthines.	1 2 1 2 3 1 3 1 2 3 4 5 6 7 8 9 (5.0, 1.3, I)	1 3 2 2 1 1 2 3 4 5 6 7 8 9 (7.0, 1.4, I)
23. Hospitalized patients with oxygen saturation less than 90 percent should receive supplemental oxygen, unless pCO2 >40 previously documented.	2 3 4 1 2 3 4 5 6 7 8 9 (8.0, 0.7, A)	1 4 4 1 2 3 4 5 6 7 8 9 (8.0, 0.6, A)
24. Hospitalized patients with pCO2 of greater than 40 should receive at least one additional blood gas measurement to evaluate response to treatment.	1 2 1 5 1 2 3 4 5 6 7 8 9 (9.0, 0.9, A)	3 2 4 1 2 3 4 5 6 7 8 9 (8.0, 0.8, A)
25. Hospitalized patients with pCO2 of greater than 40 should be monitored with pulse oximetry.	3 4 2 1 2 3 4 5 6 7 8 9 (8.0, 0.6, A)	2 5 2 1 2 3 4 5 6 7 8 9 (8.0, 0.4, A)

Scales: 1 = low validity or feasibility;   9 = high validity or feasibility.

Chapter 4
QUALITY INDICATORS FOR PERSONS WITH MODERATE TO SEVERE ASTHMA

	Validity	Feasibility
26. Patients with 2 or more hospitalizations for asthma exacerbation in the previous year should receive (or should have received) consultation with an asthma specialist.	1 1 4 2 1 1 2 3 4 5 6 7 8 9 (5.0, 1.3, I)	4 3 2 1 2 3 4 5 6 7 8 9 (7.0, 1.1, I)
27. Hospitalized patients should not receive sedative drugs (e.g., anxiolytics), except if on a ventilator, physiologically dependent on sedatives, or in alcohol withdrawal.	6 3 1 2 3 4 5 6 7 8 9 (7.0, 0.7, A)	4 3 2 1 2 3 4 5 6 7 8 9 (8.0, 0.7, A)
(FOLLOW-UP)		
28. Patients with the diagnosis of asthma should have at least 2 visits within a calendar year.	1 1 2 4 1 1 2 3 4 5 6 7 8 9 (6.0, 1.2, I)	4 3 2 1 2 3 4 5 6 7 8 9 (6.0, 0.7, A)
29. Patients whose asthma medication regimen changes (new medication added, current medication dose decreased or increased) during one visit should have a follow-up contact within 4 weeks.	1 2 1 1 2 2 1 2 3 4 5 6 7 8 9 (5.0, 1.9, I)	1 1 2 3 2 1 2 3 4 5 6 7 8 9 (6.0, 1.6, I)
30. Patients on chronic oral corticosteroids (three or more corticosteroid tapers for exacerbations in the past year, or continuous treatment with any dose prednisone, or three or more administrations of intramuscular cortiocosteroids in the past year) should have follow-up visits at least 2 times in a calendar year.	1 7 1 2 3 4 5 6 7 8 9 (7.0, 0.8, A)	1 2 5 1 1 2 3 4 5 6 7 8 9 (7.0, 0.8, I)
31. Patients seen in the emergency department with an asthma exacerbation should have a follow-up re-assessment within 72 hours.	1 2 2 3 1 1 2 3 4 5 6 7 8 9 (5.0, 1.7, I)	2 1 2 2 2 1 2 3 4 5 6 7 8 9 (5.0, 1.2, I)
32. Patients with a hospitalization for asthma exacerbation should receive outpatient follow-up contact within 14 days.	2 6 1 2 3 4 5 6 7 8 9 (7.0, 0.9, I)	1 1 4 3 1 2 3 4 5 6 7 8 9 (7.0, 0.9, A)

Scales: 1 = low validity or feasibility; 9 = high validity or feasibility.

November 1995

Chapter 5
QUALITY INDICATORS FOR BREAST MASS

(DIAGNOSIS)

	Validity	Feasibility

1. If a palpable breast mass has been detected, at least one of the following procedures should be completed within 3 months:
- fine needle aspiration,
- mammography,
- ultrasound,
- biopsy, or
- follow-up visit.

	Validity	Feasibility
	1 4 4 1 2 3 4 5 6 7 8 9 (8.0, 0.6, A)	1 1 4 3 1 2 3 4 5 6 7 8 9 (8.0, 0.7, A)

2. If a breast mass has been detected on two separate occasions, then either a biopsy or FNA or ultrasound should be performed within 3 months of the second visit.

	2 5 2 1 2 3 4 5 6 7 8 9 (8.0, 0.4, A)	1 1 4 3 1 2 3 4 5 6 7 8 9 (8.0, 0.7, A)

3. A biopsy or FNA should be performed in the following circumstances:

a. Mammography is suggestive of malignancy.

	2 3 4 1 2 3 4 5 6 7 8 9 (8.0, 0.7, A)	2 3 4 1 2 3 4 5 6 7 8 9 (8.0, 0.7, A)

b. Persistent palpable mass that is not cystic on diagnostic testing (ultrasound or mammography).

	3 3 3 1 2 3 4 5 6 7 8 9 (8.0, 0.7, A)	2 4 3 1 2 3 4 5 6 7 8 9 (8.0, 0.6, A)

4. A biopsy should be performed if FNA cannot rule out malignancy.

	2 5 2 1 2 3 4 5 6 7 8 9 (8.0, 0.4, A)	3 3 3 1 2 3 4 5 6 7 8 9 (8.0, 0.7, A)

Scales: 1 = low validity or feasibility; 9 = high validity or feasibility.

Chapter 6
QUALITY INDICATORS FOR CESAREAN DELIVERY

A. PRIOR CESAREAN DELIVERY

(TREATMENT)

	Validity	Feasibility
1. For women who have delivered by cesarean, the type of uterine incision used (transverse lower segment or vertical) should be noted in the medical record.	4 3 2 1 2 3 4 5 6 7 8 9 (8.0, 0.7, A)	2 3 3 1 1 2 3 4 5 6 7 8 9 (7.0, 1.0, A)
2. For women with a cesarean delivery in a prior pregnancy, the number and type of previous uterine scar(s) should be noted in the current delivery medical record. (If this information is not available, an attempt to locate it should be documented in the chart.)	1 3 3 2 1 2 3 4 5 6 7 8 9 (8.0, 0.8, A)	1 3 1 3 1 1 2 3 4 5 6 7 8 9 (6.0, 1.1, I)
3. Women with one prior transverse lower segment cesarean should undergo a trial of labor unless another indication for cesarean delivery is present (including refusal of a trial of labor).	1 2 3 3 1 2 3 4 5 6 7 8 9 (8.0, 0.9, A)	1 2 3 3 1 2 3 4 5 6 7 8 9 (8.0, 0.9, A)
4. Women with a prior classical vertical cesarean should have a scheduled repeat cesarean delivery.	3 4 2 1 2 3 4 5 6 7 8 9 (8.0, 0.6, A)	1 6 2 1 2 3 4 5 6 7 8 9 (8.0, 0.7, A)

B. FAILURE TO PROGRESS IN LABOR

(DIAGNOSIS)

	Validity	Feasibility
1. When the diagnosis of failure to progress in labor is made, a woman should be in the active phase of labor.	3 6 1 2 3 4 5 6 7 8 9 (8.0, 0.3, A)	2 4 3 1 2 3 4 5 6 7 8 9 (7.0, 0.6, A)
2. When the diagnosis of failure to progress in labor is made, at least two exams of cervical dilatation separated in time by at least 2 hours should have been done and recorded in the medical record.	2 7 1 2 3 4 5 6 7 8 9 (8.0, 0.2, A)	5 4 1 2 3 4 5 6 7 8 9 (7.0, 0.4, A)
3. Before a cesarean delivery is used to treat failure to progress in labor, at least two of the following therapeutic interventions should have been tried after the time of the diagnosis of FTP: - amniotomy, - oxytocin, or - ambulation.	1 3 5 1 2 3 4 5 6 7 8 9 (8.0, 0.6, A)	2 1 2 4 1 2 3 4 5 6 7 8 9 (7.0, 1.0, I)

Scales: 1 = low validity or feasibility; 9 = high validity or feasibility.

Chapter 6
QUALITY INDICATORS FOR CESAREAN DELIVERY

C. FETAL DISTRESS

(DIAGNOSIS)

	Validity	Feasibility

1. Fetuses should be monitored during active labor. The forms of monitoring are:
- intermittent auscultation with a stethoscope or doppler device, as recommended by ACOG for low risk, or
- continuous electronic fetal monitoring (EFM).

```
                      1       4 4 3 2 1              1   3 5
Validity      1 2 3 4 5 6 7 8 9          1 2 3 4 5 6 7 8 9    Feasibility
              (7.0, 0.8, A)              (8.0, 0.7, A)
```

D. ANTIBIOTIC PROPHYLAXIS

1. Women who give birth by cesarean should receive at least one dose of antibiotic prophylaxis.

```
                  2 1   3 2 1                      3 3 3
Validity  1 2 3 4 5 6 7 8 9          1 2 3 4 5 6 7 8 9    Feasibility
          (7.0, 1.0, I)              (8.0, 0.7, A)
```

2. Prophylactic antibiotic regimens should include one of the following:
- broad spectrum penicillins,
- broad spectrum cephalosporins, or
- metronidazole.

```
                        1 4 4                          5 4
Validity  1 2 3 4 5 6 7 8 9          1 2 3 4 5 6 7 8 9    Feasibility
          (8.0, 0.6, A)              (8.0, 0.4, A)
```

3. Aminoglycosides should not be used, alone or in combination, for antibiotic prophylaxis.

```
                    2 4 3                          3 2 3 1
Validity  1 2 3 4 5 6 7 8 9          1 2 3 4 5 6 7 8 9    Feasibility
          (7.0, 0.6, A)              (7.0, 0.9, I)
```

4. Prophylactic antibiotics should be administered after the umbilical cord is clamped.

```
                    2 2 5                        2 2 3 1 1
Validity  1 2 3 4 5 6 7 8 9          1 2 3 4 5 6 7 8 9    Feasibility
          (8.0, 0.7, A)              (5.0, 1.1, I)
```

Scales: 1 = low validity or feasibility; 9 = high validity or feasibility.

Chapter 7
QUALITY INDICATORS FOR CIGARETTE USE COUNSELING

	Validity	Feasibility

(SCREENING AND INITIAL EVALUATION)

1. Enrollees should have the presence or absence of tobacco
use noted in the medical record at the intake history and
physical or at least once during the course of a year.

```
                    3 4 1                        3 6
Validity      1 2 3 4 5 6 7 8 9    Feasibility  1 2 3 4 5 6 7 8 9
                 (8.0, 1.1, A)                  (8.0, 0.7, I)
```

(TREATMENT)

2. Current smokers should receive counseling to stop
smoking.

```
                  3 3 3                      2 2 2 2 1
              1 2 3 4 5 6 7 8 9          1 2 3 4 5 6 7 8 9
                 (8.0, 0.7, A)              (7.0, 1.1, I)
```

3. If counseling alone fails to help the patient quit smoking,
the patient should be offered nicotine replacement therapy (gum
or patch), except if contraindicated.

```
                1 6 2                       1 3 4 1
              1 2 3 4 5 6 7 8 9          1 2 3 4 5 6 7 8 9
                 (7.0, 0.3, A)              (7.0, 0.7, I)
```

4. Nicotine replacement should only be prescribed in conjunction
with counseling.

```
              3 2 3 1                      1 3 2 3
              1 2 3 4 5 6 7 8 9          1 2 3 4 5 6 7 8 9
                 (7.0, 0.9, I)              (6.0, 0.9, I)
```

5. Nicotine replacement should not be prescribed if the patient:

a. Is pregnant or nursing.

```
            1 1 2 2 3                        4 2 3
              1 2 3 4 5 6 7 8 9          1 2 3 4 5 6 7 8 9
                 (8.0, 1.1, A)              (8.0, 0.8, A)
```

b. Has had a myocardial infarction in past year.

```
            1 1 2 5                          5 4
              1 2 3 4 5 6 7 8 9          1 2 3 4 5 6 7 8 9
                 (8.0, 1.3, I)              (7.0, 0.4, A)
```

d. Continues to smoke.

```
          1 1 4 1 2                        2 2 3 1
              1 2 3 4 5 6 7 8 9          1 2 3 4 5 6 7 8 9
                 (6.0, 1.0, I)              (4.0, 1.6, I)
```

(FOLLOW-UP)

6. Tobacco abuse should be added to the problem list of
current smokers or addressed within one year.

```
                2 4 1                      1 1        1 6
              1 2 3 4 5 6 7 8 9          1 2 3 4 5 6 7 8 9
                 (8.0, 1.3, A)              (8.0, 1.1, A)
```

Scales: 1 = low validity or feasibility; 9 = high validity or feasibility.

Chapter 8
QUALITY INDICATORS FOR DEPRESSION

	Validity	Feasibility

(DIAGNOSIS/DETECTION)

1. Clinicians should ask about the presence or absence of depression or depressive symptoms in any person with any of the following risk factors for depression:

a. Divorce in past six months.

	Validity	Feasibility
	1 1 3 3 1	3 4 2
	1 2 3 4 5 6 7 8 9	1 2 3 4 5 6 7 8 9
	(6.0, 0.9, I)	(6.0, 0.6, A)

b. Unemployment.

	Validity	Feasibility
	1 1 5 2	2 1 3 2 1
	1 2 3 4 5 6 7 8 9	1 2 3 4 5 6 7 8 9
	(6.0, 0.6, A)	(5.0, 1.0, I)

c. History of depression.

	Validity	Feasibility
	5 4	1 8
	1 2 3 4 5 6 7 8 9	1 2 3 4 5 6 7 8 9
	(7.0, 0.4, A)	(7.0, 0.1, A)

d. Death in family in past six months.

	Validity	Feasibility
	1 6 2	1 2 3 3
	1 2 3 4 5 6 7 8 9	1 2 3 4 5 6 7 8 9
	(7.0, 0.6, A)	(6.0, 0.8, I)

e. Alcohol or other drug abuse.

	Validity	Feasibility
	1 5 2 1	1 4 3 1
	1 2 3 4 5 6 7 8 9	1 2 3 4 5 6 7 8 9
	(7.0, 0.7, A)	(6.0, 0.8, I)

f. Traumatic events.

	Validity	Feasibility
	2 3 2 2	1 2 4 1 1
	1 2 3 4 5 6 7 8 9	1 2 3 4 5 6 7 8 9
	(6.0, 0.9, I)	(6.0, 0.8, A)

2. If the diagnosis of depression is made, specific co-morbidities should be elicited and documented in the chart:

a. Presence or absence of alcohol or other drug.

	Validity	Feasibility
	5 4	2 4 3
	1 2 3 4 5 6 7 8 9	1 2 3 4 5 6 7 8 9
	(7.0, 0.4, A)	(7.0, 0.6, A)

b. Medication use.

	Validity	Feasibility
	2 7	1 1 7
	1 2 3 4 5 6 7 8 9	1 2 3 4 5 6 7 8 9
	(8.0, 0.2, A)	(8.0, 0.3, A)

c. General medical disorder(s).

	Validity	Feasibility
	2 7	4 5
	1 2 3 4 5 6 7 8 9	1 2 3 4 5 6 7 8 9
	(8.0, 0.2, A)	(8.0, 0.4, A)

(TREATMENT)

3. If co-morbidity (substance abuse, contributing medication) is present that contributes to depression, the initial treatment objective should be to remove the comorbidity or treat the medical disorder.

	Validity	Feasibility
	1 3 5	1 7 1
	1 2 3 4 5 6 7 8 9	1 2 3 4 5 6 7 8 9
	(8.0, 0.6, A)	(7.0, 0.3, A)

4. Once diagnosis of major depression has been made, treatment with anti-depressant medication and/or psychotherapy should begin within 2 weeks.

	Validity	Feasibility
	2 2 5	1 3 4
	1 2 3 4 5 6 7 8 9	1 2 3 4 5 6 7 8 9
	(8.0, 0.7, A)	(7.0, 0.9, A)

5. Presence or absence of suicidal ideation should be documented during the first or second diagnostic visit.

	Validity	Feasibility
	1 5 3	1 1 4 3
	1 2 3 4 5 6 7 8 9	1 2 3 4 5 6 7 8 9
	(8.0, 0.4, A)	(8.0, 0.7, A)

Scales: 1 = low validity or feasibility; 9 = high validity or feasibility.

Chapter 8
QUALITY INDICATORS FOR DEPRESSION

Indicator	Validity	Feasibility
6. Medication treatment visits or telephone contacts should occur at least once in the 2 weeks following initial diagnosis.	4 5 1 2 3 4 5 6 7 8 9 (7.0, 0.4, I)	1 4 3 1 1 2 3 4 5 6 7 8 9 (6.0, 0.7, I)
7. At least one of the following should occur if there is no or inadequate response to therapy for depression at 8 weeks: - referral to psychotherapist if not already seeing one, - change or increase in dose of medication if on medication, - addition of medication if only using psychotherapy, or - change in diagnosis documented in chart.	5 4 1 2 3 4 5 6 7 8 9 (7.0, 0.4, A)	8 1 1 2 3 4 5 6 7 8 9 (7.0, 0.1, A)
8. Anti-depressants should be prescribed at appropriate dosages.	1 7 1 1 2 3 4 5 6 7 8 9 (8.0, 0.2, A)	1 3 4 1 1 2 3 4 5 6 7 8 9 (8.0, 0.8, A)
9. Anti-anxiety agents should not be prescribed as a sole agent for the treatment of depression.	3 3 3 1 2 3 4 5 6 7 8 9 (7.0, 0.7, I)	4 5 1 2 3 4 5 6 7 8 9 (8.0, 0.4, A)
10. Persons who have suicidality should be asked if they have specific plans to carry out suicide.	4 5 1 2 3 4 5 6 7 8 9 (9.0, 0.4, A)	2 4 3 1 2 3 4 5 6 7 8 9 (8.0, 0.6, A)
11. Persons who have suicidality and have any of the following risk factors should be hospitalized:		
a. Psychosis.	1 3 2 3 1 2 3 4 5 6 7 8 9 (8.0, 0.9, A)	2 1 1 5 1 2 3 4 5 6 7 8 9 (8.0, 1.2, A)
b. Current alcohol or drug abuse or dependency.	1 1 1 6 1 2 3 4 5 6 7 8 9 (8.0, 1.1, A)	1 1 3 1 2 1 1 2 3 4 5 6 7 8 9 (6.0, 1.3, I)
c. Specific plans to carry out suicide (e.g., obtaining a weapon, putting affairs in order, making a suicide note).	5 4 1 2 3 4 5 6 7 8 9 (8.0, 0.4, A)	1 1 3 4 1 2 3 4 5 6 7 8 9 (8.0, 1.0, A)
(FOLLOW-UP)		
12. Once depression has resolved, follow-up visits should occur twice in a year at a minimum, while patient is still on medication, for the first year of treatment.	1 8 1 2 3 4 5 6 7 8 9 (7.0, 0.4, A)	1 1 6 1 1 2 3 4 5 6 7 8 9 (7.0, 0.4, A)
13. At each visit during which depression is discussed, degree of response/remission and side effects of medication should be assessed and documented during the first year of treatment.	1 5 3 1 2 3 4 5 6 7 8 9 (7.0, 0.8, A)	1 6 1 1 2 3 4 5 6 7 8 9 (7.0, 0.6, A)
14. Persons hospitalized for depression should have follow-up with a mental health specialist or their primary care doctor within two weeks of discharge.	1 1 2 5 1 2 3 4 5 6 7 8 9 (8.0, 0.8, A)	2 7 1 2 3 4 5 6 7 8 9 (8.0, 0.2, A)

Scales: 1 = low validity or feasibility; 9 = high validity or feasibility.

Chapter 9
QUALITY INDICATORS FOR DIABETES MELLITUS

(DIAGNOSIS)

	Validity	Feasibility

1. Patients with fasting blood sugar > 140 or postprandial blood sugar > 200 should have diabetes noted in progress notes or problem list.

```
                          1 6 2                    1 6 2
              1 2 3 4 5 6 7 8 9        1 2 3 4 5 6 7 8 9
              (8.0, 0.3, A)          . (8.0, 0.3, A)
```

2. Patients with the diagnosis of [Type I] diabetes should have:

a. Glycosylated hemoglobin or fructosamine every 6 months.

```
                        7 2                    1 4 4
              1 2 3 4 5 6 7 8 9        1 2 3 4 5 6 7 8 9
              (7.0, 0.2, A)            (7.0, 0.6, A)
```

b. Eye and visual exam (annual).

```
                1 3 4 1                1 1 3 4
              1 2 3 4 5 6 7 8 9        1 2 3 4 5 6 7 8 9
              (8.0, 0.8, A)            (7.0, 0.8, A)
```

c. Triglycerides (annual).

```
              2 1 2 3 1                  1 2 1 2 3
              1 2 3 4 5 6 7 8 9        1 2 3 4 5 6 7 8 9
              (6.0, 1.3, I)            (7.0, 1.3, I)
```

d. Total cholesterol (annual).

```
                3 1 5                      1 2  4 2
              1 2 3 4 5 6 7 8 9        1 2 3 4 5 6 7 8 9
              (7.0, 0.8, I)            (7.0, 1.0, I)
```

e. HDL cholesterol (annual).

```
              1 3 2 2 1                  1 2 1 3 2
              1 2 3 4 5 6 7 8 9        1 2 3 4 5 6 7 8 9
              (6.0, 1.0, I)            (7.0, 1.1, I)
```

f. Measurement of urine protein (annual).

```
                  4 5                      1 6 2
              1 2 3 4 5 6 7 8 9        1 2 3 4 5 6 7 8 9
              (8.0, 0.4, A)            (7.0, 0.4, A)
```

g. Examination of feet at least twice a year.

```
              1 1  2 2 3                3 2 2 2
              1 2 3 4 5 6 7 8 9        1 2 3 4 5 6 7 8 9
              (7.0, 1.6, I)            (6.0, 1.0, I)
```

h. Measurement of blood pressure at every visit.

```
              1  2 4 2                    3 4 2
              1 2 3 4 5 6 7 8 9        1 2 3 4 5 6 7 8 9
              (8.0, 0.8, A)            (8.0, 0.6, A)
```

Scales: 1 = low validity or feasibility; 9 = high validity or feasibility.

Chapter 9
QUALITY INDICATORS FOR DIABETES MELLITUS

2. Patients with the diagnosis of [Type II] diabetes should have:

Indicator	Validity	Feasibility
a. Glycosylated hemoglobin or fructosamine every 6 months.	1 2 3 4 5 6 7 8 9 (7.0, 1.2, I)	1 2 3 4 5 6 7 8 9 (7.0, 0.9, A)
b. Eye and visual exam (annual).	1 2 3 4 5 6 7 8 9 (7.0, 1.6, I)	1 2 3 4 5 6 7 8 9 (7.0, 0.8, A)
c. Triglycerides (annual).	1 2 3 4 5 6 7 8 9 (6.0, 1.3, I)	1 2 3 4 5 6 7 8 9 (7.0, 1.3, I)
d. Total cholesterol (annual).	1 2 3 4 5 6 7 8 9 (6.0, 0.8, I)	1 2 3 4 5 6 7 8 9 (7.0, 1.0, I)
e. HDL cholesterol (annual).	1 2 3 4 5 6 7 8 9 (6.0, 1.0, I)	1 2 3 4 5 6 7 8 9 (7.0, 1.1, I)
f. Measurement of urine protein (annual).	1 2 3 4 5 6 7 8 9 (7.0, 0.4, A)	1 2 3 4 5 6 7 8 9 (7.0, 0.4, A)
g. Examination of feet at least twice a year.	1 2 3 4 5 6 7 8 9 (6.0, 2.0, I)	1 2 3 4 5 6 7 8 9 (6.0, 1.0, I)
h. Measurement of blood pressure at every visit.	1 2 3 4 5 6 7 8 9 (8.0, 0.8, A)	1 2 3 4 5 6 7 8 9 (8.0, 0.6, A)
3. [Type I] patients taking insulin should monitor their glucose at home, unless documented to be unable or unwilling.	1 2 3 4 5 6 7 8 9 (8.0, 0.6, A)	1 2 3 4 5 6 7 8 9 (6.0, 1.6, I)
3. [Type II] patients taking insulin should monitor their glucose at home, unless documented to be unable or unwilling.	1 2 3 4 5 6 7 8 9 (7.0, 0.6, A)	1 2 3 4 5 6 7 8 9 (6.0, 1.7, I)
(TREATMENT) 4. Diabetics should receive dietary and exercise counseling.	1 2 3 4 5 6 7 8 9 (8.0, 0.7, A)	1 2 3 4 5 6 7 8 9 (7.0, 0.7, A)
5. Type II diabetics who have failed dietary therapy should receive oral hypoglycemic therapy.	1 2 3 4 5 6 7 8 9 (8.0, 0.6, A)	1 2 3 4 5 6 7 8 9 (8.0, 0.3, A)
6. Type II diabetics who have failed oral hypoglycemics should be offered insulin.	1 2 3 4 5 6 7 8 9 (7.0, 1.0, A)	1 2 3 4 5 6 7 8 9 (7.0, 0.6, A)

Scales: 1 = low validity or feasibility; 9 = high validity or feasibility.

Chapter 9
QUALITY INDICATORS FOR DIABETES MELLITUS

	Validity	Feasibility
7. If a hypertensive [Type I] patient without known CAD is receiving other antihypertensive therapy in the absence of ACE inhibitors or calcium channel blockers, progress note should document failure of ACE inhibitors or calcium channel blockers to control blood pressure.	4 5 1 2 3 4 5 6 7 8 9 (8.0, 0.4, A)	1 5 3 1 2 3 4 5 6 7 8 9 (7.0, 0.4, A)
7. If a hypertensive [Type II] patient without known CAD is receiving other antihypertensive therapy in the absence of ACE inhibitors or calcium channel blockers, progress note should document failure of ACE inhibitors or calcium channel blockers to control blood pressure.	4 5 1 2 3 4 5 6 7 8 9 (8.0, 0.4, A)	1 5 3 1 2 3 4 5 6 7 8 9 (7.0, 0.4, A)
(FOLLOW-UP)		
8. Patients with [Type I] diabetes should have a follow-up visit at least every 6 months.	3 6 1 2 3 4 5 6 7 8 9 (8.0, 0.3, A)	1 3 3 2 1 2 3 4 5 6 7 8 9 (8.0, 0.8, A)
8. Patients with [Type II] diabetes should have a follow-up visit at least every 6 months.	1 1 1 4 2 1 2 3 4 5 6 7 8 9 (7.0, 1.0, I)	1 3 3 2 1 2 3 4 5 6 7 8 9 (8.0, 0.8, A)

Scales: 1 = low validity or feasibility; 9 = high validity or feasibility.

Chapter 10
QUALITY INDICATORS FOR FAMILY PLANNING/CONTRACEPTION

(SCREENING)

1. A history to determine risk for unintended pregnancy should be taken yearly on women who present otherwise for routine care. In order to establish risk, the following elements of the history need to be documented:

Indicator	Validity	Feasibility
a. Menstrual status (e.g., pre- or post-menopausal, history of hysterectomy), last menstrual period, or pregnancy test.	4 4 1 1 2 3 4 5 6 7 8 9 (8.0, 0.6, A)	1 1 3 3 1 1 2 3 4 5 6 7 8 9 (7.0, 1.0, A)
b. Sexual history (presence or absence of current heterosexual intercourse).	1 5 2 1 1 2 3 4 5 6 7 8 9 (7.0, 0.6, A)	1 4 3 1 1 2 3 4 5 6 7 8 9 (6.0, 1.2, I)
c. Current contraceptive practices.	4 4 1 1 2 3 4 5 6 7 8 9 (8.0, 0.6, A)	1 2 2 4 1 2 3 4 5 6 7 8 9 (7.0, 1.0, I)
d. Desire for pregnancy.	1 1 1 2 1 1 1 1 1 2 3 4 5 6 7 8 9 (6.0, 1.8, I)	1 1 1 2 2 2 1 2 3 4 5 6 7 8 9 (5.0, 1.8, I)

(TREATMENT)

Indicator	Validity	Feasibility
2. Women at risk for unintended pregnancy should receive counseling about effective contraceptive methods.	2 5 2 1 2 3 4 5 6 7 8 9 (8.0, 0.4, A)	2 1 5 1 1 2 3 4 5 6 7 8 9 (7.0, 0.7, I)
3. The smoking status of women prescribed combination OCs should be documented in the medical record.	1 2 3 3 1 2 3 4 5 6 7 8 9 (8.0, 0.9, A)	3 3 3 1 2 3 4 5 6 7 8 9 (8.0, 0.7, A)
4. Women who smoke and are prescribed oral contraceptives should be counseled and encouraged to quit smoking.	2 3 4 1 2 3 4 5 6 7 8 9 (8.0, 0.7, A)	2 4 1 2 1 2 3 4 5 6 7 8 9 (7.0, 0.8, A)
5. Women over age 35 who smoke should not be prescribed combination oral contraceptives.	3 5 1 1 2 3 4 5 6 7 8 9 (8.0, 0.4, A)	2 3 4 1 2 3 4 5 6 7 8 9 (8.0, 0.7, A)

Scales: 1 = low validity or feasibility; 9 = high validity or feasibility.

Chapter 11
QUALITY INDICATORS FOR HEADACHE

(DIAGNOSIS)

1. Patients with new onset headache should be asked about:

	Validity	Feasibility
a. Location of the pain (e.g., frontal, bilateral).	2 1 6 1 2 3 4 5 6 7 8 9 (8.0, 0.6, A)	1 1 2 5 1 2 3 4 5 6 7 8 9 (8.0, 0.8, A)
b. Associated symptoms (e.g., aura).	3 6 1 2 3 4 5 6 7 8 9 (8.0, 0.3, A)	1 1 3 4 1 2 3 4 5 6 7 8 9 (7.0, 0.8, A)
c. Temporal profile (e.g., new onset, constant).	2 6 1 1 2 3 4 5 6 7 8 9 (8.0, 0.3, A)	1 3 5 1 2 3 4 5 6 7 8 9 (8.0, 0.6, A)
d. Severity.	1 5 3 1 2 3 4 5 6 7 8 9 (7.0, 0.6, A)	1 3 1 3 1 2 3 4 5 6 7 8 9 (6.0, 1.2, I)
e. Family history.	4 2 3 1 2 3 4 5 6 7 8 9 (7.0, 0.8, I)	1 5 2 1 2 3 4 5 6 7 8 9 (7.0, 0.9, A)
f. Aggravating or alleviating factors.	7 2 1 2 3 4 5 6 7 8 9 (7.0, 0.2, A)	1 4 3 1 2 3 4 5 6 7 8 9 (7.0, 0.8, A)

2. Patients with new onset headache should have an examination evaluating the:

	Validity	Feasibility
a. Cranial nerves.	5 3 1 1 2 3 4 5 6 7 8 9 (7.0, 0.6, A)	2 3 4 1 2 3 4 5 6 7 8 9 (7.0, 0.7, A)
b. Fundi.	3 4 2 1 2 3 4 5 6 7 8 9 (8.0, 0.6, A)	1 2 5 1 1 2 3 4 5 6 7 8 9 (8.0, 0.6, A)
c. Deep tendon reflexes.	2 3 3 1 1 2 3 4 5 6 7 8 9 (7.0, 0.8, A)	1 2 6 1 2 3 4 5 6 7 8 9 (8.0, 0.8, I)
d. Blood pressure.	1 2 5 1 1 2 3 4 5 6 7 8 9 (8.0, 0.7, A)	1 1 6 1 1 2 3 4 5 6 7 8 9 (8.0, 0.4, A)

3. CT or MRI scanning is indicated in patients with new onset headache and any of the following circumstances:

	Validity	Feasibility
a. Abnormal neurological examination,	2 6 1 1 2 3 4 5 6 7 8 9 (8.0, 0.3, A)	2 7 1 2 3 4 5 6 7 8 9 (8.0, 0.4, A)
b. Constant headache, or	1 2 3 2 1 1 2 3 4 5 6 7 8 9 (6.0, 1.0, I)	4 4 1 2 3 4 5 6 7 8 9 (6.0, 1.3, I)
c. Severe headache.	1 1 3 4 1 2 3 4 5 6 7 8 9 (7.0, 0.8, A)	1 2 6 1 2 3 4 5 6 7 8 9 (8.0, 0.8, I)

Scales: 1 = low validity or feasibility; 9 = high validity or feasibility.

Chapter 11
QUALITY INDICATORS FOR HEADACHE

	Validity	Feasibility

4. Skull X-rays should not be part of an evaluation for headache.

(TREATMENT)

```
                        7 2                        7 2
Validity:     1 2 3 4 5 6 7 8 9      Feasibility:  1 2 3 4 5 6 7 8 9
              (8.0, 0.2, A)                        (8.0, 0.2, A)
```

5. Patients with acute mild migraine or tension headache, should have tried aspirin, tylenol, or other nonsteroidal anti-inflammatory agents before being prescribed any other medication.

```
                  1     5 3                        1 1 6 1
              1 2 3 4 5 6 7 8 9                    1 2 3 4 5 6 7 8 9
              (7.0, 0.7, A)                        (7.0, 0.4, A)
```

6. For patients with acute moderate or severe migraine headache, one of the following should have been tried before being prescribed any other agent:
- parenteral ketorolac,
- subcutaneous sumatriptan,
- parenteral dihydroergotamine,
- parenteral chlorpromazine, or
- parenteral metaclopramide.

```
                1 2 2   3 1                        1 1 2 3
              1 2 3 4 5 6 7 8 9                    1 2 3 4 5 6 7 8 9
              (5.0, 1.4, I)                        (7.0, 1.0, I)
```

6. For patients with acute moderate or severe migraine headache, one of the following should have been tried before being prescribed any other agent:
- oral ketorolac,
- oral sumatriptan,
- oral dihydroergotamine,
- oral chlorpromazine, or
- oral metaclopramide.

```
                    2   5 2                        1 1 2 5
              1 2 3 4 5 6 7 8 9                    1 2 3 4 5 6 7 8 9
              (7.0, 0.7, A)                        (8.0, 0.8, A)
```

7. Recurrent moderate or severe tension headaches should be treated with a trial of tricyclic antidepressant agents, if no medical contraindications to use.

```
                1 3 2 3                            4 4 1
              1 2 3 4 5 6 7 8 9                    1 2 3 4 5 6 7 8 9
              (7.0, 0.9, I)                        (8.0, 1.0, I)
```

8. If a patient has more than 2 moderate to severe migraine headaches each month, then prophylactic treatment with one of the following agents should be offered:
- beta blockers,
- calcium channel blockers,
- tricyclic antidepressants,
- naproxen,
- aspirin,
- fluoxitene,
- valproate, or
- cyproheptadine.

```
                      5 4                              3 1 5
              1 2 3 4 5 6 7 8 9                    1 2 3 4 5 6 7 8 9
              (7.0, 0.4, A)                        (8.0, 0.8, I)
```

9. Sumatriptan and ergotamine should not be concurrently administered.

```
                    2 4 3                          1 3 3 2
              1 2 3 4 5 6 7 8 9                    1 2 3 4 5 6 7 8 9
              (8.0, 0.6, A)                        (8.0, 0.8, A)
```

10. Opioid agonists and barbiturates should not be first-line therapy for migraine or tension headaches.

```
                1   1 2 5                          1 1 4 3
              1 2 3 4 5 6 7 8 9                    1 2 3 4 5 6 7 8 9
              (8.0, 0.9, A)                        (7.0, 0.9, A)
```

Scales: 1 = low validity or feasibility; 9 = high validity or feasibility.

	Validity	Feasibility

11. Sumatriptan and ergotamine should not be given in patients
with a history of:
- uncontrolled hypertension,
- atypical chest pain, or
- ischemic heart disease or angina.

	Validity	Feasibility
	1 5 3	1 6 2
	1 2 3 4 5 6 7 8 9	1 2 3 4 5 6 7 8 9
	(8.0, 0.4, A)	(8.0, 0.3, A)

Scales: 1 = low validity or feasibility; 9 = high validity or feasibility.

Chapter 12
QUALITY INDICATORS FOR HYPERTENSION

	Validity	Feasibility

(DIAGNOSIS)

1. Systolic and diastolic blood pressure should be measured on adult women otherwise presenting for care at least once each year.

Validity:
```
            1 5 3
1 2 3 4 5 6 7 8 9
   (8.0, 0.4, A)
```
Feasibility:
```
            1 4 4
1 2 3 4 5 6 7 8 9
   (8.0, 0.6, A)
```

2. Patients with a new diagnosis of stage 1 hypertension should have at least three measurements on different days with a mean SBP > 140 and/or a mean DBP > 90.

Validity:
```
            1 6 2
1 2 3 4 5 6 7 8 9
   (7.0, 0.3, A)
```
Feasibility:
```
        4 1 4
1 2 3 4 5 6 7 8 9
   (7.0, 0.9, I)
```

3. Initial history and physical of patients with hypertension should document assessment of at least two items from each of the following groups by the third visit:

a. History: family or personal history of premature CAD, CVA, diabetes, hyperlipidemia.

Validity:
```
          5 3
1 2 3 4 5 6 7 8 9
   (7.0, 0.8, A)
```
Feasibility:
```
        1 6 2
1 2 3 4 5 6 7 8 9
   (7.0, 0.3, A)
```

b. Medication or substance use: personal history of tobacco abuse, alcohol abuse, or taking of medications that may cause hypertension.

Validity:
```
          1 8
1 2 3 4 5 6 7 8 9
   (8.0, 0.1, A)
```
Feasibility:
```
      1 1 2 5
1 2 3 4 5 6 7 8 9
   (8.0, 0.9, A)
```

c. Physical exam: examination of the fundi, heart sounds, abdomen for bruits, peripheral arterial pulses, neurologic system.

Validity:
```
      2 1 3 2
1 2 3 4 5 6 7 8 9
   (7.0, 1.8, I)
```
Feasibility:
```
      1 3 3 2
1 2 3 4 5 6 7 8 9
   (7.0, 0.9, I)
```

4. Stage 1 hypertensive women taking the following drugs may cause hypertension should have the drug discontinued (at least temporarily) before pharmacotherapy is initiated.
- oral contraceptives,
- nasal decongestants,
- appetite suppressants,
- monamine oxidase inhibitors, and
- tricyclic antidepressants.

Validity:
```
        2 3 3 1
1 2 3 4 5 6 7 8 9
   (7.0, 1.0, A)
```
Feasibility:
```
        1 5 1 1
1 2 3 4 5 6 7 8 9
   (7.0, 0.8, A)
```

Scales: 1 = low validity or feasibility; 9 = high validity or feasibility.

5. Initial laboratory tests should include the following:

	Validity	Feasibility

a. Urinalysis.	`1 1  1 1 1 4`
	`1 2 3 4 5 6 7 8 9`
	`(7.0, 1.8, I)`
		`                  2 6`
		`1 2 3 4 5 6 7 8 9`
		`(8.0, 0.9, A)`

b. Glucose.	`      2 4 1`
	`1 2 3 4 5 6 7 8 9`
	`(7.0, 1.3, I)`
		`        1 1   4 3`
		`1 2 3 4 5 6 7 8 9`
		`(7.0, 1.2, A)`

c. Potassium.	`      2 4 3`
	`1 2 3 4 5 6 7 8 9`
	`(7.0, 0.6, A)`
		`        1 4 4`
		`1 2 3 4 5 6 7 8 9`
		`(7.0, 0.6, A)`

d. Calcium.	`    4 4 1`
	`1 2 3 4 5 6 7 8 9`
	`(6.0, 0.6, A)`
		`      2   3 4`
		`1 2 3 4 5 6 7 8 9`
		`(7.0, 0.9, A)`

e. Creatinine.	`        4 5`
	`1 2 3 4 5 6 7 8 9`
	`(8.0, 0.4, A)`
		`          1 8`
		`1 2 3 4 5 6 7 8 9`
		`(8.0, 0.1, A)`

f. Uric acid.	`1 1 1 2 3 2`
	`1 2 3 4 5 6 7 8 9`
	`(5.0, 1.0, A)`
		`      1 1   3 4`
		`1 2 3 4 5 6 7 8 9`
		`(7.0, 1.2, A)`

g. Cholesterol.	`          8 1`
	`1 2 3 4 5 6 7 8 9`
	`(7.0, 0.1, A)`
		`          4 5`
		`1 2 3 4 5 6 7 8 9`
		`(8.0, 0.4, A)`

h. Triglycerides.	`  1   2 1 5`
	`1 2 3 4 5 6 7 8 9`
	`(7.0, 1.1, I)`
		`  1       5 3`
		`1 2 3 4 5 6 7 8 9`
		`(7.0, 0.8, A)`

i. Electrocardiogram.	`1 2 1   3 2`
	`1 2 3 4 5 6 7 8 9`
	`(7.0, 2.0, D)`
		`        1   2 6`
		`1 2 3 4 5 6 7 8 9`
		`(8.0, 0.9, I)`

j. Echocardiogram.	`1 2 5 1`
	`1 2 3 4 5 6 7 8 9`
	`(3.0, 0.6, A)`
		`1 3   2 1 2`
		`1 2 3 4 5 6 7 8 9`
		`(5.0, 1.9, D)`

(TREATMENT)

6. First-line treatment for [Stage 1-2] hypertension is
lifestyle modification. The medical record should indicate
counseling for at least one of the following interventions prior
to pharmacotherapy:
- weight reduction,
- increased physical activity,
- low sodium diet, or
- alcohol intake reduction.

	Validity	Feasibility

	`          3 5 1`
	`1 2 3 4 5 6 7 8 9`
	`(8.0, 0.4, A)`
		`        1 3 3  2`
		`1 2 3 4 5 6 7 8 9`
		`(7.0, 1.0, I)`

Scales: 1 = low validity or feasibility; 9 = high validity or feasibility.

Chapter 12
QUALITY INDICATORS FOR HYPERTENSION

	Validity	Feasibility

6. First-line treatment for [Stage 3] hypertension is lifestyle modification. The medical record should indicate counseling for at least one of the following interventions:
- weight reduction,
- increased physical activity,
- low sodium diet, or
- alcohol intake reduction.

Validity:
```
              1       4 2 2
1 2 3 4 5 6 7 8 9
(7.0, 1.0, A)
```
Feasibility:
```
            1     1 2 2 1 1
1 2 3 4 5 6 7 8 9
(6.0, 1.2, I)
```

7. [Stage 1-2] hypertensives whose blood pressure remains [stage 1-2] after 6 months lifestyle modification should receive pharmacotherapy.

Validity:
```
              5 3 1
1 2 3 4 5 6 7 8 9
(7.0, 0.6, A)
```
Feasibility:
```
            1 4 3 1
1 2 3 4 5 6 7 8 9
(7.0, 0.7, A)
```

7. [Stage 3 hypertensives should receive pharmacotherapy.

Validity:
```
            2 5 2
1 2 3 4 5 6 7 8 9
(8.0, 0.4, A)
```
Feasibility:
```
            2 5 2
1 2 3 4 5 6 7 8 9
(8.0, 0.4, A)
```

8. First-line pharmacotherapy for diabetics should include an ACE inhibitor or a calcium channel blocker.

Validity:
```
            5 4
1 2 3 4 5 6 7 8 9
(7.0, 0.4, A)
```
Feasibility:
```
              4 5
1 2 3 4 5 6 7 8 9
(8.0, 0.4, A)
```

(FOLLOW-UP)

9. Hypertensive patients should visit the provider at least once a year.

Validity:
```
          1 3 3 1
1 2 3 4 5 6 7 8 9
(7.0, 1.2, A)
```
Feasibility:
```
          1 1 1 3 2 1
1 2 3 4 5 6 7 8 9
(7.0, 1.1, I)
```

10. Hypertensive patients with persistent elevations of SBP > 160 or DBP > 90 should have one of the following interventions recorded in the medical record:
- change in dose or regimen of antihypertensives,
- repeated education regarding lifestyle modifications.

Validity:
```
              3 6
1 2 3 4 5 6 7 8 9
(8.0, 0.3, A)
```
Feasibility:
```
              4 5
1 2 3 4 5 6 7 8 9
(8.0, 0.4, A)
```

Scales: 1 = low validity or feasibility; 9 = high validity or feasibility.

Chapter 13
QUALITY INDICATORS FOR ACUTE LOW BACK PAIN (NON PREGNANT)

	Validity	Feasibility

(ASSESSMENT)

1. Patients presenting with acute low back pain should receive a focused medical history and physical examination. The history should include questions about at least one of the following "red flags":
- spine fracture red flags: trauma, prolonged use of steroids,
- cancer red flags: history of cancer, unexplained weight loss, immunosuppression,
- infection red flags: fever, IV drug use,
- cauda equina syndrome or rapidly progressing neurologic deficit red flags: acute onset of urinary retention or overflow incontinence, loss of anal sphincter tone or fecal incontinence, saddle anesthesia, and global progressive motor weakness in the lower limbs.

	Validity	Feasibility
	2 7	4 2 2 1
	1 2 3 4 5 6 7 8 9	1 2 3 4 5 6 7 8 9
	(8.0, 0.2, A)	(7.0, 0.9, I)

2. The examination should include neurologic screening and straight leg raising.

	Validity	Feasibility
	1 2 5 1	1 2 3
	1 2 3 4 5 6 7 8 9	1 2 3 4 5 6 7 8 9
	(8.0, 0.7, A)	(8.0, 0.8, A)

(TREATMENT)

5. Patients should not be taking any of the following medications for treatment of acute low back pain:

a. Phenylbutazone.

	Validity	Feasibility
	1 1 3 3 1	1 2 2 4
	1 2 3 4 5 6 7 8 9	1 2 3 4 5 6 7 8 9
	(7.0, 0.9, A)	(7.0, 0.9, I)

b. Dexamethasone.

	Validity	Feasibility
	1 1 1 4 2	1 1 2 5
	1 2 3 4 5 6 7 8 9	1 2 3 4 5 6 7 8 9
	(8.0, 1.2, A)	(8.0, 0.8, A)

c. Other oral steroids.

	Validity	Feasibility
	1 2 4 2	4 5
	1 2 3 4 5 6 7 8 9	1 2 3 4 5 6 7 8 9
	(8.0, 0.8, A)	(8.0, 0.4, A)

d. Colchicine.

	Validity	Feasibility
	1 2 6	1 2 6
	1 2 3 4 5 6 7 8 9	1 2 3 4 5 6 7 8 9
	(8.0, 0.8, A)	(8.0, 0.8, A)

e. Anti-depressants.

	Validity	Feasibility
	1 1 2 2 3	1 1 2 5
	1 2 3 4 5 6 7 8 9	1 2 3 4 5 6 7 8 9
	(7.0, 1.1, I)	(8.0, 0.8, A)

6. Patients should not be prescribed the following physical treatments for acute low back pain:

a. Transcutaneous electrical nerve stimulation.

	Validity	Feasibility
	2 2 4 1	2 2 4 1
	1 2 3 4 5 6 7 8 9	1 2 3 4 5 6 7 8 9
	(8.0, 0.8, A)	(8.0, 1.2, I)

b. Lumbar corsets & support belts.

	Validity	Feasibility
	1 3 2 3	2 3 1 3
	1 2 3 4 5 6 7 8 9	1 2 3 4 5 6 7 8 9
	(7.0, 0.9, I)	(6.0, 1.0, I)

Scales: 1 = low validity or feasibility; 9 = high validity or feasibility.

Chapter 13
QUALITY INDICATORS FOR ACUTE LOW BACK PAIN (NON PREGNANT)

	Validity	Feasibility
c. Spinal traction.	2 4 2 1 1 2 3 4 5 6 7 8 9 (7.0, 0.7, A)	1 1 4 3 1 2 3 4 5 6 7 8 9 (7.0, 0.7, A)
d. Biofeedback.	2 3 4 1 2 3 4 5 6 7 8 9 (6.0, 0.7, I)	3 1 4 1 1 2 3 4 5 6 7 8 9 (7.0, 0.9, I)
7. Prolonged bed rest (> 4 days) should not be recommended.	2 1 5 1 1 2 3 4 5 6 7 8 9 (8.0, 0.7, A)	2 3 3 1 1 2 3 4 5 6 7 8 9 (6.0, 0.9, I)

Scales: 1 = low validity or feasibility; 9 = high validity or feasibility.

Chapter 14
QUALITY INDICATORS FOR PRENATAL CARE

(SCREENING)

	Validity	Feasibility
ROUTINE PRENATAL CARE		
1. The first prenatal visit should occur in the first trimester.	6 3 1 2 3 4 5 6 7 8 9 (7.0, 0.3, A)	1 3 2 3 1 2 3 4 5 6 7 8 9 (7.0, 0.9, I)
2. The physician should make an accurate determination of gestational age using any of the following: a. an ultrasound in the 1st or 2nd trimester, reliable LMP and size within 2 wks indicated by dates in the 1st trimester, no 1st trimester exam, but reliable LMP & 2 of the following: size within 2 weeks of dates in 2d trimester, quickening by 20 weeks, or fetal heart tones by fetoscope before 20 weeks; or if unreliable LMP, then an ultrasound is required.	1 3 4 1 1 2 3 4 5 6 7 8 9 (8.0, 0.7, A)	1 1 2 4 1 1 2 3 4 5 6 7 8 9 (8.0, 0.9, A)
b. if unknown LMP, then an ultrasound is required.	1 8 1 2 3 4 5 6 7 8 9 (8.0, 0.1, A)	1 8 1 2 3 4 5 6 7 8 9 (8.0, 0.1, A)
3. Women should be screened for anemia at the first prenatal visit.	1 2 5 1 1 2 3 4 5 6 7 8 9 (7.0, 0.8, I)	1 3 5 1 2 3 4 5 6 7 8 9 (8.0, 0.7, A)
4. Women should be rescreened for anemia after 24 weeks.	2 1 6 1 2 3 4 5 6 7 8 9 (7.0, 1.0, I)	1 4 4 1 2 3 4 5 6 7 8 9 (7.0, 0.8, A)
SUBSTANCE ABUSE		
5. A smoking history should be obtained at the first prenatal visit.	2 3 4 1 2 3 4 5 6 7 8 9 (8.0, 0.7, A)	2 6 1 1 2 3 4 5 6 7 8 9 (8.0, 0.3, A)
6. An alcohol history should be obtained at the first prenatal visit.	3 4 2 1 2 3 4 5 6 7 8 9 (8.0, 0.6, A)	4 5 1 2 3 4 5 6 7 8 9 (8.0, 0.4, A)
7. A drug history should be obtained during the first prenatal visit.	1 2 4 2 1 2 3 4 5 6 7 8 9 (8.0, 0.7, A)	1 4 4 1 2 3 4 5 6 7 8 9 (7.0, 0.6, A)
INFECTIONS AND SEXUALLY TRANSMITTED DISEASES		
Asymptomatic Bacteriuria		
7. A history should be taken at the first prenatal visit to elicit risk factors for STDs and Hepatitis B.	1 1 7 1 2 3 4 5 6 7 8 9 (8.0, 0.3, A)	3 3 3 1 2 3 4 5 6 7 8 9 (7.0, 0.7, I)
8. Women should receive a urine screen at the first prenatal visit.	2 4 1 2 1 2 3 4 5 6 7 8 9 (7.0, 0.8, A)	1 1 6 1 1 2 3 4 5 6 7 8 9 (8.0, 0.4, A)
Rubella		
9. Women should receive a serologic test for rubella immunity before delivery.	1 5 3 1 2 3 4 5 6 7 8 9 (7.0, 0.4, A)	1 2 6 1 2 3 4 5 6 7 8 9 (8.0, 0.4, A)

Scales: 1 = low validity or feasibility; 9 = high validity or feasibility.

Chapter 14
QUALITY INDICATORS FOR PRENATAL CARE

	Validity	Feasibility

Hepatitis B Carriers

10. High risk women should be screened for HBSAg before delivery.

	Validity	Feasibility
votes	7 1 1	5 2 2
scale	1 2 3 4 5 6 7 8 9	1 2 3 4 5 6 7 8 9
	(7.0, 0.3, A)	(7.0, 0.7, A)

Syphilis

11. A non-treponemal screening test (e.g., VDRL) should be performed on high risk women at the first prenatal visit.

	Validity	Feasibility
votes	2 3 4	3 6
scale	1 2 3 4 5 6 7 8 9	1 2 3 4 5 6 7 8 9
	(7.0, 0.7, A)	(8.0, 0.3, A)

Gonorrhea

12. A cervical gonorrhea culture should be performed on high risk women at the first prenatal visit.

	Validity	Feasibility
votes	2 1 5	2 4 3
scale	1 2 3 4 5 6 7 8 9	1 2 3 4 5 6 7 8 9
	(7.0, 1.1, I)	(7.0, 0.6, A)

Chlamydia

13. Women at high risk (adolescents, unmarried, those with multiple sex partners, low SES, other STD diagnosed) should receive a cervical chlamydia culture or antigen detection at the first prenatal visit.

	Validity	Feasibility
votes	2 3 4	1 4 4
scale	1 2 3 4 5 6 7 8 9	1 2 3 4 5 6 7 8 9
	(7.0, 0.7, A)	(7.0, 0.6, A)

Human Immunodeficiency Virus

14. Pregnant women should be counseled about their individual risk for HIV infection at the first prenatal visit.

	Validity	Feasibility
votes	1 2 4 2	1 4 2 2
scale	1 2 3 4 5 6 7 8 9	1 2 3 4 5 6 7 8 9
	(8.0, 0.7, A)	(7.0, 0.8, A)

15. Pregnant women should be offered HIV testing at the first prenatal visit.

	Validity	Feasibility
votes	3 4 2	2 5 2
scale	1 2 3 4 5 6 7 8 9	1 2 3 4 5 6 7 8 9
	(8.0, 0.6, A)	(8.0, 0.4, A)

INHERITED DISORDERS

Down Syndrome

16. Women age 35 and over, or who have had a previous Down syndrome infant, should receive amniocentesis or chorionic villus sampling (CVS), or should explicitly decline such a test after genetic counseling.

	Validity	Feasibility
votes	2 5 2	1 6 2
scale	1 2 3 4 5 6 7 8 9	1 2 3 4 5 6 7 8 9
	(8.0, 0.4, A)	(8.0, 0.3, A)

Neural Tube Defects (NTDs)

17. Women should be offered AFP testing; this should be performed between 15 and 20 weeks.

	Validity	Feasibility
votes	1 2 6	1 1 7
scale	1 2 3 4 5 6 7 8 9	1 2 3 4 5 6 7 8 9
	(8.0, 0.4, A)	(8.0, 0.3, A)

18. Women who have had a previous NTD infant should receive amniocentesis or should explicitly decline such a test after counseling.

	Validity	Feasibility
votes	2 1 4 2	1 6 2
scale	1 2 3 4 5 6 7 8 9	1 2 3 4 5 6 7 8 9
	(8.0, 0.8, A)	(8.0, 0.4, A)

18. Women with a prior NTD infant should have folic acid supplementation recommended in the preconceptual period.

	Validity	Feasibility
votes	1 2 4 2	1 1 1 2 3 1
scale	1 2 3 4 5 6 7 8 9	1 2 3 4 5 6 7 8 9
	(8.0, 0.8, A)	(7.0, 1.3, I)

Scales: 1 = low validity or feasibility; 9 = high validity or feasibility.

Chapter 14
QUALITY INDICATORS FOR PRENATAL CARE

	Validity	Feasibility

Sickle Cell Disease

19. Women who are African American or have a family history of sickle cell disease should be offered screening at the first prenatal visit, if status unknown.

Validity:
```
              1 2 5 1
1 2 3 4 5 6 7 8 9
(8.0, 0.6, A)
```
Feasibility:
```
              1 4 4
1 2 3 4 5 6 7 8 9
(7.0, 0.6, A)
```

20. For women with the sickle cell trait, the baby's father should be offered screening.

Validity:
```
            2 1 5 1
1 2 3 4 5 6 7 8 9
(8.0, 0.7, A)
```
Feasibility:
```
            1 2 2 4
1 2 3 4 5 6 7 8 9
(7.0, 1.0, I)
```

Rh Isoimmunization

21. Women should receive an Rh factor and antibody screen at the first prenatal visit.

Validity:
```
              2 5 2
1 2 3 4 5 6 7 8 9
(8.0, 0.4, A)
```
Feasibility:
```
              3 5 1
1 2 3 4 5 6 7 8 9
(8.0, 0.4, A)
```

COMMON PREGNANCY COMPLICATIONS

Intrauterine Growth Retardation

22. Measurements of the symphysis-fundal height should be made at each visit from 20-32 weeks.

Validity:
```
        1 2 3 2
1 2 3 4 5 6 7 8 9
(7.0, 1.3, I)
```
Feasibility:
```
          1     5 3
1 2 3 4 5 6 7 8 9
(7.0, 0.7, A)
```

Post-term Pregnancy

23. Fetal assessment should begin at 41.5 weeks and continue until labor (spontaneous or induced) begins.

Validity:
```
          1 4 3 1
1 2 3 4 5 6 7 8 9
(7.0, 0.7, A)
```
Feasibility:
```
              1 3 5
1 2 3 4 5 6 7 8 9
(8.0, 0.6, A)
```

Pregnancy-Induced Hypertension (PIH)

24. Blood pressure measurements should be taken at each visit.

Validity:
```
            1 4 4
1 2 3 4 5 6 7 8 9
(8.0, 0.6, A)
```
Feasibility:
```
                5 4
1 2 3 4 5 6 7 8 9
(8.0, 0.4, A)
```

Gestational Diabetes Mellitus

25. A one-hour, 50g glucose challenge test should be performed on women with risk factors at 24-28 weeks.

Validity:
```
          2 1 6
1 2 3 4 5 6 7 8 9
(8.0, 0.6, A)
```
Feasibility:
```
            1 1 7
1 2 3 4 5 6 7 8 9
(8.0, 0.3, A)
```

(DIAGNOSIS)

INFECTIONS AND SEXUALLY TRANSMITTED DISEASES

Hepatitis B Carriers

26. For women carrying HBsAg, carrier status should be documented in delivery record.

Validity:
```
              7 2
1 2 3 4 5 6 7 8 9
(8.0, 0.2, A)
```
Feasibility:
```
            1 6 2
1 2 3 4 5 6 7 8 9
(8.0, 0.4, A)
```

Syphilis

27. Women whose non-treponemal tests are weakly reactive or reactive should receive a treponemal test to confirm presence of syphilis.

Validity:
```
              2 5 2
1 2 3 4 5 6 7 8 9
(8.0, 0.4, A)
```
Feasibility:
```
              2 5 2
1 2 3 4 5 6 7 8 9
(8.0, 0.4, A)
```

Scales: 1 = low validity or feasibility; 9 = high validity or feasibility.

Chapter 14
QUALITY INDICATORS FOR PRENATAL CARE

	Validity	Feasibility

INHERITED DISORDERS

Neural Tube Defects (NTDs)

28. Women with an abnormal serum AFP should receive an ultrasound to evaluate gestational age and possible multiple gestation.

Validity:
```
                    1 6 2
1 2 3 4 5 6 7 8 9
   (8.0, 0.3, A)
```
Feasibility:
```
                1 4 4
1 2 3 4 5 6 7 8 9
   (8.0, 0.6, A)
```

Sickle Cell Disease

29. Women with the sickle cell trait should be offered either amniocentesis or chorionic villus sampling, unless the baby's father is known to be negative for the sickle trait.

Validity:
```
              2 3 4
1 2 3 4 5 6 7 8 9
   (7.0, 0.7, A)
```
Feasibility:
```
              2 2 5
1 2 3 4 5 6 7 8 9
   (8.0, 0.7, A)
```

COMMON PREGNANCY COMPLICATIONS

Intrauterine Growth Retardation

30. Women whose symphysis-fundal height is 4cm less than indicated by their gestational age between 20-32 weeks should have an ultrasound.

Validity:
```
          1     3 5
1 2 3 4 5 6 7 8 9
   (8.0, 0.8, A)
```
Feasibility:
```
                2 7
1 2 3 4 5 6 7 8 9
   (8.0, 0.2, A)
```

Pregnancy-induced Hypertension (PIH)

31. For elevated BPs (systolic > 140mm Hg, or diastolic > 90mm Hg, or systolic rise > 30mm Hg, or diastolic rise > 15mm Hg), proteinuria and peripheral edema should be assessed.

Validity:
```
              6 3
1 2 3 4 5 6 7 8 9
   (8.0, 0.3, A)
```
Feasibility:
```
                1 4 4
1 2 3 4 5 6 7 8 9
   (8.0, 0.6, A)
```

32. For patients with elevated BP and either proteinuria (1+ or more) or edema (> trace), PIH diagnosis should be made.

Validity:
```
              3 5 1
1 2 3 4 5 6 7 8 9
   (8.0, 0.4, A)
```
Feasibility:
```
              3 5 1
1 2 3 4 5 6 7 8 9
   (8.0, 0.4, A)
```

Gestational Diabetes Mellitus

33. Pregnant women with abnormal glucose challenge tests (>= 140 mg/dL or 7.8 mmol/L) should have a 3-hour plasma glucose tolerance test performed.

Validity:
```
              4 4 1
1 2 3 4 5 6 7 8 9
   (8.0, 0.6, A)
```
Feasibility:
```
              2 6 1
1 2 3 4 5 6 7 8 9
   (8.0, 0.3, A)
```

(TREATMENT)

SUBSTANCE ABUSE

34. Pregnant women identified as smokers should receive counseling to stop smoking from their physician.

Validity:
```
          1 1 1 3
1 2 3 4 5 6 7 8 9
   (7.0, 0.9, A)
```
Feasibility:
```
                1 6 2
1 2 3 4 5 6 7 8 9
   (7.0, 0.6, A)
```

35. Pregnant women identified as smokers should be referred to a smoking cessation clinic, group, or counselor.

Validity:
```
      1 1 1 3 3
1 2 3 4 5 6 7 8 9
   (5.0, 1.0, A)
```
Feasibility:
```
              1 3 1 2 2
1 2 3 4 5 6 7 8 9
   (6.0, 1.2, I)
```

36. Women who indicate they use any amount of alcohol should be counseled to eliminate alcohol consumption during pregnancy and should be referred for treatment if appropriate.

Validity:
```
            4 1 4
1 2 3 4 5 6 7 8 9
   (8.0, 0.9, A)
```
Feasibility:
```
          1   3 2 2
1 2 3 4 5 6 7 8 9
   (7.0, 1.1, A)
```

37. Women who indicate they use drugs should be counseled by their physician to cease use during pregnancy and should be referred for treatment if appropriate.

Validity:
```
              2 4 3
1 2 3 4 5 6 7 8 9
   (8.0, 0.6, A)
```
Feasibility:
```
            1 1 1 4 2
1 2 3 4 5 6 7 8 9
   (8.0, 0.9, A)
```

Scales: 1 = low validity or feasibility; 9 = high validity or feasibility.

November 1995

Chapter 14
QUALITY INDICATORS FOR PRENATAL CARE

	Validity	Feasibility

INFECTIONS AND SEXUALLY TRANSMITTED DISEASES

Asymptomatic Bacteriuria

39. Pregnant women with positive cultures (> 100,000 bacteria/cc) should receive an appropriate antibiotic.

Validity:
```
              1 4 4
1 2 3 4 5 6 7 8 9
   (8.0, 0.6, A)
```
Feasibility:
```
                1 3 5
1 2 3 4 5 6 7 8 9
   (9.0, 0.6, A)
```

Rubella

40. Pregnant women not immune to rubella should receive postpartum immunization within 6 weeks.

Validity:
```
            2 4 3
1 2 3 4 5 6 7 8 9
   (8.0, 0.6, A)
```
Feasibility:
```
            2 3 4
1 2 3 4 5 6 7 8 9
   (8.0, 0.7, A)
```

Syphilis

41. Pregnant women with confirmed positive serology should be treated with penicillin, if not allergic, appropriate for the stage of disease; tetracycline and doxycycline are contraindicated.

Validity:
```
              1 3 5
1 2 3 4 5 6 7 8 9
   (9.0, 0.6, A)
```
Feasibility:
```
              5 4
1 2 3 4 5 6 7 8 9
   (8.0, 0.4, A)
```

Gonorrhea

42. Pregnant women with positive cultures should receive appropriate treatment.

Validity:
```
            6 3
1 2 3 4 5 6 7 8 9
   (8.0, 0.3, A)
```
Feasibility:
```
            7 2
1 2 3 4 5 6 7 8 9
   (8.0, 0.2, A)
```

Human Immunodeficiency Virus

43. Pregnant women known to be HIV positive with CD4+ counts of 200 or greater should be offered treatment with zidovudine during pregnancy and intrapartum.

Validity:
```
              6 3
1 2 3 4 5 6 7 8 9
   (8.0, 0.3, A)
```
Feasibility:
```
              6 3
1 2 3 4 5 6 7 8 9
   (8.0, 0.3, A)
```

INHERITED DISORDERS

Down Syndrome

44. Pregnant women whose amniocentesis shows infant with abnormal karyotype should receive additional counseling.

Validity:
```
            5 4
1 2 3 4 5 6 7 8 9
   (8.0, 0.4, A)
```
Feasibility:
```
            2 4 3
1 2 3 4 5 6 7 8 9
   (8.0, 0.6, A)
```

Neural Tube Defects (NTDs)

45. Pregnant women with abnormal serum AFP for gestational age and normal ultrasound should be offered an amniocentesis and counseling.

Validity:
```
        3 2 3 1
1 2 3 4 5 6 7 8 9
   (7.0, 0.9, I)
```
Feasibility:
```
            6 3
1 2 3 4 5 6 7 8 9
   (7.0, 0.3, A)
```

46. Pregnant women whose amniotic fluid AFP shows infant with probable NTD should be offered additional counseling.

Validity:
```
          1 6 2
1 2 3 4 5 6 7 8 9
   (8.0, 0.3, A)
```
Feasibility:
```
            2 7
1 2 3 4 5 6 7 8 9
   (8.0, 0.2, A)
```

Sickle Cell Disease

47. Pregnant women whose amniocentesis shows an infant with sickle cell disease should be offered counseling.

Validity:
```
          3 4 2
1 2 3 4 5 6 7 8 9
   (8.0, 0.6, A)
```
Feasibility:
```
          4 4 1
1 2 3 4 5 6 7 8 9
   (8.0, 0.6, A)
```

Rh Isoimmunization

48. Pregnant women who are Rh negative should receive Rhogam between 26 and 30 weeks antenatally and postpartum.

Validity:
```
          2 4 3
1 2 3 4 5 6 7 8 9
   (8.0, 0.6, A)
```
Feasibility:
```
              5 4
1 2 3 4 5 6 7 8 9
   (8.0, 0.4, A)
```

Scales: 1 = low validity or feasibility; 9 = high validity or feasibility.

Chapter 14
QUALITY INDICATORS FOR PRENATAL CARE

	Validity	Feasibility

COMMON PREGNANCY COMPLICATIONS

Post-Term Pregnancy

49. Labor should be induced when monitoring shows non-reassuring fetal status or oligohydramnios.

Validity	Feasibility
5 3 1 1 2 3 4 5 6 7 8 9 (7.0, 0.6, A)	2 6 1 1 2 3 4 5 6 7 8 9 (8.0, 0.3, A)

50. Pregnancies with reliable dates should not extend beyond 44 weeks.

Validity	Feasibility
5 4 1 2 3 4 5 6 7 8 9 (8.0, 0.4, A)	5 4 1 2 3 4 5 6 7 8 9 (8.0, 0.4, A)

Pregnancy-Induced Hypertension (PIH)

51. If PIH diagnosed and patient is not admitted, bedrest should be recommended & a return visit should occur w/in 1 week.

Validity	Feasibility
1 1 6 1 2 3 4 5 6 7 8 9 (8.0, 0.9, A)	1 1 6 1 2 3 4 5 6 7 8 9 (8.0, 0.8, A)

52. If PIH diagnosed and pregnancy is at term (>= 37 weeks), either labor should be induced or delivery by cesarean section should take place.

Validity	Feasibility
2 5 1 2 3 4 5 6 7 8 9 (8.0, 0.7, A)	1 2 6 1 2 3 4 5 6 7 8 9 (8.0, 0.4, A)

53. If severe PIH is diagnosed by any of the following: (systolic > 160 mm Hg, diastolic > 110 mm Hg, 3-4+ proteinuria, pulmonary edema, oliguria, RUQ pain or seizures), patient should be admitted to induce labor or deliver by cesarean section.

Validity	Feasibility
6 3 1 2 3 4 5 6 7 8 9 (8.0, 0.3, A)	4 5 1 2 3 4 5 6 7 8 9 (9.0, 0.4, A)

Gestational Diabetes Mellitus

54. Pregnant women with abnormal 3-hour glucose tolerance tests should receive dietary counseling and have glucose monitoring.

Validity	Feasibility
1 4 3 1 1 2 3 4 5 6 7 8 9 (7.0, 0.7, A)	1 2 2 3 1 1 2 3 4 5 6 7 8 9 (7.0, 1.0, I)

55. Pregnant women on dietary therapy, with 2 or more consecutive abnormal fasting (> 105 mg/dL) or postprandial (> 120 mg/dL one-hour post), plasma glucose tests should be placed on insulin therapy.

Validity	Feasibility
1 2 3 3 1 2 3 4 5 6 7 8 9 (7.0, 0.8, I)	2 5 2 1 2 3 4 5 6 7 8 9 (7.0, 0.4, A)

56. An oral agent should not be used in diabetic pregnant women.

Validity	Feasibility
6 3 1 2 3 4 5 6 7 8 9 (8.0, 0.3, A)	6 3 1 2 3 4 5 6 7 8 9 (8.0, 0.3, A)

(FOLLOW-UP)

INFECTIONS AND SEXUALLY TRANSMITTED DISEASES

Asymptomatic Bacteriuria

57. Women treated for positive cultures should receive a post-treatment follow-up culture within one month of completing treatment.

Validity	Feasibility
1 1 3 3 1 1 2 3 4 5 6 7 8 9 (7.0, 0.9, A)	4 5 1 2 3 4 5 6 7 8 9 (8.0, 0.4, A)

Syphilis

58. Women diagnosed with syphilis in pregnancy should be followed up with monthly serology and retreated if necessary.

Validity	Feasibility
2 7 1 2 3 4 5 6 7 8 9 (8.0, 0.2, A)	2 7 1 2 3 4 5 6 7 8 9 (8.0, 0.2, A)

Scales: 1 = low validity or feasibility; 9 = high validity or feasibility.

Chapter 14
QUALITY INDICATORS FOR PRENATAL CARE

	Validity	Feasibility

Gonorrhea

59. Women with positive cultures should receive a post-treatment follow-up culture 2 weeks after treatment is completed.

Validity:
```
        1   1 3 3 1
1 2 3 4 5 6 7 8 9
   (7.0, 1.0, A)
```
Feasibility:
```
              1 3 4 1
1 2 3 4 5 6 7 8 9
   (8.0, 0.8, A)
```

Chlamydia

60. Women with positive cultures should receive a post-treatment follow-up culture 4-7 days after treatment is completed.

Validity:
```
      1 1 3 3 1
1 2 3 4 5 6 7 8 9
   (7.0, 0.9, A)
```
Feasibility:
```
1           5 3
1 2 3 4 5 6 7 8 9
   (7.0, 0.9, A)
```

COMMON PREGNANCY COMPLICATIONS

Gestational Diabetes Mellitus

61. Women with abnormal 3-hour plasma glucose tolerance tests who are an dietary therapy should have biweekly fasting or postprandial glucose tests.

Validity:
```
        1 3 4 1
1 2 3 4 5 6 7 8 9
   (7.0, 0.7, I)
```
Feasibility:
```
        2 1 2 4
1 2 3 4 5 6 7 8 9
   (7.0, 1.0, I)
```

Scales: 1 = low validity or feasibility;   9 = high validity or feasibility.

Chapter 15
QUALITY INDICATORS FOR CORTIOCOSTEROIDS
FOR FETAL MATURATION IN LABOR

(TREATMENT)

	Validity	Feasibility
1. Women admitted to the hospital with labor, between 24 and 34 weeks gestation, and without ruptured membranes, should receive antenatal steroids, even if delivery is anticipated in less than 24 hours.	2 5 2 1 2 3 4 5 6 7 8 9 (8.0, 0.4, A)	1 5 3 1 2 3 4 5 6 7 8 9 (8.0, 0.4, A)
2. Steroid treatment should consist of either: - betamethasone 12 mg. IM q24h x 2, or - dexamethasone 6 mg. IM q12h x 4.	1 8 1 2 3 4 5 6 7 8 9 (8.0, 0.1, A)	1 7 1 1 2 3 4 5 6 7 8 9 (8.0, 0.2, A)
3. Women admitted to the hospital at 24-32 weeks gestation with ruptured membranes should receive antenatal steroid administration.	1 2 5 1 1 2 3 4 5 6 7 8 9 (7.0, 0.6, I)	4 4 1 1 2 3 4 5 6 7 8 9 (8.0, 0.6, A)

Scales: 1 = low validity or feasibility; 9 = high validity or feasibility.

Chapter 16
QUALITY INDICATORS FOR ROUTINE PREVENTIVE CARE

	Validity	Feasibility

Immunizations

1. Notation of date that a patient received a tetanus/diphtheria booster within the last ten years should be included in the medical record.
   - Validity: 1 1 2 5   1 2 3 4 5 6 7 8 9   (8.0, 0.8, A)
   - Feasibility: 1 2 3 2 1   1 2 3 4 5 6 7 8 9   (6.0, 0.9, I)

2. Women should receive a yearly influenza vaccine if they have:

   a. Asthma.
   - Validity: 6 2 1   1 2 3 4 5 6 7 8 9   (7.0, 0.4, A)
   - Feasibility: 6 3   1 2 3 4 5 6 7 8 9   (7.0, 0.3, A)

   b. Chronic obstructive pulmonary disease.
   - Validity: 1 2 5 1   1 2 3 4 5 6 7 8 9   (8.0, 0.6, A)
   - Feasibility: 4 5   1 2 3 4 5 6 7 8 9   (8.0, 0.4, A)

   c. Chronic cardivascular disorders.
   - Validity: 3 4 1 1   1 2 3 4 5 6 7 8 9   (7.0, 0.7, I)
   - Feasibility: 6 3   1 2 3 4 5 6 7 8 9   (7.0, 0.3, A)

   d. Diabetes mellitus.
   - Validity: 3 3 2 1   1 2 3 4 5 6 7 8 9   (7.0, 0.8, I)
   - Feasibility: 1 5 3   1 2 3 4 5 6 7 8 9   (7.0, 0.4, A)

   e. Renal failure.
   - Validity: 2 2 4 1   1 2 3 4 5 6 7 8 9   (8.0, 0.8, A)
   - Feasibility: 5 4   1 2 3 4 5 6 7 8 9   (7.0, 0.4, A)

   f. Hemoglobinopathies (e.g., sickle cell disease).
   - Validity: 2 2 4 1   1 2 3 4 5 6 7 8 9   (8.0, 0.8, A)
   - Feasibility: 5 4   1 2 3 4 5 6 7 8 9   (7.0, 0.4, A)

   g. Immunosuppression.
   - Validity: 1 2 2 4   1 2 3 4 5 6 7 8 9   (8.0, 0.9, A)
   - Feasibility: 3 3 3   1 2 3 4 5 6 7 8 9   (8.0, 0.7, A)

Sexually Transmitted Diseases and HIV Prevention

3. A sexual history should be documented in the chart.
   - Validity: 1 3 4 1   1 2 3 4 5 6 7 8 9   (8.0, 0.8, A)
   - Feasibility: 1 2 3 2 1   1 2 3 4 5 6 7 8 9   (7.0, 1.1, I)

4. Patients who have ever been sexually active with men should be asked the following questions:

   a. If they currently have a single sexual partner.
   - Validity: 1 1 6   1 2 3 4 5 6 7 8 9   (7.0, 0.9, I)
   - Feasibility: 2 2 3 1   1 2 3 4 5 6 7 8 9   (5.0, 1.7, I)

   b. If they have had more than 2 sexual partners in the past 6 months.
   - Validity: 1 2 4 1   1 2 3 4 5 6 7 8 9   (7.0, 1.4, I)
   - Feasibility: 2 2 3 1   1 2 3 4 5 6 7 8 9   (5.0, 1.9, D)

   c. If they have had a history of any STDs.
   - Validity: 2 1 3 2   1 2 3 4 5 6 7 8 9   (7.0, 1.3, I)
   - Feasibility: 2 2 3 1   1 2 3 4 5 6 7 8 9   (6.0, 1.3, I)

   d. If they or their partner(s) have had more than 1 partner.
   - Validity: 2 1 1 1 2 1   1 2 3 4 5 6 7 8 9   (5.0, 1.9, I)
   - Feasibility: 3 1 2 2 1   1 2 3 4 5 6 7 8 9   (5.0, 2.2, I)

5. Patients should be asked about current or past use of intravenous drugs at least once.
   - Validity: 1 3 4   1 2 3 4 5 6 7 8 9   (7.0, 1.0, A)
   - Feasibility: 2 1 2 4   1 2 3 4 5 6 7 8 9   (6.0, 1.7, I)

Scales: 1 = low validity or feasibility; 9 = high validity or feasibility.

Chapter 16
QUALITY INDICATORS FOR ROUTINE PREVENTIVE CARE

	Validity	Feasibility
6. Patients who are sexually active with men and not in a monogamous relationship, have had more than 2 male sexual partners in the past six months, have a history of STDs, or have used intravenous drugs, should be counseled regarding the prevention and transmission of HIV and other STDs.	1 2 3 4 5 6 7 8 9 (8.0, 0.8, A)	1 2 3 4 5 6 7 8 9 (7.0, 0.3, I)

Obesity Counseling

	Validity	Feasibility
7. The medical record should include measurements of height and weight at least once.	1 2 3 4 5 6 7 8 9 (7.0, 1.3, I)	1 2 3 4 5 6 7 8 9 (7.0, 0.8, A)

Seat Belt Use Counseling

	Validity	Feasibility
8. Patients should receive counseling regarding the use of seat belts on at least one occasion.	1 2 3 4 5 6 7 8 9 (7.0, 0.8, A)	1 2 3 4 5 6 7 8 9 (5.0, 1.4, I)

Breast Examination

	Validity	Feasibility
9. A clinical breast exam should be performed on women aged 40 to 50 at least once every three years during a routine visit.	1 2 3 4 5 6 7 8 9 (8.0, 1.3, I)	1 2 3 4 5 6 7 8 9 (8.0, 0.4, A)

Hyperlipidemia Screening

	Validity	Feasibility
10. As a screen for familial hypercholesterolemia, the medical record should indicate that adult women have undergone a cholesterol measurement at sometime in their lives.	1 2 3 4 5 6 7 8 9 (8.0, 0.8, A)	1 2 3 4 5 6 7 8 9 (8.0, 0.9, A)
11. In women with known cardiac risk factors including hypertension, smoking, diabetes, family history of myocardial infarction or familial hypercholesterolemia in a first degree relative, the medical record should indicate a serum cholesterol and triglycerides level in the last 5 years.	1 2 3 4 5 6 7 8 9 (8.0, 0.4, A)	1 2 3 4 5 6 7 8 9 (8.0, 0.4, A)

Cervical Cancer Screening

	Validity	Feasibility
12. The medical record should contain the date and result of the last Pap smear.	1 2 3 4 5 6 7 8 9 (8.0, 0.3, A)	1 2 3 4 5 6 7 8 9 (8.0, 0.8, A)
13. Women who have not had a Pap smear within the last 3 years should have one performed (unless never sexually active or have had a hysterectomy).	1 2 3 4 5 6 7 8 9 (8.0, 0.3, A)	1 2 3 4 5 6 7 8 9 (8.0, 0.3, A)
14. Women who have not had 3 consecutive normal smears and who have not had a Pap smear within the last year should have one performed.	1 2 3 4 5 6 7 8 9 (7.0, 1.0, A)	1 2 3 4 5 6 7 8 9 (8.0, 1.2, I)
15. Women with a history of cervical dysplasia or carcinoma-in-situ who have not had a Pap smear within the last year should have one performed.	1 2 3 4 5 6 7 8 9 (8.0, 0.3, A)	1 2 3 4 5 6 7 8 9 (8.0, 0.4, A)
16. Women with severely abnormal Pap smear should have colposcopy performed.	1 2 3 4 5 6 7 8 9 (9.0, 0.4, A)	1 2 3 4 5 6 7 8 9 (8.0, 0.6, A)

Scales: 1 = low validity or feasibility; 9 = high validity or feasibility.

November 1995

Chapter 16
QUALITY INDICATORS FOR ROUTINE PREVENTIVE CARE

	Validity	Feasibility

17. If a woman has a Pap smear that is not normal but is not severely abnormal, then one of the following should occur within 6 months of the initial Pap: 1) repeat Pap smear; or 2) colposcopy.

```
                    6 1 1              2 3 3 1
1 2 3 4 5 6 7 8 9    1 2 3 4 5 6 7 8 9
    (7.0, 0.7, A)        (7.0, 1.0, A)
```

18. Women with a Pap smear that is not normal but is not severely abnormal, and who have had the abnormality documented on at least 2 Pap smears in a 2-year period, should have colposcopy performed.

```
            1  5 1 2            2  2 3 2
1 2 3 4 5 6 7 8 9    1 2 3 4 5 6 7 8 9
    (7.0, 0.8, A)        (8.0, 1.1, A)
```

19. Patients who are seen for acute care, but have not been seen for routine care within the last 3 years should be referred for or have received a routine care visit within 3 months.

```
        3 4 1 1        1  1 2 2 3
1 2 3 4 5 6 7 8 9    1 2 3 4 5 6 7 8 9
    (8.0, 1.2, A)        (6.0, 1.3, I)
```

Scales: 1 = low validity or feasibility; 9 = high validity or feasibility.

Chapter 17
QUALITY INDICATORS FOR UPPER RESPIRATORY INFECTIONS

	Validity	Feasibility

(DIAGNOSIS)

Pharyngitis

1. If a patient presents with a complaint of sore throat, the medical history should document presence or absence of previous episodes of rheumatic fever.

```
            1   4 2 2                    1 1 2 3 1 1
1 2 3 4 5 6 7 8 9            1 2 3 4 5 6 7 8 9
   (4.0, 0.9, A)               (4.0, 1.1, I)
```

2. History/physical exam should document presence or absence of:

a. Fever.

```
        1     1 5 2                    1       3 1 4
1 2 3 4 5 6 7 8 9            1 2 3 4 5 6 7 8 9
   (7.0, 0.8, A)               (7.0, 1.2, I)
```

b. Tonsillar exudate.

```
        1     1 4 3                  1 1     1 2 4
1 2 3 4 5 6 7 8 9            1 2 3 4 5 6 7 8 9
   (7.0, 0.9, A)               (7.0, 1.3, I)
```

c. Anterior cervical adenopathy.

```
      1 1     5 2                  1 1 1     3 3
1 2 3 4 5 6 7 8 9            1 2 3 4 5 6 7 8 9
   (7.0, 1.0, A)               (7.0, 1.4, I)
```

Bronchitis/Cough

3. The history of patients presenting with cough of less than 3 weeks duration should document presence or absence of preceding viral infection (e.g., common cold, influenza).

```
            3 2 4                    2 1 3 1 2
1 2 3 4 5 6 7 8 9            1 2 3 4 5 6 7 8 9
   (6.0, 0.8, I)               (5.0, 1.1, I)
```

4. The history of patients presenting with cough of less than 3 weeks duration should document presence or absence of fever and shortness of breath (dyspnea).

```
            2 5 2                    1 4 3 1
1 2 3 4 5 6 7 8 9            1 2 3 4 5 6 7 8 9
   (7.0, 0.4, A)               (6.0, 0.7, I)
```

5. Patients presenting with acute cough should receive a physical examination of the chest for evidence of pneumonia.

```
              2 6 1                  1 1 2 4 1
1 2 3 4 5 6 7 8 9            1 2 3 4 5 6 7 8 9
   (8.0, 0.3, A)               (8.0, 0.9, A)
```

6. Patients presenting with acute cough and with evidence of consolidation on physical exam of the chest (dullness to percussion, egophony, etc.) should receive a chest x-ray to look for evidence of pneumonia.

```
        3 3 1 2                    1 1 3   2 2
1 2 3 4 5 6 7 8 9            1 2 3 4 5 6 7 8 9
   (4.0, 0.9, I)               (5.0, 1.4, I)
```

Scales: 1 = low validity or feasibility;   9 = high validity or feasibility.

Chapter 17
QUALITY INDICATORS FOR UPPER RESPIRATORY INFECTIONS

	Validity	Feasibility

Nasal Congestion

7. If a patient presents with the complaint of nasal congestion and/or rhinorrhea not attributed to the common cold, the history should include:

a. Seasonality of symptoms.

Validity:
```
        2 4 1 2
1 2 3 4 5 6 7 8 9
     (5.0, 0.8, A)
```
Feasibility:
```
      2 3 2 1
1 2 3 4 5 6 7 8 9
     (4.0, 1.1, I)
```

b. Presence or absence of sneezing.

Validity:
```
      2 5 1 1
1 2 3 4 5 6 7 8 9
     (5.0, 0.6, A)
```
Feasibility:
```
    1 1 3 1 3
1 2 3 4 5 6 7 8 9
     (3.0, 1.1, I)
```

c. Facial pain.

Validity:
```
      2 2 2 3
1 2 3 4 5 6 7 8 9
     (6.0, 1.0, I)
```
Feasibility:
```
      2 3 2 1
1 2 3 4 5 6 7 8 9
     (4.0, 1.1, I)
```

d. Fever.

Validity:
```
    2       4 3
1 2 3 4 5 6 7 8 9
     (7.0, 1.0, A)
```
Feasibility:
```
  1 1 1 1 2 3
1 2 3 4 5 6 7 8 9
     (7.0, 1.4, I)
```

e. Specific irritants.

Validity:
```
    1 2 2 4
1 2 3 4 5 6 7 8 9
     (5.0, 0.9, A)
```
Feasibility:
```
  1 1 2 2 2 1
1 2 3 4 5 6 7 8 9
     (4.0, 1.3, I)
```

f. Use of topical nasal decongestants.

Validity:
```
    1 3 3 1 1
1 2 3 4 5 6 7 8 9
     (6.0, 0.9, A)
```
Feasibility:
```
      1 2 3 2
1 2 3 4 5 6 7 8 9
     (5.0, 1.3, I)
```

Acute Sinusitis

8. If the diagnosis of acute sinusitis is made, symptoms should be present for a duration of less than 3 weeks (e.g., fever, malaise, cough, nasal congestion, purulent nasal discharge, ear pain or blockage, post-nasal drip, dental pain, headache, or facial pain).

Validity:
```
        2 1 5 1
1 2 3 4 5 6 7 8 9
     (7.0, 0.7, I)
```
Feasibility:
```
        3 2 3 1
1 2 3 4 5 6 7 8 9
     (6.0, 0.9, I)
```

(TREATMENT)

Pharyngitis

9. Patients with sore throat and fever, tonsillar exudate and anterior cervical adenopathy should receive immediate treatment for presumed streptococcal infection.

Validity:
```
1 1   2 3 2
1 2 3 4 5 6 7 8 9
     (7.0, 1.6, I)
```
Feasibility:
```
      1 2 1 3 2
1 2 3 4 5 6 7 8 9
     (7.0, 1.1, I)
```

10. Treatment of streptococcal throat infection should be with penicillin V, amoxicillin or erythromycin for 10 days; or with a single injection of benzathine penicillin.

Validity:
```
      1 1 7
1 2 3 4 5 6 7 8 9
     (8.0, 0.4, A)
```
Feasibility:
```
    1 2 5 1
1 2 3 4 5 6 7 8 9
     (8.0, 0.7, A)
```

11. If an antibiotic is NOT prescribed with the diagnosis of sore throat, a throat culture or rapid antigen test should be obtained if any of the following are present:
- fever,
- tonsillar exudate, or
- anterior cervical adenopathy.

Validity:
```
      7 1
1 2 3 4 5 6 7 8 9
     (7.0, 0.8, A)
```
Feasibility:
```
      6 2
1 2 3 4 5 6 7 8 9
     (7.0, 0.8, A)
```

Scales: 1 = low validity or feasibility; 9 = high validity or feasibility.

Chapter 17
QUALITY INDICATORS FOR UPPER RESPIRATORY INFECTIONS

	Validity	Feasibility

Bronchitis/Cough

14. If the history documents cigarette smoking in a patient with acute cough, encouragement to stop smoking should be documented.

Validity:
```
    2         5 1 1
1 2 3 4 5 6 7 8 9
(7.0, 1.2, A)
```
Feasibility:
```
1 1 1       4 1
1 2 3 4 5 6 7 8 9
(7.0, 1.9, I)
```

Influenza

15. Women with asthma, chronic obstructive pulmonary disease, chronic cardiovascular disorders, diabetes mellitus, renal failure, hemoglobinopathies (e.g., sickle cell disease) or immunosuppresssion, who present with symptoms of influenza within the first 48 hours should be considered for treatment with amantadine or rimantadine.

Validity:
```
        3 3 3
1 2 3 4 5 6 7 8 9
(7.0, 0.7, I)
```
Feasibility:
```
        1 3 2 3
1 2 3 4 5 6 7 8 9
(7.0, 1.4, I)
```

Nasal Congestion

16. If topical nasal decongestants are prescribed, duration of treatment should be for no longer than 4 days.

Validity:
```
    1 3 4 1
1 2 3 4 5 6 7 8 9
(7.0, 0.7,.I)
```
Feasibility:
```
    1 3 2 3
1 2 3 4 5 6 7 8 9
(6.0, 1.4, I)
```

16. Patients with nasal congestion and/or cough without a concurrent diagnosis of sinusitis, bronchitis or pneumonia should not be prescribed antibiotics.

Validity:
```
        1 2 6
1 2 3 4 5 6 7 8 9
(8.0, 0.4, A)
```
Feasibility:
```
        1 1 4 3
1 2 3 4 5 6 7 8 9
(7.0, 0.7, A)
```

Acute Sinusitis

17. Treatment for acute sinusitis should be with antibiotics for at least 10 days.

Validity:
```
    1   5 3
1 2 3 4 5 6 7 8 9
(7.0, 0.6, A)
```
Feasibility:
```
            7 2
1 2 3 4 5 6 7 8 9
(7.0, 0.2, A)
```

18. Treament for acute sinusitis should include a systemic or topical nasal decongestant.

Validity:
```
1 1 1 2 3 1
1 2 3 4 5 6 7 8 9
(5.0, 1.2, I)
```
Feasibility:
```
        4 3 2
1 2 3 4 5 6 7 8 9
(6.0, 0.7, A)
```

19. If topical nasal decongestants are prescribed, duration of treatment should be for no longer than 4 days.

Validity:
```
    2 6   1
1 2 3 4 5 6 7 8 9
(6.0, 0.4, A)
```
Feasibility:
```
1   2 2 3 1
1 2 3 4 5 6 7 8 9
(5.0, 1.1, A)
```

21. In the absence of symptoms of allergic rhinitis (thin, watery rhinorrhea, and sneezing), antihistamines should not be prescribed for acute sinusitis.

Validity:
```
1 1 1 5 1
1 2 3 4 5 6 7 8 9
(6.0, 0.8, A)
```
Feasibility:
```
        3 5 1
1 2 3 4 5 6 7 8 9
(6.0, 0.4, A)
```

22. If symptoms fail to improve after first course of antibiotic treatment, therapy with another antibiotic for at least 10 days should be instituted.

Validity:
```
    1   3 4 1
1 2 3 4 5 6 7 8 9
(7.0, 0.8, I)
```
Feasibility:
```
            8 1
1 2 3 4 5 6 7 8 9
(7.0, 0.1, A)
```

23. If the patient does not improve after two courses of antibiotics, referral to an otolaryngologist or for a diagnostic test (CT, x-ray, ultrasound of the sinuses) is indicated.

Validity:
```
        1 7 1
1 2 3 4 5 6 7 8 9
(7.0, 0.2, A)
```
Feasibility:
```
    1 5 3
1 2 3 4 5 6 7 8 9
(6.0, 0.4, I)
```

Chronic Sinusitis

24. If a diagnosis of chronic sinusitis is made, the patient should be treated with at least 3 weeks of antibiotics.

Validity:
```
        5 4
1 2 3 4 5 6 7 8 9
(7.0, 0.4, A)
```
Feasibility:
```
    1 7 1
1 2 3 4 5 6 7 8 9
(7.0, 0.3, A)
```

25. If patient has repeated symptoms after 2 separate 3-week trials of antibiotics, a referral to an otolaryngologist or for a diagnostic test is indicated.

Validity:
```
1 1 1 4 2
1 2 3 4 5 6 7 8 9
(7.0, 0.9, I)
```
Feasibility:
```
    4 3 2
1 2 3 4 5 6 7 8 9
(7.0, 0.7, I)
```

Scales: 1 = low validity or feasibility;   9 = high validity or feasibility.

November 1995

Chapter 17
QUALITY INDICATORS FOR UPPER RESPIRATORY INFECTIONS

	Validity	Feasibility

26. If topical nasal decongestants are prescribed, duration of treatment should be for no longer than 4 days.

```
                    1     3 4 1              2 5 2
              1 2 3 4 5 6 7 8 9      1 2 3 4 5 6 7 8 9
                (7.0, 0.8, I)        (6.0, 0.4, A)
```

27. In the absence of symptoms of allergic rhinitis (thin, watery rhinorrhea, and sneezing), antihistamines should not be prescribed.

```
              1 2 1 2 2 1            2 2 1 1 3
              1 2 3 4 5 6 7 8 9      1 2 3 4 5 6 7 8 9
                (6.0, 1.3, I)        (5.0, 1.4, I)
```

Scales: 1 = low validity or feasibility; 9 = high validity or feasibility.

Chapter 18
QUALITY INDICATORS FOR URINARY TRACT INFECTION

(DIAGNOSIS)

Indicator	Validity	Feasibility
1. In women presenting with dysuria, presence or absence of fever and flank pain should be elicited.	1 2 3 4 5 6 7 8 9 (8.0, 0.6, A)	1 2 3 4 5 6 7 8 9 (8.0, 0.7, A)
2. In women presenting with dysuria, a history of vaginal discharge should be elicited.	1 2 3 4 5 6 7 8 9 (8.0, 1.4, I)	1 2 3 4 5 6 7 8 9 (3.0, 2.0, D)
3. If a woman presents with dysuria and a complaint of vaginal discharge, a speculum exam and microscopic examination of discharge (if any) should be performed (e.g., KOH and saline wet mount).	1 2 3 4 5 6 7 8 9 (7.0, 0.6, A)	1 2 3 4 5 6 7 8 9 (7.0, 0.6, A)
4. Women presenting with dysuria should be asked about the possibility of concurrent pregnancy (e.g., date of LMP) or be given a pregnancy test.	1 2 3 4 5 6 7 8 9 (7.0, 0.3, A)	1 2 3 4 5 6 7 8 9 (7.0, 1.0, I)
5. A urinalysis or dipstick should be performed on women in whom urinary tract infection is suspected.	1 2 3 4 5 6 7 8 9 (7.0, 0.8, I)	1 2 3 4 5 6 7 8 9 (7.0, 0.9, A)
6. A urine culture should be obtained for women who have dysuria and any one of the following:		
a. "Several" (three or more) infections in the past year.	1 2 3 4 5 6 7 8 9 (8.0, 0.8, A)	1 2 3 4 5 6 7 8 9 (8.0, 1.1, A)
b. Diabetes or immunocompromised state.	1 2 3 4 5 6 7 8 9 (8.0, 0.6, A)	1 2 3 4 5 6 7 8 9 (8.0, 0.4, A)
c. Fever, chills and/or flank pain.	1 2 3 4 5 6 7 8 9 (8.0, 1.3, I)	1 2 3 4 5 6 7 8 9 (8.0, 0.8, A)
d. Suspected diagnosis of pyelonephritis.	1 2 3 4 5 6 7 8 9 (8.0, 1.0, I)	1 2 3 4 5 6 7 8 9 (8.0, 1.0, A)
e. Structural or functional anomalies of the urinary tract.	1 2 3 4 5 6 7 8 9 (8.0, 0.4, A)	1 2 3 4 5 6 7 8 9 (7.0, 0.6, A)
f. Pregnancy.	1 2 3 4 5 6 7 8 9 (8.0, 0.7, A)	1 2 3 4 5 6 7 8 9 (8.0, 0.4, A)
g. A relapse of symptoms, if no culture previously obtained.	1 2 3 4 5 6 7 8 9 (8.0, 0.2, A)	1 2 3 4 5 6 7 8 9 (8.0, 0.2, A)
h. A recent hospitalization.	1 2 3 4 5 6 7 8 9 (6.0, 1.9, I)	1 2 3 4 5 6 7 8 9 (6.0, 1.6, I)
h. A recent invasive procedure.	1 2 3 4 5 6 7 8 9 (8.0, 1.0, I)	1 2 3 4 5 6 7 8 9 (7.0, 1.6, I)

Scales: 1 = low validity or feasibility; 9 = high validity or feasibility.

Chapter 18
QUALITY INDICATORS FOR URINARY TRACT INFECTION

(TREATMENT)

	Validity	Feasibility

7. If the patient has dysuria and a clear catch urinalysis shows more than 5 WBC per high-power field, the patient should receive treatment with antimicrobials.

```
Validity                        Feasibility
        1     8                             4 4 1
1 2 3 4 5 6 7 8 9               1 2 3 4 5 6 7 8 9
(8.0, 0.3, A)                  (8.0, 0.6, A)
```

8. If a diagnosis of UTI (upper or lower tract) has been made, the patient should be treated with antimicrobial therapy.

```
          1 1 7                             4 3 2
1 2 3 4 5 6 7 8 9               1 2 3 4 5 6 7 8 9
(8.0, 0.3, A)                  (8.0, 0.7, A)
```

9. Trimethoprim-sulfamethoxazole should be used as a first-line agent in outpatients with uncomplicated lower tract infection unless there is:

a. Documented history of allergy or pregnancy.

```
          1 1 7                           1 2 6
1 2 3 4 5 6 7 8 9               1 2 3 4 5 6 7 8 9
(8.0, 0.3, A)                  (8.0, 0.4, A)
```

10. Treatment with antimicrobials for uncomplicated lower tract infection should not exceed 7 days.

```
          3 4 2                         2 1 2 4
1 2 3 4 5 6 7 8 9               1 2 3 4 5 6 7 8 9
(7.0, 0.6, I)                  (7.0, 1.3, I)
```

11. At least 10 days of antimicrobial therapy should be prescribed for a suspected upper tract infection (pyelonephritis).

```
        1 1 2 4 1                        1 1 6 1
1 2 3 4 5 6 7 8 9               1 2 3 4 5 6 7 8 9
(8.0, 0.9, A)                  (8.0, 0.9, A)
```

12. A patient with known or suspected upper tract infection who has uncontrolled vomiting in the office or ER should receive parenteral antibiotics.

```
            2 7                             1 8
1 2 3 4 5 6 7 8 9               1 2 3 4 5 6 7 8 9
(8.0, 0.2, A)                  (8.0, 0.1, A)
```

13. A pregnant patient with pyelonephritis should receive parenteral antibiotics.

```
              4 5                           1 4 4
1 2 3 4 5 6 7 8 9               1 2 3 4 5 6 7 8 9
(9.0, 0.4, A)                  (8.0, 0.6, A)
```

14. Regimens of at least 7 days should be used for patients with complicated lower tract infections, that is, those with:

a. Diabetes.

```
            4 5                           1 5 2 1
1 2 3 4 5 6 7 8 9               1 2 3 4 5 6 7 8 9
(8.0, 0.4, A)                  (7.0, 0.7, A)
```

b. Functional or structural anomaly of the urinary tract.

```
            5 4                           1 7 1
1 2 3 4 5 6 7 8 9               1 2 3 4 5 6 7 8 9
(7.0, 0.4, A)                  (7.0, 0.3, A)
```

c. Symptoms for longer than 7 days.

```
    1 1 1 1 3 2                          1 3 4 1
1 2 3 4 5 6 7 8 9               1 2 3 4 5 6 7 8 9
(7.0, 1.3, I)                  (7.0, 1.2, I)
```

d. Urinary tract infection in past month.

```
          2 3 4                         2 1 4 2
1 2 3 4 5 6 7 8 9               1 2 3 4 5 6 7 8 9
(7.0, 0.9, A)                  (7.0, 0.8, I)
```

e. Use of diaphragm.

```
  2 2 1 1 2 1                        2 2 3 1 1
1 2 3 4 5 6 7 8 9               1 2 3 4 5 6 7 8 9
(4.0, 1.7, I)                  (6.0, 1.2, I)
```

f. Pregnancy.

```
            4 5                         1 1 4 3
1 2 3 4 5 6 7 8 9               1 2 3 4 5 6 7 8 9
(8.0, 0.4, A)                  (7.0, 0.7, A)
```

Scales: 1 = low validity or feasibility; 9 = high validity or feasibility.

Chapter 18
QUALITY INDICATORS FOR URINARY TRACT INFECTION

(FOLLOW-UP)

	Validity	Feasibility

15. For [upper tract infection], a repeat culture should be obtained within 2 weeks of finishing treatment.

```
                    3   2 3                      2 3 1 3
1                   6   7 8 9                    6 7 8 9
1 2 3 4 5 6 7 8 9            1 2 3 4 5 6 7 8 9
   (7.0, 1.7, I)                (6.0, 1.0, I)
```

15. For [complicated lower tract infection], a repeat culture should be obtained within 2 weeks of finishing treatment.

```
             2 2 3 2                        2 4 1 2
1 2 3 4 5 6 7 8 9            1 2 3 4 5 6 7 8 9
   (7.0, 0.9, I)                (6.0, 0.8, I)
```

Scales: 1 = low validity or feasibility; 9 = high validity or feasibility.

Chapter 19
QUALITY INDICATORS FOR VAGINITIS
AND SEXUALLY TRANSMITTED DISEASES

	Validity	Feasibility

(DIAGNOSIS)

Vaginitis

1. In women presenting with a chief complaint of vaginal discharge, the practitioner should perform a speculum exam to determine if the discharge has a cervical or vaginal source.

Validity: 1 1 4 3 — 1 2 3 4 5 6 7 8 9 (7.0, 0.7, A)
Feasibility: 2 1 2 4 — 1 2 3 4 5 6 7 8 9 (7.0, 1.0, I)

2. At a minimum, the following tests should be performed on the vaginal discharge: normal saline wet mount for clue cells and trichomads; KOH wet mount for yeast hyphae.

Validity: 2 2 2 1 2 — 1 2 3 4 5 6 7 8 9 (6.0, 1.2, I)
Feasibility: 1 1 3 1 3 — 1 2 3 4 5 6 7 8 9 (6.0, 1.1, I)

3. A sexual history should be obtained from women presenting with a chief complaint of vaginal discharge. The history should include:

a. Number of male sexual partners in previous 6 months.

Validity: 1 1 7 — 1 2 3 4 5 6 7 8 9 (7.0, 0.3, A)
Feasibility: 5 3 1 — 1 2 3 4 5 6 7 8 9 (5.0, 0.6, A)

b. Absence or presence of symptoms in partners.

Validity: 2 2 5 — 1 2 3 4 5 6 7 8 9 (7.0, 1.1, I)
Feasibility: 1 5 3 — 1 2 3 4 5 6 7 8 9 (5.0, 0.4, A)

c. Use of condoms.

Validity: 3 3 2 1 — 1 2 3 4 5 6 7 8 9 (6.0, 0.8, I)
Feasibility: 4 5 — 1 2 3 4 5 6 7 8 9 (6.0, 0.4, A)

d. Prior history of sexually transmitted diseases.

Validity: 1 1 2 3 2 — 1 2 3 4 5 6 7 8 9 (7.0, 1.0, I)
Feasibility: 1 5 1 2 — 1 2 3 4 5 6 7 8 9 (6.0, 0.7, I)

4. If three of the following four criteria are met, a diagnosis of bacterial vaginosis or gardnerella vaginosis should be made:
- pH greater than 4.5,
- positive whiff test,
- clue cells on wet mount, and
- thin homogenous discharge.

Validity: 4 5 — 1 2 3 4 5 6 7 8 9 (8.0, 0.4, A)
Feasibility: 4 4 — 1 2 3 4 5 6 7 8 9 (7.0, 1.0, A)

Cervicitis

5. Routine testing for gonorrhea and chlamydia trachomatis (culture and antigen detection, respectively) should be performed with the routine pelvic exam for women with multiple male sexual partners (more than 1 in previous 6 months).

Validity: 4 3 2 — 1 2 3 4 5 6 7 8 9 (7.0, 0.7, I)
Feasibility: 1 4 1 3 — 1 2 3 4 5 6 7 8 9 (6.0, 0.9, I)

Pelvic Inflammatory Disease (PID)

6. If a patient is given the diagnosis of PID, a speculum and bimanual pelvic exam should have been performed.

Validity: 4 5 — 1 2 3 4 5 6 7 8 9 (9.0, 0.4, A)
Feasibility: 3 6 — 1 2 3 4 5 6 7 8 9 (9.0, 0.3, A)

7. If a patient is given the diagnosis of PID, at least 2 of the following signs should be present on physical exam:
- lower abdominal tenderness,
- adnexal tenderness, and
- cervical motion tenderness.

Validity: 2 7 — 1 2 3 4 5 6 7 8 9 (8.0, 0.2, A)
Feasibility: 2 7 — 1 2 3 4 5 6 7 8 9 (8.0, 0.2, A)

Scales: 1 = low validity or feasibility; 9 = high validity or feasibility.

Chapter 19
QUALITY INDICATORS FOR VAGINITIS
AND SEXUALLY TRANSMITTED DISEASES

	Validity	Feasibility

STD - General

8. If a patient presents with an initial infection of any sexually transmitted disease, HIV testing should be discussed and offered.

	Validity	Feasibility
	1 7 1 1 2 3 4 5 6 7 8 9 (7.0, 0.4, A)	1 1 3 1 1 2 3 4 5 6 7 8 9 (6.0, 0.9, I)

STD--General

9. If a patient presents with any sexually transmitted disease (gonorrhea, chlamydia, trachomatis, herpes, chancroid, syphilis) a non-treponemal test (VDRL or RPR) for syphilis should be obtained.

	Validity	Feasibility
	2 4 2 1 1 2 3 4 5 6 7 8 9 (7.0, 0.7, A)	1 2 2 3 1 1 2 3 4 5 6 7 8 9 (7.0, 1.0, I)

(TREATMENT)

Vaginitis

10. Treatment for bacterial vaginosis should be with metronidazole (orally or vaginally) or clindamycin (orally or vaginally).

	Validity	Feasibility
	2 6 1 1 2 3 4 5 6 7 8 9 (8.0, 0.3, A)	3 5 1 1 2 3 4 5 6 7 8 9 (8.0, 0.4, A)

11. Treatment for T. vaginalis should be with oral metronidazole in the absence of allergy to metronidazole or first trimester pregnancy.

	Validity	Feasibility
	3 5 1 1 2 3 4 5 6 7 8 9 (8.0, 0.4, A)	4 4 1 1 2 3 4 5 6 7 8 9 (8.0, 0.6, A)

12. Treatment for non-recurrent (three or fewer episodes in previous year) yeast vaginitis should be with topical "azole" preparations (e.g., clotrimazole, butoconazole, etc.) or fluconazole.

	Validity	Feasibility
	3 5 1 1 2 3 4 5 6 7 8 9 (8.0, 0.4, A)	5 2 1 1 2 3 4 5 6 7 8 9 (7.0, 0.8, A)

Cervicitis

13. Women treated for gonorrhea should also be treated for chlamydia.

	Validity	Feasibility
	2 6 1 1 2 3 4 5 6 7 8 9 (8.0, 0.3, A)	2 5 2 1 2 3 4 5 6 7 8 9 (8.0, 0.4, A)

Pelvic Inflammatory Disease (PID)

14. Patients with PID and any of the following conditions should receive parenteral antibiotics:

c. Pelvic abscess is present or suspected.

	Validity	Feasibility
	5 4 1 2 3 4 5 6 7 8 9 (8.0, 0.4, A)	5 4 1 2 3 4 5 6 7 8 9 (8.0, 0.4, A)

d. The patient is pregnant.

	Validity	Feasibility
	2 4 3 1 2 3 4 5 6 7 8 9 (8.0, 0.6, A)	1 5 3 1 2 3 4 5 6 7 8 9 (8.0, 0.6, A)

f. The patient has HIV infection.

	Validity	Feasibility
	2 5 2 1 2 3 4 5 6 7 8 9 (8.0, 0.4, A)	2 3 4 1 2 3 4 5 6 7 8 9 (8.0, 0.7, A)

g. Uncontrolled nausea and vomiting.

	Validity	Feasibility
	2 6 1 1 2 3 4 5 6 7 8 9 (8.0, 0.3, A)	7 2 1 2 3 4 5 6 7 8 9 (8.0, 0.2, A)

i. The patient does not improve within 72 hours of starting therapy.

	Validity	Feasibility
	1 5 3 1 2 3 4 5 6 7 8 9 (7.0, 0.6, A)	3 1 5 1 2 3 4 5 6 7 8 9 (8.0, 1.1, I)

Scales: 1 = low validity or feasibility;   9 = high validity or feasibility.

Chapter 19
QUALITY INDICATORS FOR VAGINITIS
AND SEXUALLY TRANSMITTED DISEASES

	Validity	Feasibility
15. Total antibiotic therapy for PID should be for no less than 10 days (inpatient, if applicable, plus outpatient).	4 5 1 2 3 4 5 6 7 8 9 (8.0, 0.4, A)	2 3 4 1 2 3 4 5 6 7 8 9 (7.0, 0.9, A)

Genital Ulcers

	Validity	Feasibility
16. Patients with genital herpes should be counseled regarding reducing the risk of transmission to sexual partners.	1 2 5 1 1 2 3 4 5 6 7 8 9 (8.0, 0.6, A)	2 3 3 1 1 2 3 4 5 6 7 8 9 (6.0, 1.2, I)
17. In the absence of allergy, patients with chancroid should be treated with azithromycin, ceftriaxone, or erythromycin.	2 5 2 1 2 3 4 5 6 7 8 9 (8.0, 0.4, A)	2 6 1 1 2 3 4 5 6 7 8 9 (8.0, 0.3, A)
18. In the absence of allergy, patients with primary and secondary syphilis should be treated with benzathine penicillin G (IM).	1 4 4 1 2 3 4 5 6 7 8 9 (8.0, 0.6, A)	2 3 4 1 2 3 4 5 6 7 8 9 (8.0, 0.7, A)
19. If a patient has a primary ulcer consistent with syphilis, treatment for syphilis should be initiated before laboratory testing is back.	1 1 7 1 2 3 4 5 6 7 8 9 (8.0, 0.7, A)	1 1 2 4 1 1 2 3 4 5 6 7 8 9 (8.0, 1.2, A)

STD--General

	Validity	Feasibility
20. Sexual partners of patients with new diagnoses of gonorrhea, chlamydia, chancroid and primary or secondary syphilis should be referred for treatment.	2 4 3 1 2 3 4 5 6 7 8 9 (8.0, 0.6, A)	1 1 2 2 1 2 1 2 3 4 5 6 7 8 9 (7.0, 1.3, I)

(FOLLOW-UP)

Pelvic Inflammatory Disease (PID)

	Validity	Feasibility
21. Patients receiving outpatient therapy for PID should receive a follow-up contact within 72 hours of diagnosis.	7 2 1 2 3 4 5 6 7 8 9 (7.0, 0.2, A)	2 5 2 1 2 3 4 5 6 7 8 9 (7.0, 0.7, A)
22. Patients being treated for PID should have a microbiological re-examination (e.g., cultures) within 2 weeks of completing therapy.	2 2 1 1 1 1 1 1 2 3 4 5 6 7 8 9 (3.0, 1.8, I)	1 1 1 2 4 1 2 3 4 5 6 7 8 9 (5.0, 1.3, A)

Genital Ulcers

	Validity	Feasibility
23. Patients receiving treatment for chancroid should be re-examined within 10 days of treatment initiation to assess clinical improvement.	2 5 2 1 2 3 4 5 6 7 8 9 (7.0, 0.4, A)	1 3 2 3 1 2 3 4 5 6 7 8 9 (7.0, 0.9, I)
24. Patients with primary or secondary syphilis should be re-examined clinically and serologically within 6 months after treatment.	2 7 1 2 3 4 5 6 7 8 9 (8.0, 0.2, A)	1 2 1 5 1 2 3 4 5 6 7 8 9 (8.0, 0.9, I)
25. Patients with an initial diagnosis of HPV should have a speculum examination and a pap smear (unless a pap smear had been done in the past year).	2 6 1 1 2 3 4 5 6 7 8 9 (7.0, 0.4, A)	1 3 4 1 1 2 3 4 5 6 7 8 9 (7.0, 0.8, I)

Scales: 1 = low validity or feasibility;   9 = high validity or feasibility.

November 1995

Chapter 19
QUALITY INDICATORS FOR VAGINITIS
AND SEXUALLY TRANSMITTED DISEASES

	Validity	Feasibility

26. Patients with an initial diagnosis of HPV should be counseled regarding:

a. Smoking.

```
        1 1 1 2 1 1 1 1                    3 3   2 1
1 2 3 4 5 6 7 8 9              1 2 3 4 5 6 7 8 9
  (5.0, 1.8, I)                  (6.0, 1.1, I)
```

b. Contraceptive options.

```
        1 1 1 2 3                    1   7     1
1 2 3 4 5 6 7 8 9              1 2 3 4 5 6 7 8 9
  (4.0, 1.6, I)                  (5.0, 0.8, A)
```

Scales: 1 = low validity or feasibility; 9 = high validity or feasibility.

Chapter 20
QUALITY INDICATORS FOR PRESCRIPTION OF MEDICATIONS

Note: There is no text chapter corresponding to the indicators in this section.

	Validity	Feasibility
1. At the time someone is prescribed a medication, there should be a notation in the chart stating what medications, if any, the person is allergic to.	1 7 1 1 2 3 4 5 6 7 8 9 (8.0, 0.4, A)	3 5 1 1 2 3 4 5 6 7 8 9 (8.0, 0.4, A)
2. The chart should have a clearly specified place to mark medication allergies.	1 2 4 2 1 2 3 4 5 6 7 8 9 (8.0, 0.8, A)	1 2 4 2 1 2 3 4 5 6 7 8 9 (8.0, 0.8, A)
3. All allergies found in the chart must be listed in the allergy list discussed in the preceding indicator.	1 1 7 1 2 3 4 5 6 7 8 9 (8.0, 0.4, A)	1 1 2 3 2 1 2 3 4 5 6 7 8 9 (8.0, 1.1, A)
4. People with an allergy to a medication should only receive it if they have a notation in their chart stating why.	1 5 3 1 2 3 4 5 6 7 8 9 (8.0, 0.4, A)	4 1 4 1 2 3 4 5 6 7 8 9 (8.0, 0.9, A)
5. If a medication that is a known teratogen is prescribed, the medical record should contain documentation of at least one of the following: - effective contraception (sterilization, OCPs, depo, Norplant, IUD, hysterectomy, lesbian), - LMP, - negative pregnancy test.	3 3 3 1 2 3 4 5 6 7 8 9 (8.0, 0.7, A)	1 2 4 2 1 2 3 4 5 6 7 8 9 (8.0, 0.7, A)

Scales: 1 = low validity or feasibility; 9 = high validity or feasibility.

1

APPENDIX C: CROSSWALK TABLE OF ORIGINAL AND FINAL INDICATORS

Chapter 1 — Acne

Original Indicator	Modified Indicator	Comments
(DIAGNOSIS)	(DIAGNOSIS)	
1. For patients presenting with acne, the following history should be documented in their chart: a. location of lesions (back, face, neck, chest); b. aggravating factors (stress, seasons, cosmetics, creams); c. menstrual history and premenstrual worsening of acne; d. previous treatments; and e. medications and drug use	1. For patients presenting with **a chief complaint of** acne, the following history should be documented in their chart: **a.** location of lesions (back, face, neck, chest); -- b. aggravating factors (stress, seasons, cosmetics, creams); -- c. menstrual history and premenstrual worsening of acne; **b.** previous treatments; and **c.** medications and drug use	Added chief complaint to clarify that acne history should only be taken if main problem. •MODIFIED• **Dropped (b) aggravating factors and (c) menstrual history and premenstrual worsening due to low validity score from panelists.**
(TREATMENT)	(TREATMENT)	
2. If oral antibiotics are prescribed, there must be documentation of moderate to severe acne (papules and pustules).	2. If oral antibiotics are prescribed, there must be documentation of moderate to severe acne, **papules and/or pustules must be present.**	Definition of moderate to severe acne was difficult to operationalize.
3. If tetracycline is prescribed, there must be documentation of the last menstrual period or a negative pregnancy test for women of child-bearing age.	--	•DELETED•
4. If isotretinoin is prescribed, there must be documentation of severe acne (papules, pustules, cysts and nodules) and a failure of previous therapy.	3. If isotretinoin is prescribed, there must be documentation of cysts and/or nodules.	Definition of severe acne was difficult to operationalize.
5. If isotretinoin is prescribed, a negative pregnancy test should be obtained within two weeks of start of therapy.	4. If isotretinoin is prescribed, a negative pregnancy test should be obtained within two weeks of start of therapy.	•UNCHANGED•
6. If isotretinoin is prescribed, there should be documentation that counseling regarding use of an effective means of contraception (including abstinence) was provided.	5. If isotretinoin is prescribed, there should be documentation that counseling regarding **the necessity of** use of effective means of contraception (including abstinence) was provided.	Panelists felt that wording should reflect joint responsibility of provider and patient to prevent pregnancy.
(FOLLOW-UP)	(FOLLOW-UP)	
7. If isotretinoin is prescribed, monthly pregnancy tests should be performed.	-- If isotretinoin is prescribed, monthly pregnancy tests should be performed.	•UNCHANGED• •DROPPED• due to low validity score from panelists.
8. If isotretinoin is prescribed, monthly liver function tests should be performed.	6. If isotretinoin is prescribed, monthly liver function tests should be performed **for three months.**	PDR recommends monitoring until levels are stable. Panelists determined three months was sufficient.
9. •NEW•	-- **If isotretinoin is prescribed, monthly triglyceride levels should be performed for three months.**	•NEW• Based on PDR recommendation. •DROPPED• due to low validity score from panelists.

Chapter 2 — Alcohol Dependence

Original Indicator	Modified Indicator	Comments
(DIAGNOSIS)	**(DIAGNOSIS)**	
Screening	*Screening*	
1. New patients should be screened for problem drinking. This should include an assessment of at least one of the following: a. Quantity (e.g., drinks per day) b. Binge drinking (e.g., more than 5 drinks in a day in the last month).	1. New patients should be screened for problem drinking. This should include an assessment of at least one of the following: a. Quantity (e.g., drinks per day) **and/or frequency** b. Binge drinking (e.g., more than 5 drinks in a day in the last month).	Frequency added to (a) because threshold is lower for women.
Initial Assessment	*Initial Assessment*	
2. The record should indicate more detailed screening for dependence, tolerance of psychoactive effects, loss of control and consequences of use (examples include but are not confined to the following questionnaires: CAGE, MAST, HSS, AUDIT, SAAST, and SMAST), if the medical record indicates any of the following: a. Patient drinks more than 2 drinks each day. b. Patient drinks more than 11 drinks per week. c. Patient drinks more than 5 drinks in a day in the last month.	2. The record should indicate more detailed screening for dependence, tolerance of psychoactive effects, loss of control and consequences of use (examples include but are not confined to the following questionnaires: CAGE, MAST, HSS, AUDIT, SAAST, and SMAST), if the medical record indicates any of the following: a. Patient drinks more than 2 drinks each day. b. Patient drinks more than 11 drinks per week. c. Patient drinks more than 5 drinks in a day in the last month.	**•UNCHANGED•**
(TREATMENT)	**(TREATMENT)**	
3. Patients diagnosed with alcohol dependence should be referred for further treatment to at least one of the following: • Inpatient rehabilitation program • Outpatient rehabilitation program • Mutual help group (e.g., AA) • Supportive psychotherapy • Aversion therapy	3. Patients diagnosed with alcohol dependence should be referred for further treatment to at least one of the following: • Inpatient rehabilitation program • Outpatient rehabilitation program • Mutual help group (e.g., AA) • **Substance abuse counseling** • Aversion therapy	Psychotherapy deleted because panel did not think effective treatment. Changed to substance abuse counseling so that a wide range of counseling would apply.
(FOLLOW-UP)	**(FOLLOW-UP)**	
4. Regular or binge drinkers (as defined above) should be advised to decrease their drinking.	4. Regular or binge drinkers (as defined above) should be advised to decrease their drinking.	**•UNCHANGED•**
5. Providers should reassess the alcohol intake of patients who report regular or binge drinking at every visit.	5. Providers should reassess the alcohol intake of patients who report regular or binge drinking at **the next routine health** visit.	Reassessment at every visit was too burdensome. More important to reassess at the next visit.

Chapter 3 — Allergic Rhinitis

Original Indicator	Modified Indicator	Comments
(DIAGNOSIS)	**(DIAGNOSIS)**	
1. If a diagnosis of allergic rhinitis is made, the search for a specific allergen by history should be documented in the chart (for initial history).	1. If a diagnosis of allergic rhinitis is made, the search for a specific allergen by history should be documented in the chart (for initial history).	•UNCHANGED•
2. If a diagnosis of allergic rhinitis is made, history should include whether the patient uses any topical or systemic nasal decongestants.	2. If a diagnosis of allergic rhinitis is made, history should include whether the patient uses any topical or ~~systemic~~ nasal decongestants.	Systemic deleted because it was a typographical error in original.
(TREATMENT)	**(TREATMENT)**	
3. Treatment for allergic rhinitis should include at least one of the following: antihistamine, nasal steroids, nasal cromolyn.	3. Treatment for allergic rhinitis should include at least one of the following: **allergen avoidance,** antihistamine, nasal steroids, nasal cromolyn.	Allergen avoidance added because panel felt it was a common and appropriate treatment.
4. If topical or systemic nasal decongestants are prescribed, duration of treatment should be for no longer than 4 days.	4. If topical or ~~systemic~~ nasal decongestants are prescribed, duration of treatment should be for no longer than 4 days.	Systemic deleted because it was a typographical error in original.

Chapter 4 — Asthma [persons with moderate to severe]

	Original Indicator		Modified Indicator	Comments
	(DIAGNOSIS)	1.	**(DIAGNOSIS)**	
1.	Patients with the diagnosis of asthma should have had some historical evaluation of asthma precipitants (environmental exposures, exercise, allergens) within six months (before or after) of diagnosis.	1.	Patients with the diagnosis of asthma should have had some historical evaluation of asthma precipitants (environmental exposures, exercise, allergens) within six months (before or after) of diagnosis.	• UNCHANGED•
2.	Patients with the diagnosis of asthma should have baseline spirometry performed within six months of diagnosis.	2.	Patients with the diagnosis of asthma should have baseline spirometry **or peak flow** performed within six months of diagnosis.	Peak flow is also an adequate measure of control in known asthmatics.
3.	Peak expiratory flow rate (PEFR) or FEV1 should be measured in patients with chronic asthma at least annually.	3.	Peak expiratory flow rate (PEFR) or FEV1 should be measured in patients with chronic asthma at least annually.	• UNCHANGED•
	(TREATMENT)		**(TREATMENT)**	
	Chronic — Treatment		*Chronic — Treatment*	
4.	Patients with the diagnosis of asthma should have been prescribed a beta$_2$-agonist inhaler for symptomatic relief of exacerbations to use as needed.	4.	Patients with the diagnosis of asthma should have been prescribed a beta$_2$-agonist inhaler for symptomatic relief of exacerbations to use as needed.	• UNCHANGED•
5.	Patients who report using a beta$_2$-agonist inhaler more than 3 times per day on a daily basis (not only during an exacerbation) should be prescribed a longer acting bronchodilator (theophylline) and/or an anti-inflammatory agent (inhaled corticosteroids, cromolyn).	5.	Patients who report using a beta$_2$-agonist inhaler more than 3 times per day on a daily basis (not only during an exacerbation) should be prescribed a longer acting bronchodilator (theophylline) and/or an anti-inflammatory agent (inhaled corticosteroids, cromolyn).	• UNCHANGED•
6.	Patients with asthma should not receive beta-blocker medications (e.g., atenolol, propanalol).	6.	Patients with asthma should not receive beta-blocker medications (e.g., atenolol, propanalol).	• UNCHANGED•
7.	Asthmatic patients who require systemic steroids in the past should have documented current or past inhaled steroid use.	7.	Asthmatic patients who require systemic steroids in the past should have documented current or past inhaled steroid use.	Wording changed to clarify the intent of the indicator
8.	Patients on theophylline should have at least one serum theophylline level determination per year.	8.	Patients on **chronic** theophylline **[dose > 600 mg/day]** should have at least one serum theophylline level determination per year.	Chronic added to justify monitoring levels. Dose added to operationalize chronic.
9.	Patients with the diagnosis of asthma should have a documented flu vaccination in the fall/winter of the previous year (September - January).	9.	Patients with the diagnosis of asthma should have a documented flu vaccination in the fall/winter of the previous year (September - January).	• UNCHANGED• Note: Duplicate of Ch. 16 indicator #2a.
10.	Patients with the diagnosis of asthma should have a pneumococcal vaccination documented in the chart.	10.	Patients with the diagnosis of asthma should have a pneumococcal vaccination documented in the chart.	• UNCHANGED•
	Flare-up — Diagnosis and Treatment		*Flare-up — Diagnosis and Treatment*	
11.	Patients presenting to the physician's office with an asthma exacerbation or historical worsening of asthma symptoms should be evaluated with PEFR or forced expiratory volume at 1 second (FEV$_1$).	11.	Patients presenting to the physician's office with an asthma exacerbation or historical worsening of asthma symptoms should be evaluated with PEFR or forced expiratory volume at 1 second (FEV$_1$).	• UNCHANGED•
12.	At the time of an exacerbation, patients on theophylline should have theophylline level measured.	12.	At the time of an exacerbation, patients on theophylline should have theophylline level measured.	• UNCHANGED•
13.	A physical exam of the chest should be performed in patients presenting with an asthma exacerbation.	13.	A physical exam of the chest should be performed in patients presenting with an asthma exacerbation **in the physician's office or emergency room.**	Wording added to improve operationalization of indicator.

	Original Indicator		Modified Indicator	Comments
14.	Patients presenting to the physician's office or ER with an FEV_1 or $PEFR \leq 70\%$ of baseline (or predicted) should be treated with beta$_2$-agonists before discharge.	14.	Patients presenting to the physician's office or ER with an FEV_1 or $PEFR \leq 70\%$ of baseline (or predicted) should be treated with beta$_2$-agonists before discharge.	•UNCHANGED•
15.	Patients who receive treatment with beta$_2$-agonists in the physician's office or ER for $FEV_1 < 70\%$ of baseline (or predicted) should have an FEV_1 or PEFR repeated prior to discharge.	15.	Patients who receive treatment with beta$_2$-agonists in the physician's office or ER for $FEV_1 < 70\%$ of baseline (or predicted) should have an FEV_1 or PEFR repeated prior to discharge.	•UNCHANGED•
16.	Patients with an FEV_1 or $PEFR \leq 70\%$ of baseline (or predicted) after treatment for asthma exacerbation in the physician's office should be placed on an oral corticosteroid taper.	16.	Patients with an FEV_1 or $PEFR \leq 70\%$ of baseline (or predicted) after treatment for asthma exacerbation in the physician's office should be placed on an oral corticosteroid taper.	•UNCHANGED•
17.	Patients who have a PEFR or $FEV_1 \leq 40\%$ of baseline (or predicted) after treatment with beta$_2$-agonists should be admitted to the hospital.	17.	Patients who have a PEFR or $FEV_1 \leq 40\%$ of baseline (or predicted) after treatment with beta$_2$-agonists should **not be discharged from ER.**	Panelists felt modified wording was clearer.
	Hospital — Treatment and Diagnosis		**Hospital — Treatment and Diagnosis**	
18.	Patients admitted to the hospital for asthma exacerbation should have oxygen saturation measured.	18.	Patients admitted to the hospital for asthma exacerbation should have oxygen saturation measured.	•UNCHANGED•
19.	Hospitalized patients with PEFR or FEV_1 less than 25 percent of predicted or personal best should receive arterial blood gas measurement.	19.	Hospitalized patients with PEFR or FEV_1 less than 25 percent of predicted or personal best should receive arterial blood gas measurement.	•UNCHANGED•
20.	Hospitalized patients should receive systemic steroids (either PO or IV).	20.	Hospitalized patients should receive systemic steroids (either PO or IV).	•UNCHANGED•
21.	Hospitalized patients should receive treatment with beta$_2$-agonists.	21.	Hospitalized patients should receive treatment with beta$_2$-agonists.	•UNCHANGED•
22.	Hospitalized patients should receive treatment with methylxanthines.	--	Hospitalized patients should receive treatment with methylxanthines.	•UNCHANGED• •**DROPPED• due to low validity score from panelists.**
23.	Hospitalized patients with oxygen saturation less than 90 percent should receive supplemental oxygen.	22.	Hospitalized patients with oxygen saturation less than 90 percent should receive supplemental oxygen, **unless $pCO_2 > 40$ is previously documented.**	Avoids mandating oxygen therapy in patients who retain CO_2.
24.	Hospitalized patients with pCO_2 of greater than 40 should receive at least one additional blood gas measurement to evaluate response to treatment.	23.	Hospitalized patients with pCO_2 of greater than 40 should receive at least one additional blood gas measurement to evaluate response to treatment **unless $pCO_2 > 40$ is previously documented.**	Wording added to improve operationalization of indicator.
25.	Hospitalized patients with pCO_2 of greater than 40 should be monitored in an intensive care setting.	24.	Hospitalized patients with pCO_2 of greater than 40 should be monitored **with pulse oximetry unless $pCO_2 > 40$ is previously documented.**	Original indicator was too strict. Not all patients with $pCO_2 > 40$ need to be in ICU. Wording added (unless $pCO_2 > 40...$) to improve operationalization of indicator.
26.	Patients with 2 or more hospitalizations for asthma exacerbation in the previous year should receive (or should have received) consultation with an asthma specialist.	--	Patients with 2 or more hospitalizations for asthma exacerbation in the previous year should receive (or should have received) consultation with an asthma specialist.	•UNCHANGED• •**DROPPED• due to low validity score from panelists.**

Women's Quality Indicators

cont'd

	Original Indicator	Modified Indicator	Comments
27.	Hospitalized patients should not receive sedative drugs (e.g., anxiolytics).	25. Hospitalized patients should not receive sedative drugs (e.g., anxiolytics), **except if on a ventilator, physiologically dependent on sedatives, or in alcohol withdrawal.**	Panelists felt exceptions were necessary in order to retain original indicator.
	(FOLLOW-UP)	(FOLLOW-UP)	
28.	Patients with the diagnosis of asthma should have at least 2 visits within a calendar year.	-- Patients with the diagnosis of asthma should have at least 2 visits within a calendar year.	•**UNCHANGED**• •**DROPPED• due to low validity score from panelists.**
29.	Patients whose asthma medication regimen changes (new medication added, current medication dose decreased or increased) during one visit should have a follow-up visit within 4 weeks.	-- Patients whose asthma medication regimen changes (new medication added, current medication dose decreased or increased) during one visit should have a follow-up **contact** within 4 weeks.	Visit changed to contact so that telephone consult would be an acceptable form of follow-up. •**DROPPED• due to low validity scores from panelists.**
30.	Patients on chronic oral corticosteroids (three or more corticosteroid tapers for exacerbations in the past year, or continuous treatment with any dose prednisone, or three or more administrations of intramuscular corticosteroids in the past year) should have follow-up visits at least 4 times in a calendar year.	26. Patients on chronic oral corticosteroids (three or more corticosteroid tapers for exacerbations in the past year, or continuous treatment with any dose prednisone, or three or more administrations of intramuscular corticosteroids in the past year) should have follow-up visits at least **2** times in a calendar year.	Panelists felt 2 follow-up visits would be sufficient.
31.	Patients seen in the emergency department with an asthma exacerbation should have a follow-up re-assessment within 72 hours.	-- Patients seen in the emergency department with an asthma exacerbation should have a follow-up re-assessment within 72 hours.	•**UNCHANGED**• •**DROPPED• due to low validity score from panelists.**
32.	Patients with a hospitalization for asthma exacerbation should receive outpatient follow-up within 14 days.	27. Patients with a hospitalization for asthma exacerbation should receive outpatient follow-up **contact** within 14 days.	Contact added so that telephone consult would be an acceptable form of follow-up.

Women's Quality Indicators

Chapter 5 — Breast Mass

	Original Indicator		Modified Indicator	Comments
1.	If a palpable breast mass has been detected, at least one of the following procedures should be completed within 6 months: • Fine needle aspiration • Mammography • Ultrasound • Biopsy • Follow-up visit	1.	If a palpable breast mass has been detected, at least one of the following procedures should be completed within 3 months: • Fine needle aspiration, • Mammography, • Ultrasound, • Biopsy, or • Follow-up visit	Follow-up procedure should be completed within 3 months of detection rather than 6 months to prevent intervening metastasis.
2.	If a breast mass has been detected on two separate occasions, then either a biopsy or FNA should be performed within 6 months of the second visit.	2.	If a breast mass has been detected on two separate occasions, then either a biopsy or FNA **or ultrasound** should be performed within **3** months of the second visit.	Ultrasound is an acceptable initial diagnostic test. Follow-up procedure should be completed within 3 months of detection rather than 6 months to prevent intervening metastasis.
3.	•NEW•	3.	**A biopsy or FNA should be performed in the following circumstances:** a. **Mammography is suggestive of malignancy** b. **Persistent palpable mass that is not cystic on diagnostic testing (ultrasound or mammography).**	•NEW• Additional indicator for subsequent diagnostic tests.
4.	•NEW•	4.	**A biopsy should be performed if FNA cannot rule out malignancy.**	•NEW• Additional indicator for subsequent diagnostic tests.

Chapter 6 — Cesarean Delivery

	Original Indicator		Modified Indicator	Comments
	A. Prior Cesarean Delivery		**A. Prior Cesarean Delivery**	
	(TREATMENT)		(TREATMENT)	
1.	For women who have delivered by cesarean, the type of uterine incision used (transverse lower segment or vertical) should be noted in the medical record.	1.	For women who have delivered by cesarean, the type of uterine incision used (transverse lower segment or vertical) should be noted in the medical record.	•UNCHANGED• Note: This indicator applies to a cesarean section delivery that occurred during the study period, not to a prior cesarean section as the section heading implies.
2.	For women with a cesarean delivery in a prior pregnancy, the number and type of previous uterine scar(s) should be noted in the current delivery medical record. (If this information is not available, an attempt to locate it should be documented in the chart.)	2.	For women with a cesarean delivery in a prior pregnancy, the number and type of previous uterine scar(s) should be noted in the current delivery medical record. (If this information is not available, an attempt to locate it should be documented in the chart.)	•UNCHANGED•
3.	Women with one prior transverse lower segment cesarean should undergo a trial of labor unless another indication for cesarean delivery is present.	3.	Women with one prior transverse lower segment cesarean should undergo a trial of labor unless another indication for cesarean delivery is present **(including refusal of a trial of labor).**	Women can not be forced to undergo a trial of labor if they do not desire it.
4.	Women with a prior vertical cesarean should have a scheduled repeat cesarean delivery.	4.	Women with a prior **classical** vertical cesarean should have a scheduled repeat cesarean delivery.	Classical added because incidence of uterine rupture is highest with this type of vertical incision.
	(DIAGNOSIS)		(DIAGNOSIS)	
	B. Failure To Progress In Labor		**B. Failure To Progress In Labor**	
1.	When the diagnosis of failure to progress in labor is made, a woman should be in the active phase of labor.	5.	When the diagnosis of failure to progress in labor is made, a woman should be in the active phase of labor.	•UNCHANGED•
2.	When the diagnosis of failure to progress in labor is made, at least two exams of cervical dilatation separated in time by at least 2 hours should have been done and recorded in the medical record.	6.	When the diagnosis of failure to progress in labor is made, at least two exams of cervical dilatation separated in time by at least 2 hours should have been done and recorded in the medical record.	•UNCHANGED•
	(TREATMENT)		(TREATMENT)	
3.	Before a cesarean delivery is used to treat failure to progress in labor, at least one of the following therapeutic interventions should have been tried after the time of the diagnosis of FTP: • Amniotomy • Oxytocin • Ambulation	7.	Before a cesarean delivery is used to treat failure to progress in labor, at least **two** of the following therapeutic interventions should have been tried after the time of the diagnosis of FTP: • Amniotomy, • Oxytocin, or • Ambulation.	Changed to two of the following because more should be done before going to a C-section.
	C. Fetal Distress		**C. Fetal Distress**	
	(DIAGNOSIS)		(DIAGNOSIS)	

cont'd

	Original Indicator	Modified Indicator	Comments
1.	Fetuses should be monitored during active labor. The forms of monitoring are: • intermittent auscultation with a stethoscope or doppler device, or • continuous electronic fetal monitoring (EFM).	--	Fetuses should be monitored during active labor. The forms of monitoring are: • intermittent auscultation with a stethoscope or doppler device **as recommended by ACOG for low risk**, or • continuous electronic fetal monitoring (EFM).	ACOG minimum standard is every 30 minutes during first stage of labor for low risk. Added to define intermittent. **DROPPED due to operationalization difficulties.**
	D. Antibiotic Prophylaxis (TREATMENT)		***D. Antibiotic Prophylaxis*** (TREATMENT)	
1.	Women who give birth by cesarean should receive at least one dose of antibiotic prophylaxis.	8.	Women who give birth by cesarean should receive at least one dose of antibiotic prophylaxis.	•**UNCHANGED•**
2.	Prophylactic antibiotic regimens should include one of the following: • broad spectrum penicillins, • broad spectrum cephalosporins, or • metronidazole.	9.	Prophylactic antibiotic regimens should include one of the following: • broad spectrum penicillins, • broad spectrum cephalosporins, or • metronidazole.	•**UNCHANGED•**
3.	Aminoglycosides should not be used, alone or in combination, for antibiotic prophylaxis.	10.	Aminoglycosides should not be used, alone or in combination, for antibiotic prophylaxis.	•**UNCHANGED•**
4.	Prophylactic antibiotics should be administered after the umbilical cord is clamped.	--	Prophylactic antibiotics should be administered after the umbilical cord is clamped.	•**DROPPED due to operationalization difficulties**

Chapter 7 — Cigarette Use Counseling

Original Indicator		Modified Indicator		Comments
(SCREENING)		(SCREENING)		
1.	Enrollees should have the presence or absence of tobacco use noted in the medical record at the intake history and physical or at least once during the course of a year.	1.	Enrollees should have the presence or absence of tobacco use noted in the medical record at the intake history and physical or at least once during the course of a year.	•UNCHANGED•
(TREATMENT)		(TREATMENT)		
2.	Current smokers should receive counseling to stop smoking.	2.	Current smokers should receive counseling to stop smoking.	•UNCHANGED•
3.	If counseling alone fails to help the patient quit smoking, the patient should be offered nicotine replacement therapy (gum or patch).	3.	If counseling alone fails to help the patient quit smoking, the patient should be offered nicotine replacement therapy (gum or patch), **except if contraindicated.**	Added because there are contraindications to nicotine replacement in some patients (see indicator #5 below).
4.	Nicotine replacement should only be prescribed in conjunction with counseling.	4.	Nicotine replacement should only be prescribed in conjunction with counseling.	•UNCHANGED•
5.	Nicotine replacement should not be prescribed if the patient:	5.	Nicotine replacement should not be prescribed if the patient:	Nicotine gum may worsen TMJ disease, but panelists felt that (c) should be deleted because patient would self-discontinue gum if painful.
	a. is pregnant or nursing	**a.**	is pregnant or nursing	
	b. has had a myocardial infarction in past year	**b.**	has had a myocardial infarction in past year	•MODIFIED•
	c. has temporomandibular joint disease	--	c. has temporomandibular joint disease	
	d. continues to smoke	--	d. continues to smoke	**Dropped (d) continues to smoke due to low validity score from panelists.**
(FOLLOW-UP)		(FOLLOW-UP)		
6.	Tobacco abuse should be added to the problem list of all current smokers or addressed within one year.	6.	Tobacco abuse should be added to the problem list of all current smokers or addressed within one year.	•UNCHANGED•

Chapter 8 — Depression

Original Indicator		Modified Indicator		Comments
(SCREENING)		**(SCREENING)**		
1.	Clinicians should ask about the presence or absence of depression or depressive symptoms in any person with any of the following risk factors for depression:	1.	Clinicians should ask about the presence or absence of depression or depressive symptoms in any person with any of the following risk factors for depression:	Panelists felt there were a variety of other risk factors for depression. The category "traumatic events" was added to cover some of these other events.
	a. divorce in past six months,	--	a. divorce in past six months,	
	b. unemployment,	--	b. unemployment,	**•MODIFIED•**
	c. history of depression,	a.	c. history of depression,	
	d. death in family in past six months, or	b.	d. death in family in past six months, ~~or~~	Dropped (a) divorce in past 6 months, (b) unemployment, and (f) traumatic events due to low validity scores from panelists.
	e. alcohol or other drug abuse.	c.	e. alcohol or other drug abuse, **or**	
		--	f. **traumatic events.**	
(DIAGNOSIS)		**(DIAGNOSIS)**		
2.	If the diagnosis of depression is made, specific co-morbidities should be elicited and documented in the chart:	2.	If the diagnosis of depression is made, specific co-morbidities should be elicited and documented in the chart:	Wording changed to clarify that substance abuse includes both drugs and alcohol.
	a. presence or absence of substance abuse;	a.	a. presence or absence of **alcohol or other drug** abuse;	
	b. medication use; and	b.	b. medication use; and	
	c. general medical disorder(s).	c.	c. general medical disorder(s).	
(TREATMENT)		**(TREATMENT)**		
3.	If co-morbidity (substance abuse, contributing medication) is present that contributes to depression, the initial treatment objective should be to remove the comorbidity or treat the medical disorder.	--	If co-morbidity (substance abuse, contributing medication) is present that contributes to depression, the initial treatment objective should be to remove the comorbidity or treat the medical disorder.	**•UNCHANGED•** **DROPPED due to operationalization difficulties**
4.	Once diagnosis of major depression has been made, treatment with anti-depressant medication and/or psychotherapy should begin within 2 weeks.	3.	Once diagnosis of major depression has been made, treatment with anti-depressant medication and/or psychotherapy should begin within 2 weeks.	**•UNCHANGED•**
5.	Presence or absence of suicidal ideation should be documented during the first or second diagnostic visit.	4.	Presence or absence of suicidal ideation should be documented during the first or second diagnostic visit.	**•UNCHANGED•**
6.	Medication treatment visits or telephone contacts should occur weekly for a minimum of 4 weeks.	5.	Medication treatment visits or telephone contacts should occur **at least once in the 2 weeks following initial diagnosis.**	Weekly for 4 weeks was too often.
7.	At least one of the following should occur if there is no or incomplete response to therapy for depression at 6 weeks: • Referral to psychotherapist, if not already seeing one; • Change or increase in dose of medication, if on medication; • Addition of medication, if only using psychotherapy • Change in diagnosis documented in chart	6.	At least one of the following should occur if there is no or **inadequate** response to therapy for depression at **8 weeks:** • Referral to psychotherapist, if not already seeing one; • Change or increase in dose of medication, if on medication; • Addition of medication, if only using psychotherapy; **or** • Change in diagnosis documented in chart	Incomplete changed to inadequate for clarification. Timeframe changed from 6 to 8 weeks because the panelists agreed that it often takes 8 weeks to see an effect of treatment.
8.	Anti-depressants should be prescribed at appropriate dosages.	7.	Anti-depressants should be prescribed at appropriate dosages.	**•UNCHANGED•**
9.	Anti-anxiety agents should generally NOT be used (except alprazolam).	8.	Anti-anxiety agents should **not be prescribed as a sole agent for the treatment of depression.**	Can be used if depression and anxiety co-exist.
10.	Persons who have suicidality should be asked if they have specific plans to carry out suicide.	9.	Persons who have suicidality should be asked if they have specific plans to carry out suicide.	**•UNCHANGED•**

cont'd

	Original Indicator		Modified Indicator	Comments
11.	Persons who have suicidality and have any of the following risk factors should be hospitalized: a. psychosis b. current alcohol or drug abuse c. specific plans to carry out suicide (e.g., obtaining a weapon, putting affairs in order, making a suicide note). (FOLLOW-UP)	10.	Persons who have suicidality and have any of the following risk factors should be hospitalized: a. psychosis b. current alcohol or drug abuse **or dependency.** c. specific plans to carry out suicide (e.g., obtaining a weapon, putting affairs in order, making a suicide note). (FOLLOW-UP)	Dependency added to broaden indicator.
12.	Once depression has resolved, follow-up visits should occur every 16 weeks at a minimum, while patient is still on medication, for the first year of treatment.	--	Once depression has resolved, follow-up visits should occur **twice in a year** at a minimum, while patient is still on medication, for the first year of treatment.	Panelists felt 4 times a year was too often and not standard practice. **DROPPED due to operationalization difficulties**
13.	At each visit during which depression is discussed, degree of response/remission and side effects of medication should be assessed and documented during the first year of treatment.	11.	At each visit during which depression is discussed, degree of response/remission and side effects of medication should be assessed and documented during the first year of treatment.	•UNCHANGED•
14.	Persons hospitalized for depression should have follow-up with a mental health specialist or their primary care doctor within two weeks of discharge.	12.	Persons hospitalized for depression should have follow-up with a mental health specialist or their primary care doctor within two weeks of discharge.	•UNCHANGED•

Women's Quality Indicators

Chapter 9 — Diabetes Mellitus

Original Indicator	Modified Indicator	Comments
(DIAGNOSIS)	(DIAGNOSIS)	
1. Patients with fasting blood sugar >140 or postprandial blood sugar >200 should have diabetes noted in progress notes or problem list.	1. Patients with fasting blood sugar ≥140 or postprandial blood sugar ≥200 should have diabetes noted in progress notes or problem list.	•UNCHANGED•
2. Patients with the diagnosis of diabetes should have:	2. Patients with the diagnosis of [Type I] diabetes should have:	Panelists wanted to rate Type I and Type II diabetes separately.
a. Glycosylated hemoglobin every 6 months.	a. Glycosylated hemoglobin or fructosamine every 6 months.	Fructosamine added to (a) because it is also an acceptable form of monitoring.
b. Eye and visual exam (annual).	b. Eye and visual exam (annual).	
c. Triglycerides (annual).	-- c. Triglycerides (annual).	
d. Total cholesterol (annual).	c. Total cholesterol (annual).	
e. HDL cholesterol (annual).	-- d. HDL cholesterol (annual).	Full urinalysis not necessary for (f). Only urine protein needed.
f. Urinalysis (annual).	d. f. Measurement of urine protein (annual).	Examination of feet at every visit was a typographic error in original (g), so it was changed to twice a year.
g. Examination of feet at every visit.	e. g. Examination of feet at least twice a year.	
h. Measurement of blood pressure at every visit.	f. h. Measurement of blood pressure at every visit.	•MODIFIED•
		Dropped (c) triglycerides and (e) HDL cholesterol because of low validity scores by panelists.

cont'd

	Original Indicator		Modified Indicator	Comments
2.5	•NEW•	3.	Patients with the diagnosis of [Type II] diabetes should have:	•NEW•
				Panelists wanted to rate Type I and Type II diabetes separately.
		a.	a. Glycosylated hemoglobin or fructosamine every 6 months.	Fructosamine added to (a) because it is also an acceptable form of monitoring.
		b.	b. Eye and visual exam (annual).	
		--	c. Triglycerides (annual).	Full urinalysis not necessary for (f). Only urine protein needed.
		--	d. Total cholesterol (annual).	
		--	e. HDL cholesterol (annual).	Examination of feet at every visit was a typographic error in original (g), so it was changed to twice a year.
		c.	f. Measurement of urine protein (annual).	
		--	g. Examination of feet at least twice a year.	•MODIFIED•
		d.	h. Measurement of blood pressure at every visit.	Dropped (c) triglycerides, (d) total cholesterol, (e) HDL cholesterol, and (g) feet examination because of low validity scores by panelists.
3.a	Patients taking insulin should monitor their glucose at home.	4.	[Type-I] Patients taking insulin should monitor their glucose at home unless documented to be unable or unwilling.	Panelists rated Type I and Type II diabetes separately.
				Panelists felt that some patients refuse to take insulin or cannot self-administer it, and that this should be considered in the indicator.
3.b	•NEW•	--	[Type II] Patients taking insulin should monitor their glucose at home unless documented to be unable or unwilling.	•NEW•
				Panelists rated Type I and Type II diabetes separately.
				Panelists felt that some patients refuse to take insulin or cannot self-administer it, and that this should be considered in the indicator.
				Recombined wtih modified indicator #4, but Type I and Type II diabetes will be scored separately.
	(TREATMENT)		(TREATMENT)	
4.	Diabetics should receive dietary and exercise counseling.	5.	Diabetics should receive dietary and exercise counseling.	•UNCHANGED•
5.	Type II diabetics who have failed dietary therapy should receive oral hypoglycemic therapy.	6.	Type II diabetics who have failed dietary therapy should receive oral hypoglycemic therapy.	•UNCHANGED•

Women's Quality Indicators

-415-

cont'd

	Original Indicator		Modified Indicator	Comments
6.	Type II diabetics who have failed oral hypoglycemics should be offered insulin.	7.	Type II diabetics who have failed oral hypoglycemics should be offered insulin.	•UNCHANGED•
7.a	If patient is receiving other antihypertensive therapy in the absence of ACE inhibitors or calcium channel blockers, progress note should document failure of ACE inhibitors and calcium channel blockers to control blood pressure.	--	If **a hypertensive [Type I]** patient **without known CAD** is receiving other antihypertensive therapy in the absence of ACE inhibitors or calcium channel blockers, progress note should document failure of ACE inhibitors and calcium channel blockers to control blood pressure.	Panelists wanted to rate Type I and Type II separately. Added wording to allow other antihypertensives in patient with both CAD and DM. **DROPPED because similar to indicator Ch. #12.10 and operationalization difficulties.**
7.b	•NEW•	--	If **a hypertensive [Type II] patient without known CAD is receiving other antihypertensive therapy in the absence of ACE inhibitors or calcium channel blockers, progress note should document failure of ACE inhibitors and calcium channel blockers to control blood pressure.**	•NEW• Panelists wanted to rate Type I and Type II separately. Added wording to allow other antihypertensives in patient with both CAD and DM. **DROPPED because similar to indicator Ch. #12.10 and operationalization difficulties.**
	(FOLLOW-UP)		(FOLLOW-UP)	
8.	Patients with diabetes should have a follow-up visit at least every 6 months.	8.	Patients with [~~Type I~~]-diabetes should have a follow-up visit at least every 6 months.	Panelists wanted to rate Type I and Type II diabetes separately.
8.b	•NEW•	--	**Patients with [Type II] diabetes should have a follow-up visit at least every 6 months.**	•NEW• Panelists wanted to rate Type I and Type II diabetes separately. **Recombined wtih modified indicator #8, but Type I and Type II diabetes will be scored separately.**

Chapter 10 — Family Planning/Contraception

Original Indicator	Modified Indicator	Comments
(SCREENING)	(SCREENING)	
1. A history to determine risk for unintended pregnancy should be taken yearly on all women. In order to establish risk, the following elements of the history need to be documented:	1. A history to determine risk for unintended pregnancy should be taken yearly on all women **who present otherwise for routine care.** In order to establish risk, the following elements of the history need to be documented:	Wording changed to clarify that the indicator applies only to those women that present for routine care.
a. Menstrual status (e.g., pre- or post-menopausal, history of hysterectomy, etc.), last menstrual period, or pregnancy test;	a. Menstrual status (e.g., pre- or post-menopausal, history of hysterectomy, etc.), last menstrual period, or pregnancy test;	Wording changed in (b) to clarify that documentation of heterosexual intercourse is necessary to establish risk for unintended pregnancy.
b. Sexual history (presence or absence of current sexual intercourse);	**b.** Sexual history (presence or absence of current **heterosexual** intercourse); and	•**MODIFIED•**
c. Current contraceptive practices; and	**c.** Current contraceptive practices	
d. Desire for pregnancy	-- d. Desire for pregnancy	Dropped (d) desire for pregnancy due to low validity scores by panelists.
(TREATMENT)	(TREATMENT)	
2. Women at risk for unintended pregnancy should receive counseling about effective contraceptive methods.	2. Women at risk for unintended pregnancy should receive counseling about effective contraceptive methods.	•**UNCHANGED•**
3. The smoking status of women prescribed combination OCs should be documented in the medical record.	3. The smoking status of women prescribed combination OCs should be documented in the medical record.	•**UNCHANGED•**
4. Women who smoke and are prescribed oral contraceptives should be counseled and encouraged to quit smoking.	4. Women who smoke and are prescribed oral contraceptives should be counseled and encouraged to quit smoking.	•**UNCHANGED•**
5. Women over age 35 who smoke should not be prescribed combination oral contraceptives.	5. Women over age 35 who smoke should not be prescribed combination oral contraceptives.	•**UNCHANGED•**

Chapter 11 — Headache

Original Indicator	Modified Indicator	Comments
(DIAGNOSIS)	**(DIAGNOSIS)**	
1. Patients with new onset headache should be asked about: a. Location of the pain (e.g., frontal, bilateral); b. Associated symptoms (e.g., aura); c. Temporal profile (e.g., new onset, constant); d. Severity; and e. Family history	1. Patients with new onset headache should be asked about: a. Location of the pain (e.g., frontal, bilateral); b. Associated symptoms (e.g., aura); c. Temporal profile (e.g., new onset, constant); d. Severity; and e. Family history f. **Aggravating or alleviating factors**	Panelists agreed that factors that contribute to or relieve headaches should also be documented for new onset headaches.
2. Patients with new onset headache should have a neurological examination evaluating the: a. Cranial nerves, b. Fundi, and c. Deep tendon reflexes.	2. Patients with new onset headache should have an neurological examination evaluating the: a. Cranial nerves, b. Fundi, c. Deep tendon reflexes, **and** d. **Blood pressure.**	Panelists felt the exam should extend beyond the neurologic exam to include bp because very high bp could be the cause of headaches.
3. CT or MRI scanning is indicated in patients with new onset headache and any of the following circumstances: a. Abnormal neurological examination, b. constant headache, or c. severe headache.	3. CT or MRI scanning is indicated in patients with new onset headache and any of the following circumstances: a. Abnormal neurological examination, -- b. constant headache, or **b.** c. severe headache.	•UNCHANGED• •MODIFIED• Dropped (b) constant headache due to low validity scores by panelists.
4. Skull X-rays should not be part of an evaluation for headache.	4. Skull X-rays should not be part of an evaluation for headache.	•UNCHANGED•
(TREATMENT)	**(TREATMENT)**	
5. Patients with acute mild migraine or tension headache should receive aspirin, tylenol, or other nonsteroidal anti-inflammatory agents before being prescribed any other medication.	5. Patients with acute mild migraine or tension headache should **have tried** aspirin, tylenol, or other nonsteroidal anti-inflammatory agents before being prescribed any other medication.	Wording changed to have tried since these are available OTC.
6.a Patients with acute moderate or severe migraine headache should receive one of the following before being prescribed any other agent: • intramuscular ketorolac, • subcutaneous sumatriptan, • intravenous dihydroergotamine, • intravenous chlorpromazine, or • Intravenous metaclopramide.	-- For patients with acute moderate or severe migraine headache, one of the following **should have been tried** before being prescribed any other agent: • **parenteral** ketorolac, • subcutaneous sumatriptan, • **parenteral** dihydroergotamine, • **parenteral** chlorpromazine, or • **parenteral** metaclopramide.	Wording changed to clarify wording of original indicator. Panelists wanted to rate a separate strategy for allowing either oral or parenteral treatment. •DROPPED• due to low validity score from panelists.
6.b •NEW•	6. **For patients with acute moderate or severe migraine headache, one of the following should have been tried before being prescribed any other agent:** • oral ketorolac, • oral sumatriptan, • oral dihydroergotamine. • oral chlorpromazine. or • oral metoclopramide.	•NEW• Panelists wanted to rate a separate strategy for allowing either oral or parenteral treatment.

cont'd

	Original Indicator		Modified Indicator	Comments
7.	Recurrent moderate or severe tension headaches should be treated with a trial of tricyclic antidepressant agents.	7.	Recurrent moderate or severe tension headaches should be treated with a trial of tricyclic antidepressant agents, **if no medical contraindications to use.**	There are contraindications to use of tricyclic antidepressants in some patients.
8.	If a patient has more than 2 migraine headaches each month, then prophylactic treatment is indicated with one of the following agents: • beta blockers, • calcium channel blockers, • tricyclic antidepressants, • naproxen, • aspirin, • fluoxitene, • valproate, or • cyproheptadine.	8.	If a patient has more than 2 **moderate to severe** migraine headaches each month, then prophylactic treatment is indicated with one of the following agents **should be offered:** • beta blockers, • calcium channel blockers, • tricyclic antidepressants, • naproxen, • aspirin, • fluoxetine, • valproate, or • cyproheptadine.	Panelists felt these this indicator applied only to moderate to severe migraines. Wording changed to clarify original indicator.
9.	Sumatriptan and ergotamine should not be concurrently administered.	9.	Sumatriptan and ergotamine should not be concurrently administered.	•UNCHANGED•
10.	Opioid agonists and barbiturates should not be first-line therapy for migraine or tension headaches.	10.	Opioid agonists and barbiturates should not be first-line therapy for migraine or tension headaches.	•UNCHANGED•
11.	Sumatriptan and ergotamine should not be given in patients with a history of: • uncontrolled hypertension, • atypical chest pain, or • ischemic heart disease or angina.	11.	Sumatriptan and ergotamine should not be given in patients with a history of: • uncontrolled hypertension, • atypical chest pain, or • ischemic heart disease or angina.	•UNCHANGED•

Women's Quality Indicators

Chapter 12 — Hypertension

Original Indicator	Modified Indicator	Comments
(DIAGNOSIS)	(DIAGNOSIS)	
1. Systolic and diastolic blood pressure should be measured on adult women otherwise presenting for care at least once each year.	1. Systolic and diastolic blood pressure should be measured on adult women otherwise presenting for care at least once each year.	•UNCHANGED•
2. Patients with a new diagnosis of stage 1-3 hypertension should have at least three measurements on different days with a mean SBP≥140 and/or a mean DBP≥90.	2. Patients with a new diagnosis of stage 1-3 hypertension should have at least three measurements on different days with a mean SBP≥140 and/or a mean DBP≥90.	•UNCHANGED•
3. Initial history and physical of patients with hypertension should document assessment of at least two items from each of the following groups by the third visit: a. Family or personal history of premature CAD, CVA, diabetes, hyperlipidemia. b. Personal history of tobacco abuse, alcohol abuse, or taking of medications known to cause hypertension. c. Examination of the fundi, heart sounds, abdomen for bruits, peripheral arterial pulses, neurologic system.	3. Initial history and physical of patients with hypertension should document assessment of at least two items from each of the following groups by the third visit: a. **History:** Family or personal history of premature CAD, CVA, diabetes, hyperlipidemia. b. **Medication or substance use:** Personal history of tobacco abuse, alcohol abuse, or taking of medications **that may** cause hypertension. c. **Physical exam:** Examination of the fundi, heart sounds, abdomen for bruits, peripheral arterial pulses, neurologic system.	Wording changed to clarify original indicator.
4. Stage 1 hypertensive women taking drugs known to cause hypertension should have the drug discontinued (at least temporarily) before pharmacotherapy is initiated. • oral contraceptives, • steroids, • nasal decongestants, • appetite suppressants, • cyclosporine, • monamine oxidase inhibitors, • tricyclic antidepressants, and • erythropoietin.	4. Stage 1 hypertensive women taking drugs **that may** cause hypertension should have the drug discontinued (at least temporarily) before pharmacotherapy is initiated. • oral contraceptives, • steroids, • nasal decongestants, • appetite suppressants, • cyclosporine, • monamine oxidase inhibitors, **and** • tricyclic antidepressants, • erythropoietin.	Rare but efficacious treatments that may cause hypertension were deleted.
5. Initial laboratory tests should include the following: a. Urinalysis, b. Glucose, c. Potassium, d. Calcium, e. Creatinine, f. Uric acid, g. Cholesterol, h. Triglyceride, i. Electrocardiogram, and j. Echocardiogram.	5. Initial laboratory tests should include the following: **a.** Urinalysis, **b.** Glucose, **c.** Potassium, -- **d.** Calcium, **e.** Creatinine, -- **f.** Uric acid, **g.** Cholesterol, **h.** Triglyceride, -- **i.** Electrocardiogram, and -- **j.** Echocardiogram.	•MODIFIED• **Dropped (d) calcium, (f) uric acid, and (j) echocardiogram due to low validity scores from panelists.** **Dropped (i) electrocardiogram due to disagreement among panelists.**

cont'd

Original Indicator	Modified Indicator	Comments
(TREATMENT)	(TREATMENT)	
6a. First-line treatment for Stage 1-3 hypertension is lifestyle modification. The medical record should indicate counseling for at least one of the following interventions prior to pharmacotherapy: • weight reduction, • increased physical activity, • low sodium diet, or • alcohol intake reduction.	6. First-line treatment for [Stage 1-2] hypertension is lifestyle modification. The medical record should indicate counseling for at least one of the following interventions prior to pharmacotherapy: • weight reduction, • increased physical activity, • low sodium diet, or • alcohol intake reduction.	Panelists wanted to rate Stage 1-2 separately from Stage 3 hypertension.
6b. •NEW•	7. First-line treatment for [Stage 3] hypertension is lifestyle modification. The medical record should indicate counseling for at least one of the following interventions prior to pharmacotherapy: • weight reduction, • increased physical activity, • low sodium diet, or • alcohol intake reduction.	•NEW• Panelists wanted to rate Stage 1-2 separately from Stage 3 hypertension. Pharmacotherapy for Stage 3 hypertensives should not be withheld for other forms of interventions.
7. First-line pharmacotherapy for Stage 1-3 hypertension is monotherapy with thiazide diuretics or beta blockers. The medical record should show failure on one of these agents or a contraindication before initiation of therapy with other agents.	8. [Stage 1-2] hypertensives whose blood pressure remains [Stage 1-2] after 6 months lifestyle modification should receive pharmacotherapy.	Panelists did not agree that thiazide diuretics or beta blockers had to be used for Stage 1-2. They decided to separate out indicators for Stage 1-2 and Stage 3. Stage 1-2 should first try lifestyle modifications.
7.b •NEW•	9. [Stage 3] hypertensives should receive pharmacotherapy.	•NEW• Stage 3 hypertensives should receive pharmacotherapy right away in addition to lifestyle modifications.
8. First-line pharmacotherapy for diabetics should include an ACE inhibitor or a calcium channel blocker.	10. First-line pharmacotherapy for diabetics should include an ACE inhibitor or a calcium channel blocker.	•UNCHANGED•
(FOLLOW-UP)	(FOLLOW-UP)	
9. Hypertensive patients should visit the physician at least twice each year.	11. Hypertensive patients should visit the provider at least once each year.	Changed to provider so other health professionals were acceptable. Panelists also agreed a minimum of one visit per year was sufficient.
10. Hypertensive patients with persistent elevations of SBP>160 or DBP>90 should have one of the following interventions recorded in the medical record: • Change in dose or regimen of antihypertensives, or • Repeated education regarding lifestyle modifications.	---	•UNCHANGED• •DROPPED• due to difficulties in operationalization.
10.b •NEW•	12. Patients with average blood pressure of >140 systolic and/or >90 diastolic, as determined on at least three separate visits, should have a diagnosis of hypertension documented in their record.	•NEW• Added by staff after panel meeting.

Chapter 13 — Low Back Pain (Acute) [nonpregnant]

	Original Indicator	Modified Indicator	Comments
	(ASSESSMENT) (DIAGNOSIS)	(ASSESSMENT) (DIAGNOSIS)	
1.	Patients presenting with acute low back pain should receive a focused medical history and physical examination. The history should include questions about at least one of the following "red flags": • Spine fracture red flags: trauma, prolonged use of steroids; • Cancer red flags: history of cancer, unexplained weight loss, immunosuppression; • Infection red flags: fever, IV drug use; or • Cauda equina syndrome or rapidly progressing neurologic deficit red flags: acute onset of urinary retention or overflow incontinence, loss of anal sphincter tone or fecal incontinence, saddle anesthesia, and global progressive motor weakness in the lower limbs.	1. Patients presenting with acute low back pain should receive a focused medical history and physical examination. The history should include questions about at least one of the following "red flags": • Spine fracture red flags: trauma, prolonged use of steroids; • Cancer red flags: history of cancer, unexplained weight loss, immunosuppression; • Infection red flags: fever, IV drug use; or • Cauda equina syndrome or rapidly progressing neurologic deficit red flags: acute onset of urinary retention or overflow incontinence, loss of anal sphincter tone or fecal incontinence, saddle anesthesia, and global progressive motor weakness in the lower limbs.	•UNCHANGED•
2.	The examination should include neurologic screening and straight leg raising.	2. The examination should include neurologic screening and straight leg raising.	•UNCHANGED•
3.	If no red flags identified, diagnostic testing should not be undertaken in first 4 weeks of symptoms.	--	•DELETED• Panelists wished to allow prompt and aggressive treatment.
	(TREATMENT)	(TREATMENT)	
4.	If the patient is placed on medication for acute low back pain not due to spine fracture, cancer, infection, or cauda equina syndrome, one of the following should be used as a first-line agent: acetaminophen or NSAIDs.	--	•DELETED• Panelists wished to allow other treatments.
5.	Patients should not be taking any of the following medications for treatment of acute low back pain: a. phenylbutazone b. dexamethasone c. other oral steroids d. colchicine e. anti-depressants	3. Patients should not be taking any of the following medications for treatment of acute low back pain: a. phenylbutazone b. dexamethasone c. other oral steroids d. colchicine e. anti-depressants	•UNCHANGED•
6.	Patients should not be receiving the following physical treatments for acute low back pain: a. transcutaneous electrical nerve stimulation b. lumbar corsets & support belts c. spinal traction d. biofeedback	4. Patients should not be **prescribed** the following physical treatments for acute low back pain: **a.** transcutaneous electrical nerve stimulation **b.** lumbar corsets & support belts **c.** spinal traction -- biofeedback	Many patients use these treatments on their own. Changed to reflect that these treatments should not be prescribed by physician. •MODIFIED• Dropped (d) biofeedback due to low validity score from panelists.
7.	Patients should not be on prolonged bed rest (> 4 days).	5. Prolonged bed rest (> 4 days) **should not be recommended.**	Many patients use bedrest on their own. Changed to reflect that bedrest should not be prescribed by physician.

Chapter 14 — Prenatal Care

	Original Indicator		Modified Indicator	Comments
	(SCREENING)		**(SCREENING)**	
	Routine Prenatal Care		***Routine Prenatal Care***	
1.	The first prenatal visit should occur in the first trimester.	1.	The first prenatal visit should occur in the first trimester.	•UNCHANGED•
2.	The physician should make an accurate determination of gestational age using:	2.	The physician should make an accurate determination of gestational age using **any one of the following**:	Panelists wanted to rate (a) and (b) separately.
	• An ultrasound in the 1st or 2nd trimester, or	a.	• An ultrasound in the 1st or 2nd trimester; or	Wording changed to clarify the original indicator.
	• Reliable LMP and size within 2 wks indicated by dates in the 1st trimester, or		• Reliable LMP and size within 2 wks indicated by dates in the 1st trimester; or	
	• No 1st trimester exam, but reliable LMP & 2 of the following: 1) size w/in 2 wks. of dates in 2d trimester; 2) quickening by 20 wks.; 3) fetal heart tones by fetoscope before 20 weeks, or		• No 1st trimester exam, but reliable LMP & 2 of the following: 1) size w/in 2 wks. of dates in 2d trimester, 2) quickening by 20 wks., 3) fetal heart tones by fetoscope before 20 weeks; or	
	• If unreliable LMP, then an ultrasound is required.	b.	• If **unknown** LMP, then an ultrasound is required.	
3.	Pregnant women should be screened for anemia at the first prenatal visit.	3.	Pregnant women should be screened for anemia at the first prenatal visit.	•UNCHANGED•
4.	Pregnant women should be rescreened for anemia after 24 weeks.	4.	Pregnant women should be rescreened for anemia after 24 weeks.	•UNCHANGED•
	Substance Abuse		***Substance Abuse***	
5.	A smoking history should be obtained at the first prenatal visit.	5.	A smoking history should be obtained at the first prenatal visit.	•UNCHANGED•
6.	An alcohol history should be obtained at the first prenatal visit.	6.	An alcohol history should be obtained at the first prenatal visit.	•UNCHANGED•
7.	A drug history should be obtained during the first prenatal visit.	7.	A drug history should be obtained during the first prenatal visit.	•UNCHANGED•
	Infections and Sexually Transmitted Diseases (STDs)		***Infections and Sexually Transmitted Diseases (STDs)***	
7.5	•NEW•	8.	**A history should be taken at the first prenatal visit to elicit risk factors for STDs and Hepatitis B.**	•NEW• Added because panelists felt this indicator was important for assessment of quality of prenatal care.
	Asymptomatic Bacteriuria		***Asymptomatic Bacteriuria***	
8.	Women should receive a urine culture at the first prenatal visit.	9.	Women should receive a urine **screen** at the first prenatal visit.	A full culture is not necessary according to the literature. A urine screen is sufficient.
	Rubella		***Rubella***	
9.	Women should receive a serologic test for rubella immunity before delivery.	10.	Women should receive a serologic test for rubella immunity before delivery.	•UNCHANGED•
	Hepatitis B Carriers		***Hepatitis B Carriers***	
10.	Women should be screened for HBsAg before delivery.	11.	Women should be screened for HBsAg before delivery.	•UNCHANGED•
	Syphilis		***Syphilis***	Panelists preferred to only screen women at risk, but this change was impossible to operationalize.

Women's Quality Indicators

	Original Indicator		Modified Indicator	Comments
11.	A non-treponemal screening test (e.g., VDRC) should be performed on women at the first prenatal visit.	12.	A non-treponemal screening test (e.g., VDRL) should be performed on women at the first prenatal visit.	VDRC changed to VDRL to correct a typographical error in the original indicator. Panelists preferred to only screen women at risk, but this change was impossible to operationalize.
	Gonorrhea		*Gonorrhea*	
12.	A cervical gonorrhea culture should be performed on women at the first prenatal visit.	13.	A cervical gonorrhea culture should be performed on women at the first prenatal visit.	•UNCHANGED• Panelists preferred to only screen women at risk, but this change was impossible to operationalize.
	Chlamydia		*Chlamydia*	
13.	Women at high risk (adolescents, unmarried, those with multiple sex partners, low SES, other STD diagnosed) should receive a cervical chlamydia culture or antigen detection at the first prenatal visit.	14.	Women at high risk (adolescents, unmarried, those with multiple sex partners, low SES, other STD diagnosed) should receive a cervical chlamydia culture or antigen detection at the first prenatal visit.	•UNCHANGED•
	Human Immunodeficiency Virus		*Human Immunodeficiency Virus*	
14.	Pregnant women should be counseled about their individual risk for HIV infection at the first prenatal visit.	15.	Pregnant women should be counseled about their individual risk for HIV infection at the first prenatal visit.	•UNCHANGED•
15.	Pregnant women should be offered HIV testing at the first prenatal visit.	16.	Pregnant women should be offered HIV testing at the first prenatal visit.	•UNCHANGED•
	Inherited Disorders		***Inherited Disorders***	
	Down Syndrome		*Down Syndrome*	
16.	Women age 35 and over, or who have had a previous Down syndrome infant, should receive amniocentesis or chorionic villus sampling (CVS), or should explicitly decline such a test after genetic counseling.	17.	Women age 35 and over, or who have had a previous Down syndrome infant, should receive amniocentesis or chorionic villus sampling (CVS), or should explicitly decline such a test after genetic counseling.	•UNCHANGED•
	Neural Tube Defects (NTDs)		*Neural Tube Defects (NTDs)*	
17.	Women under age 35 should be offered serum AFP; this should be performed between 15 and 20 weeks.	18.	Women ~~under age 35~~ should be offered serum AFP **testing**; this should be performed between 15 and 20 weeks.	All women, regardless of age, should be offered an AFP test.
18.	Women who have had a previous NTD infant should receive amniocentesis or should explicitly decline such a test after genetic counseling.	19.	Women who have had a previous NTD infant should receive amniocentesis or should explicitly decline such a test after ~~genetic counseling~~.	Panelists felt that genetic counseling was not necessary.
18.5	•NEW•	20.	**Women with a prior NTD infant should have folic acid supplementation recommended in the preconceptual period.**	•NEW• Panelists felt this indicator should be added because of recent studies showing benefit of folic acid.
	Sickle Cell Disease		*Sickle Cell Disease*	
19.	Women who are African American or have a family history of sickle cell disease should be screened at the first prenatal visit.	21.	Women who are African American or have a family history of sickle cell disease should be **offered screening** at the first prenatal visit, if **status unknown**.	Medical record should indicate that screening was offered. Women cannot be forced to undergo the test.
20.	For women with the sickle cell trait, the baby's father should be screened.	22.	For women with the sickle cell trait, the baby's father should be **offered screening**.	Medical record should indicate that screening was offered. Women cannot be forced to undergo the test.
	Rh Isoimmunization		*Rh Isoimmunization*	

Women's Quality Indicators

cont'd

Original Indicator	Modified Indicator	Comments
21. Women should receive an Rh factor and antibody screen at the first prenatal visit.	23. Women should receive an Rh factor and antibody screen at the first prenatal visit.	•UNCHANGED•
Common Pregnancy Complications	*Common Pregnancy Complications*	
Intrauterine Growth Retardation	*Intrauterine Growth Retardation*	
22. Measurements of the symphysis-fundal height should be made at each visit from 20-32 weeks.	24. Measurements of the symphysis-fundal height should be made at each visit from 20-32 weeks.	•UNCHANGED•
Post-term Pregnancy	*Post-term Pregnancy*	
23. Weekly fetal monitoring should begin at 41.5 weeks and continue until labor (spontaneous or induced) begins.	25. Weekly Fetal **assessment** should begin at 41.5 weeks and continue until labor (spontaneous or induced) begins.	Weekly deleted because many practitioners will not allow a women to go beyond 42 weeks. Assessment need not include continuous or intermittent monitoring of heart rate.
Pregnancy-Induced Hypertension (PIH)	*Pregnancy-Induced Hypertension (PIH)*	
24. Blood pressure measurements should be taken at each visit.	26. Blood pressure measurements should be taken at each visit.	•UNCHANGED•
Gestational Diabetes Mellitus	*Gestational Diabetes Mellitus*	
25. A one-hour, 50g glucose challenge test should be performed on women with risk factors at 24-28 weeks.	27. A one-hour, 50g glucose challenge test should be performed on women with risk factors at 24-28 weeks.	•UNCHANGED•
(DIAGNOSIS)	(DIAGNOSIS)	
Infections and STDs	*Infections and STDs*	
Hepatitis B Carriers	*Hepatitis B Carriers*	
26. For women carrying HBsAg, carrier status should be documented in delivery record.	28. For women carrying HBsAg, carrier status should be documented in delivery record.	•UNCHANGED•
Syphilis	*Syphilis*	
27. Women whose non-treponemal tests are weakly reactive or reactive should receive a treponemal test to confirm presence of syphilis.	29. Women whose non-treponemal tests are weakly reactive or reactive should receive a treponemal test to confirm presence of syphilis.	•UNCHANGED•
Inherited Disorders	*Inherited Disorders*	
Neural Tube Defects (NTDs)	*Neural Tube Defects (NTDs)*	
28. Women with an abnormal serum AFP should receive an ultrasound to evaluate gestational age and possible multiple gestation.	30. Women with an abnormal serum AFP should receive an ultrasound to evaluate gestational age and possible multiple gestation.	•UNCHANGED•
Sickle Cell Disease	*Sickle Cell Disease*	
29. Women with the sickle cell trait should receive either amniocentesis or chorionic villus sampling, unless the baby's father is known to be negative for the sickle trait.	31. Women with the sickle cell trait should **be offered** either amniocentesis or chorionic villus sampling, unless the baby's father is known to be negative for the sickle trait.	Medical record should indicate that screening was offered. Women cannot be forced to undergo the test.
Common Pregnancy Complications	*Common Pregnancy Complications*	
Intrauterine Growth Retardation	*Intrauterine Growth Retardation*	
30. Women whose symphysis-fundal height is 4 cm less than indicated by their gestational age between 20-32 weeks should have an ultrasound.	32. Women whose symphysis-fundal height is 4 cm less than indicated by their gestational age between 20-32 weeks should have an ultrasound.	•UNCHANGED•
Pregnancy-Induced Hypertension (PIH)	*Pregnancy-Induced Hypertension (PIH)*	

cont'd

Original Indicator	Modified Indicator	Comments
31. For elevated BPs (systolic > 140mm Hg, OR systolic rise >30mm Hg or diastolic rise > 15mm Hg), proteinuria and peripheral edema should be assessed.	33. **In women without a prior diagnosis of chronic hypertension, who have** elevated BPs (systolic > 140mm Hg **at 20 weeks or later,** or diastolic > 90mm Hg **at 20 weeks or later,** OR systolic rise >30mm Hg or diastolic rise > 15mm Hg), proteinuria and peripheral edema should be assessed.	Women with chronic hypertension were excluded to be comparable with the prior RAND study of prenatal care. "At 20 weeks or later" was added because PIH is not very common prior to 20 weeks.
32. For patients with elevated BP and either proteinuria (1+ or more) or edema (> trace), PIH diagnosis should be made.	34. **In women without a prior diagnosis of chronic hypertension, who have** elevated BP and either proteinuria (1+ or more) or edema (> trace), PIH diagnosis should be made.	Women with chronic hypertension were excluded to be comparable with the prior RAND study of prenatal care.
Gestational Diabetes Mellitus	*Gestational Diabetes Mellitus*	
33. Pregnant women with abnormal glucose challenge tests (≥140 mg/dL or 7.8 mmol/L) should have a 3-hour plasma glucose tolerance test performed.	35. Pregnant women with abnormal glucose challenge tests (≥140 mg/dL or 7.8 mmol/L) should have a 3-hour plasma glucose tolerance test performed.	•UNCHANGED•
(TREATMENT) *Substance Use*	(TREATMENT) *Substance Use*	
34. Pregnant women identified as smokers should receive counseling to stop smoking from their physician.	36. Pregnant women identified as smokers should receive counseling to stop smoking from their physician.	•UNCHANGED•
35. Pregnant women identified as smokers should be referred to a smoking cessation clinic, group, or counselor.	-- Pregnant women identified as smokers should be referred to a smoking cessation clinic, group, or counselor.	•UNCHANGED• •DROPPED• due to low validity score from panelists.
36. Pregnant women who indicate they use any amount of alcohol should be counseled to eliminate alcohol consumption during pregnancy.	37. Pregnant women who indicate they use any amount of alcohol should be counseled to eliminate alcohol consumption during pregnancy **and should be referred for treatment if appropriate.**	Referral necessary if practitioner feels abuse is excessive.
37. Pregnant women who indicate they use cocaine or heroin should be counseled by their physician to cease use during pregnancy.	38. Pregnant women who indicate they use **drugs** should be counseled by their physician to cease use during pregnancy **and should be referred for treatment if appropriate.**	Changed to include drug use of any kind. Merged with original indicator #38.
38. Pregnant women who indicate they use drugs should be referred to a drug treatment clinic, group, or counselor.	--	•DELETED• Merged with original indicator #37.
Infections and Sexually Transmitted Diseases *Asymptomatic Bacteriuria*	*Infections and Sexually Transmitted Diseases* *Asymptomatic Bacteriuria*	
39. Pregnant women with positive cultures (>100,000 bacteria/cc) should receive an appropriate antibiotic.	39. Pregnant women with positive cultures (>100,000 bacteria/cc) should receive an appropriate antibiotic.	•UNCHANGED•
Rubella	*Rubella*	
40. Pregnant women not immune to rubella should receive postpartum immunization.	40. Pregnant women not immune to rubella should receive postpartum immunization **within 6 weeks.**	Timeframe added for operationalization.
Syphilis	*Syphilis*	
41. Pregnant women with confirmed positive serology should be treated with penicillin appropriate for the stage of disease; tetracycline and doxycycline are contraindicated.	41. Pregnant women with confirmed positive serology should be treated with penicillin, **if not allergic,** appropriate for the stage of disease; tetracycline and doxycycline are contraindicated.	Penicillin is contraindicated in some patients.
Gonorrhea	*Gonorrhea*	

Women's Quality Indicators

cont'd

	Original Indicator		Modified Indicator	Comments
42.	Pregnant women with positive cultures should be treated as recommended by the PHS Guidelines on STD (250 mg IM once of ceftriaxone and erythromycin base 500 mg orally 4x/day for 7 days).	42.	Pregnant women with positive cultures should **receive appropriate treatment.**	Panelists did not want to stipulate the exact treatment, so the indicator was changed to allow more general operationalization.
	Human Immunodeficiency Virus		*Human Immunodeficiency Virus*	
43.	Pregnant women known to be HIV positive with CD4+ counts of 200 or greater should be treated with zidovudine during pregnancy and intrapartum.	43.	Pregnant women known to be HIV positive with CD4+ counts of 200 or greater should be **offered treatment** with zidovudine during pregnancy and intrapartum	Medical record should indicate that screening was offered. Women cannot be forced to undergo the treatment.
	Inherited Disorders		*Inherited Disorders*	
	Down Syndrome		*Down Syndrome*	
44.	Pregnant women whose amniocentesis shows infant with abnormal karyotype should receive additional genetic counseling.	44.	Pregnant women whose amniocentesis shows infant with abnormal karyotype should receive additional genetic counseling.	Genetic counseling not necessary. Any appropriate counseling is sufficient.
	Neural Tube Defects (NTDs)		*Neural Tube Defects (NTDs)*	
45.	Pregnant women with abnormal serum AFP and normal ultrasound should be offered an amniocentesis and genetic counseling.	45.	Pregnant women with abnormal serum AFP **for gestational age** and normal ultrasound should be offered an amniocentesis and genetic counseling.	Added gestational age for clarification. "Genetic counseling not necessary. Any appropriate counseling is sufficient.
46.	Pregnant women whose amniotic fluid AFP shows infant with probable NTD should be offered additional genetic counseling.	46.	Pregnant women whose amniotic fluid AFP shows infant with probable NTD should be offered additional genetic counseling.	Genetic counseling not necessary. Any appropriate counseling is sufficient.
	Sickle Cell Disease		*Sickle Cell Disease*	
47.	Pregnant women whose amniocentesis shows an infant with sickle cell disease should be offered genetic counseling.	47.	Pregnant women whose amniocentesis shows an infant with sickle cell disease should be offered genetic counseling.	Genetic counseling not necessary. Any appropriate counseling is sufficient.
	Rh Isoimmunization		*Rh Isoimmunization*	
48.	Pregnant women who are Rh negative should receive Rhogam between 26 and 30 weeks antenatally and postpartum.	48.	Pregnant women who are Rh negative should receive Rhogam between 26 and 30 weeks antenatally and postpartum.	•UNCHANGED•
	Common Pregnancy Complications		***Common Pregnancy Complications***	
	Post-Term Pregnancy		*Post-Term Pregnancy*	
49.	Labor should be induced when fetus shows signs of distress or oligohydramnios.	49.	Labor should be induced when **monitoring** shows **non-reassuring fetal status** or oligohydramnios.	Wording changed to clarify original indicator.
50.	Pregnancies with reliable dates should not extend beyond 44 weeks.	50.	Pregnancies with reliable dates should not extend beyond 44 weeks.	•UNCHANGED•
	Pregnancy-Induced Hypertension (PIH)		*Pregnancy-Induced Hypertension (PIH)*	
51.	If PIH diagnosed and patient is not admitted, bedrest should be recommended & a return visit should occur w/in 1 week.	51.	If PIH diagnosed and patient is not admitted, bedrest should be recommended & a return visit should occur w/in 1 week.	•UNCHANGED•
52.	If PIH diagnosed and pregnancy is at term (≥ 37 weeks), either labor should be induced or delivery by cesarean section should take place.	52.	If PIH diagnosed and pregnancy is at term (≥ 37 weeks), either labor should be induced or delivery by cesarean section should take place.	•UNCHANGED•
53.	If severe PIH is diagnosed by any of the following: systolic >160 mm Hg, diastolic >110 mm Hg, 3-4+ proteinuria, pulmonary edema, oliguria, RUQ pain or seizures, then patient should be admitted to induce labor or deliver by cesarean section.	53.	If severe PIH is diagnosed by any of the following: systolic >160 mm Hg, diastolic >110 mm Hg, 3-4+ proteinuria, pulmonary edema, oliguria, RUQ pain or seizures, then patient should be admitted to induce labor or deliver by cesarean section.	•UNCHANGED•

Women's Quality Indicators

	Original Indicator		Modified Indicator	Comments
	Gestational Diabetes Mellitus		*Gestational Diabetes Mellitus*	
54.	Pregnant women with abnormal 3-hour glucose tolerance tests should receive dietary counseling from a dietician.	54.	Pregnant women with abnormal 3-hour glucose tolerance tests should receive dietary counseling **and have glucose monitoring.**	Panelists felt glucose monitoring was necessary in addition to dietary counseling.
55.	Pregnant women on dietary therapy with 2 or more consecutive abnormal fasting (>105 mg/dL) or postprandial (>120 mg/dL one-hour post) plasma glucose tests should be placed on insulin therapy.	55.	Pregnant women on dietary therapy with 2 or more consecutive abnormal fasting (>105 mg/dL) or postprandial (>120 mg/dL one-hour post) plasma glucose tests should be placed on insulin therapy.	•UNCHANGED•
56.	An oral agent should not be used in diabetic pregnant women.	56.	An oral agent should not be used in diabetic pregnant women.	•UNCHANGED•
	(FOLLOW-UP)		**(FOLLOW-UP)**	
	Infections and Sexually Transmitted Diseases		***Infections and Sexually Transmitted Diseases***	
	Asymptomatic Bacteriuria		*Asymptomatic Bacteriuria*	
57.	Women treated for positive cultures should receive a post-treatment follow-up culture within one month of completing treatment.	57.	Women treated for positive cultures should receive a post-treatment follow-up culture within one month of completing treatment.	•UNCHANGED•
	Syphilis		*Syphilis*	
58.	Women diagnosed with syphilis in pregnancy should be followed up with monthly serology and retreated if necessary.	58.	Women diagnosed with syphilis in pregnancy should be followed up with monthly serology and retreated if necessary.	•UNCHANGED•
	Gonorrhea		*Gonorrhea*	
59.	Women with positive cultures should receive a post-treatment follow-up culture 4-7 days after treatment is completed.	59.	Women with positive cultures should receive a post-treatment follow-up culture **2 weeks** after treatment is completed.	Changed to 2 weeks because studies show that some cultures still show up positive 7-10 days after treatment.
	Chlamydia		*Chlamydia*	
60.	Women with positive cultures should receive a post-treatment follow-up culture 4-7 days after treatment is completed.	60.	Women with positive cultures should receive a post-treatment follow-up culture 4-7 days after treatment is completed.	•UNCHANGED•
	Common Pregnancy Complications		***Common Pregnancy Complications***	
	Gestational Diabetes Mellitus		*Gestational Diabetes Mellitus*	
61.	Women with abnormal 3-hour plasma glucose tolerance tests who are on dietary therapy should have biweekly fasting or postprandial glucose tests.	61.	Women with abnormal 3-hour plasma glucose tolerance tests who are on dietary therapy should have biweekly fasting or postprandial glucose tests.	•UNCHANGED•

Chapter 15 — Corticosteroids for Fetal Maturation in Labor

Original Indicator	Modified Indicator	Comments
(TREATMENT)	(TREATMENT)	
1. Women admitted to the hospital with labor, between 24 and 34 weeks gestation and without ruptured membranes, should receive antenatal steroids, even if delivery is anticipated in less than 24 hours.	1. Women admitted to the hospital with labor, between 24 and 34 weeks gestation and without ruptured membranes, should receive antenatal steroids, even if delivery is anticipated in less than 24 hours.	•UNCHANGED•
2. Steroid treatment should consist of either: • Betamethasone 12 mg. IM q24h x 2, or • Dexamethasone 6 mg. IM q12h x 4.	2. Steroid treatment **for women admitted in labor without ruptured membranes between 24 and 34 weeks gestation** should consist of either: • Betamethasone 12 mg. IM q24h x 2, or • Dexamethasone 6 mg. IM q12h x 4.	Indicator reworded during operationalization to clarify the eligible population
3. Women admitted to the hospital at 24-32 weeks gestation with ruptured membranes should receive antenatal steroid administration.	3. Women admitted to the hospital at 24-32 weeks gestation with ruptured membranes should receive antenatal steroid administration.	•UNCHANGED•
•NEW•	4. **Steroid treatment for women admitted with ruptured membranes between 24 and 32 weeks gestation should consist of either:** • **Betamethasone 12 mg. IM q24h x 2, or** • **Dexamethasone 6 mg. IM q12h x 4.**	Indicator added during operationalization to clarify the eligible population of original indicator #2

Chapter 16 — Routine Preventive Care

	Original Indicator		Modified Indicator	Comments
	Immunizations		*Immunizations*	
1.	Notation of date that a patient received a tetanus/diphtheria booster within the last ten years should be included in the medical record.	1.	Notation of date that a patient received a tetanus/diphtheria booster within the last ten years should be included in the medical record.	•UNCHANGED•
2.	Women with any of the following conditions should receive a yearly influenza vaccine: a. Asthma. b. Chronic obstructive pulmonary disease. c. Chronic cardiovascular disorders. d. Diabetes mellitus. e. Renal failure. f. Hemoglobinopathies (e.g., sickle cell disease). g. Immunosuppression.	2.	Women with any of the following conditions should receive a yearly influenza vaccine: a. Asthma. b. Chronic obstructive pulmonary disease. c. Chronic cardiovascular disorders. d. Diabetes mellitus. e. Renal failure. f. Hemoglobinopathies (e.g., sickle cell disease). g. Immunosuppression.	•UNCHANGED•
	Sexually Transmitted Diseases and HIV Prevention		*Sexually Transmitted Diseases and HIV Prevention*	
3.	Patients should be asked if they have ever been sexually active.	3.	**A sexual history should be documented in the chart.**	Wording changed to clarify original indicator.
4.	Patients who have ever been sexually active should be asked the following questions: a. If they currently have a single sexual partner. b. If they have had more than 2 sexual partners in the past 6 months. c. If they have had a history of any STDs.	4.	Patients who have ever been sexually active **with men** should be asked the following questions: a. If they currently have a single sexual partner. b. If they have had more than 2 sexual partners in the past 6 months. c. If they have had a history of any STDs. d. **If they or their partner(s) have had more than 1 partner.**	Wording changed to reflect indicator refers to heterosexual sexual activity. (d) added because panelists felt that more than one partner ever was a risk factor for STDs and HIV. •MODIFIED• **Dropped (d) more than 1 partner due to low validity score from panelists.**
5.	Patients should be asked about current or past use of intravenous drugs at least once.	5.	Patients should be asked about current or past use of intravenous drugs at least once.	•UNCHANGED•
6.	Patients who are sexually active and not in a monogamous relationship, have had more than 2 sexual partners in the past six months, have a history of STDs, or have used intravenous drugs, should be counseled regarding the prevention and transmission of HIV and other STDs.	6.	Patients who are sexually active **with men** and not in a monogamous relationship, have had more than 2 **male** sexual partners in the past six months, have a history of STDs, or have used intravenous drugs, should be counseled regarding the prevention and transmission of HIV and other STDs.	Clarification that the indicator refers to heterosexual relations.
	Obesity Counseling		*Obesity Counseling*	
7.	The medical record should include measurements of height and weight at least once.	7.	The medical record should include measurements of height and weight at least once.	•UNCHANGED•
	Seat Belt Use Counseling		*Seat Belt Use Counseling*	
8.	Patients should receive counseling regarding the use of seat belts on at least one occasion.	8.	Patients should receive counseling regarding the use of seat belts on at least one occasion.	•UNCHANGED•
	Breast Examination		*Breast Examination*	

cont'd

Original Indicator	Modified Indicator	Comments
9. A clinical breast exam should be performed on women aged 40 to 50 at least once every three years during a routine visit for a pelvic exam.	9. A clinical breast exam should be performed on women aged 40 to 50 at least once every three years during a routine visit for a pelvic exam.	Practitioners should perform a clinical breast exam during any routine visit, not only for a routine pelvic exam.
Hyperlipidemia Screening	*Hyperlipidemia Screening*	
10. As a screen for familial hypercholesterolemia, the medical record should indicate that adult women have undergone a cholesterol measurement at sometime in their lives.	10. As a screen for familial hypercholesterolemia, the medical record should indicate that adult women have undergone a cholesterol measurement at sometime in their lives.	•UNCHANGED•
11. In women with known cardiac risk factors including hypertension, smoking, diabetes, family history of myocardial infarction or familial hypercholesterolemia in a first degree relative, the medical record should indicate a serum cholesterol and triglycerides level in the last 5 years.	11. In women with known cardiac risk factors including hypertension, smoking, diabetes, family history of myocardial infarction or familial hypercholesterolemia in a first degree relative, the medical record should indicate a serum cholesterol and triglycerides level in the last 5 years.	•UNCHANGED•
Cervical Cancer Screening	*Cervical Cancer Screening*	
12. The medical record should contain the date and result of the last Pap smear.	12. The medical record should contain the date and result of the last Pap smear.	•UNCHANGED•
13. Women who have not had a Pap smear within the last 3 years should have one performed (unless never sexually active or have had a hysterectomy).	13. Women who have not had a Pap smear within the last 3 years should have one performed (unless never sexually active or have had a hysterectomy).	•UNCHANGED•
14. Women who have not had 3 consecutive normal smears and who have not had a Pap smear within the last year should have one performed.	14. Women who have not had 3 consecutive normal smears and who have not had a Pap smear within the last year should have one performed.	•UNCHANGED•
15. Women with a history of cervical dysplasia or carcinoma-in-situ who have not had a Pap smear within the last year should have one performed.	15. Women with a history of cervical dysplasia or carcinoma-in-situ who have not had a Pap smear within the last year should have one performed.	•UNCHANGED•
16. Women with severely abnormal Pap smear should have colposcopy performed.	16. Women with severely abnormal Pap smear should have colposcopy performed.	•UNCHANGED•
17. If a woman has a Pap smear that is not severely abnormal, then one of the following should occur within 1 year of the initial Pap: 1) repeat Pap smear; or 2) colposcopy.	17. If a woman has a Pap smear that is not severely abnormal, then one of the following should occur within **6 months** of the initial Pap: 1) repeat Pap smear; or 2) colposcopy.	Panelists felt that follow-up within one year was too long a time period so it was changed to 6 months.
18. Women with a Pap smear that is not normal but is not severely abnormal, and who have had the abnormality documented on at least 2 Pap smears in a 2-year period, should have colposcopy performed.	18. Women with a Pap smear that is not normal but is not severely abnormal, and who have had the abnormality documented on at least 2 Pap smears in a 2-year period, should have colposcopy performed.	•UNCHANGED•
19. •NEW•	19. **Patients who are seen for acute care, but have not been seen for routine care within the last 3 years should be referred for or have received a routine care visit within 3 months.**	•NEW• Acute care is an opportunity to assess need for cervical cancer screening.